CASE STUDIES

Stahl's Essential Psychopharmacology
Volume 5

CASE STUDIES: Stahl's Essential Psychopharmacology

Volume 5

Edited by

Nevena V. Radonjić

SUNY Upstate Medical University, Syracuse, NY, USA

Thomas L. Schwartz

SUNY Upstate Medical University, Syracuse, NY, USA

Stephen M. Stahl

University of California at San Diego, CA, USA
University of Cambridge, Cambridge, UK

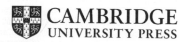

CAMBRIDGE
UNIVERSITY PRESS

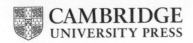

Shaftesbury Road, Cambridge CB2 8EA, United Kingdom

One Liberty Plaza, 20th Floor, New York, NY 10006, USA

477 Williamstown Road, Port Melbourne, VIC 3207, Australia

314–321, 3rd Floor, Plot 3, Splendor Forum, Jasola District Centre,
New Delhi – 110025, India

103 Penang Road, #05–06/07, Visioncrest Commercial, Singapore 238467

Cambridge University Press is part of Cambridge University Press & Assessment,
a department of the University of Cambridge.

We share the University's mission to contribute to society through the pursuit of
education, learning, and research at the highest international levels of excellence.

www.cambridge.org
Information on this title: www.cambridge.org/9781108463614

DOI: 10.1017/9781108623872

© Cambridge University Press & Assessment 2024

First published 2024

Printed in Mexico by Litográfica Ingramex, S.A. de C.V.

A catalogue record for this publication is available from the British Library.

Library of Congress Cataloging-in-Publication Data
Names: Radonjić, Nevena V., editor. | Schwartz, Thomas L., editor. |
    Stahl, Stephen M., 1951– editor. | Stahl, Stephen M., 1951– Case
    studies.
Title: Case studies : Stahl's essential psychopharmacology. Volume 5 /
    edited by Nevena V. Radonjić, Thomas L. Schwartz, Stephen M. Stahl.
Other titles: Case studies (Radonjić) | Stahl's essential
    psychopharmacology
Description: Cambridge, United Kingdom ; New York, NY : Cambridge
    University Press, 2023. | Preceded by Case studies : Stahl's essential
    psychopharmacology / Stephen M. Stahl. 2011. | Includes bibliographical
    references and index.
Identifiers: LCCN 2023027267 (print) | LCCN 2023027268 (ebook) | ISBN
    9781108463614 (v. 5 ; paperback) | ISBN 9781108623872 (v. 5 ; ebook)
Subjects: MESH: Mental Disorders – drug therapy | Psychotropic
    Drugs – therapeutic use | Psychopharmacology – methods | Case Reports |
    Examination Questions
Classification: LCC RC454 (print) | LCC RC454 (ebook) | NLM WM 18.2 |
    DDC 616.89–dc23/eng/20230726
LC record available at https://lccn.loc.gov/2023027267
LC ebook record available at https://lccn.loc.gov/2023027268

ISBN 978-1-108-46361-4 Paperback

Contents

Introduction

Following on from the success of the launch volume of *Case Studies* in 2011, we are very pleased to present a fifth collection of new clinical cases. *Stahl's Essential Psychopharmacology* started in 1996 as a textbook (currently in its fifth edition) on how psychotropic drugs work. It expanded to a companion Prescriber's Guide in 2005 (currently in its eighth edition) on how to prescribe psychotropic drugs. In 2008, a website was added (www.cambridge.org/core/publications/collections/stahl-online) with both of these books available online in combination with several more, including an *Illustrated* series of books covering specialty topics in psychopharmacology. The *Case Studies* shows how to apply the concepts presented in these previous books to real patients in a clinical practice setting.

Why a case book? For practitioners, it is necessary to know the science and application of psychopharmacology – namely, both the mechanism of action of psychotropic drugs and the evidence-based data on how to prescribe them – but this is not sufficient to become a master clinician. Many patients are beyond the data and are excluded from randomized controlled trials. Thus, a true clinical expert also needs to develop the art of psychopharmacology: namely, how to listen, educate, destigmatize, mix psychotherapy with medications, and use intuition to select and combine medications. The art of psychopharmacology is especially important when confronting the frequent situations where there is no evidence on which to base a clinical decision.

What do you do when there is no evidence? The short answer is to combine the science with the art of psychopharmacology. The best way to learn this is probably by seeing individual patients. Here we hope you will join us and peer over our shoulders to observe 28 complex cases from our own clinical practice.

Each case is anonymized in identifying details, but incorporates real case outcomes that are not fictionalized. Sometimes more than one case is combined into a single case. Hopefully, you will recognize many of these patients as similar to those you have seen in your own practice (although they will not be exactly the same patient, as the identifying historical details are changed here to comply with disclosure standards, and many patients can look very much like many other patients you know, which is why you may find this teaching approach effective for your clinical practice).

We have presented cases from our clinical practice for many years online (e.g., in the master psychopharmacology program of the Neuroscience Education Institute [NEI] at neiglobal.com) and in live courses (especially at the annual NEI Psychopharmacology Congress). Over the years, we have been fortunate to have many young psychiatrists from our universities, and indeed from all over the world, sit in on our practices to observe these cases, and now we attempt to bring this information to you in the form of a fifth case book.

The cases are presented in a novel written format in order to follow consultations over time, with different categories of information designated by different background colors and explanatory icons. For those of you familiar with *The Prescriber's Guide*, this layout will be recognizable. Included in the case book, however, are many unique sections as well; for example, presenting what was on the author's mind at various points during the management of the case, and also questions along the way for you to ask yourself in order to develop an action plan.

Additionally, these cases incorporate ideas from the recent changes in maintenance of certification standards by the American Board of Psychiatry and Neurology for those of you interested in recertification in psychiatry. Thus, there is a section on Performance in Practice (called here "Confessions of a psychopharmacologist"). This is a short section at the end of every case, looking back and seeing what could have been done better in retrospect. Another section of most cases is a short psychopharmacology lesson or tutorial, called the "Two-minute tutorial," with background information, tables, and figures from literature relevant to the case in hand.

Drugs are listed by their generic and brand names for ease of learning. Indexes are included at the back of the book for your convenience. Lists of icons and abbreviations are provided in the front of the book. Finally, this fifth collection updates the reader on the newest psychotropic drugs and their uses, and adopts the language of DSM-5.

The case-based approach is how this book attempts to complement "evidence-based prescribing" from other books in the *Essential Psychopharmacology* series, plus the literature, with "prescribing-based evidence" derived from empiric experience. It is certainly important to know the data from randomized controlled trials, but after knowing all this information, case-based clinical experience supplements that data. The old saying that applies here is that wisdom is what you learn *after* you know it all; and so, too, for studying cases after seeing the data.

A note of caution: we are not so naïve as to think that there are not potential pitfalls to the centuries-old tradition of case-based teaching. Thus, we think it is a good idea to point some of them out here in order to try to avoid these traps. Do not ignore the "law of small numbers" by basing broad predictions on narrow samples or even a single case.

Do not ignore the fact that if something is easy to recall, particularly when associated with a significant emotional event, we tend to think it happens more often than it does.

Do not forget the recency effect, namely, the tendency to think that something that has just been observed happens more often than it does.

According to editorialists[1], when moving away from evidence-based medicine to case-based medicine, it is also important to avoid:

- Eloquence or elegance-based medicine
- Vehemence-based medicine
- Providence-based medicine
- Diffidence-based medicine
- Nervousness-based medicine
- Confidence-based medicine

We have been counseled by colleagues and trainees that perhaps the most important pitfall for me to try to avoid in this book is "eminence-based medicine," and to remember specifically that:

- Radiance of gray hair is not proportional to an understanding of the facts
- Eloquence, smoothness of the tongue, and sartorial elegance cannot change reality
- Qualifications and past accomplishments do not signify a privileged access to the truth
- Experts almost always have conflicts of interest
- Clinical acumen is not measured in frequent flier miles

Thus, it is with all humility as practicing psychiatrists that we invite you to walk a mile in our shoes: experience the fascination, the disappointments, the thrills, and the learnings that result from observing cases in the real world.

Dr. Schwartz would like to thank all of those whose goal it is to teach clinicians to become better treaters of their patients, given our common goal is to improve their symptoms and reduce their suffering.

Dr. Radonjić would like to sincerely thank Dr. Thomas Schwartz, SUNY Upstate, for providing mentorship, support, and constructive feedback in the process of writing this manuscript, and Dr. Stephen Stahl for valuable input and guidance that elevated the quality of the case studies. Special thanks to Dr. Nada Zečević, University of Connecticut, and Dr. Nataša Petronijević, University of Belgrade, for continuous support during academic development. Finally, Dr. Radonjić would like to express gratitude to her family for modeling and instilling a love for research, teaching, and education.

Nevena V. Radonjić, MD, PhD

Thomas L. Schwartz, MD

Stephen M. Stahl, MD, PhD

References

1 Isaccs D, Fitzgerald D. Seven alternatives to evidence based medicine. *BMJ* 1999; 319:7225

Contributors

Melissa Abbuhl, MD, Norton College of Medicine at SUNY Upstate Medical University
Cecilia Albers, MD, University of Missouri School of Medicine
Fairouz Ali, MD, Norton College of Medicine at SUNY Upstate Medical University
Jaclyn Blaauboer, MD, Norton College of Medicine at SUNY Upstate Medical University
Elena Capello, MD, Norton College of Medicine at SUNY Upstate Medical University
Shiyu Chen, MD, Norton College of Medicine at SUNY Upstate Medical University
Brian Coringrato, DO, Norton College of Medicine at SUNY Upstate Medical University
Christopher Damiani, DO, Norton College of Medicine at SUNY Upstate Medical University
Sharon Ekure, MD, Norton College of Medicine at SUNY Upstate Medical University
James Gilfert, MD, Norton College of Medicine at SUNY Upstate Medical University
Hassaan Gomaa, MD, Pennsylvania State College of Medicine
Daniel Jackson, MD, Norton College of Medicine at SUNY Upstate Medical University
Muslim Khan, MD, Norton College of Medicine at SUNY Upstate Medical University
Kathryn Meyers, MD, Norton College of Medicine at SUNY Upstate Medical University
Christina Mihai, MD, Weill Cornell School of Medicine
Sutanaya Pal, MD, Norton College of Medicine at SUNY Upstate Medical University
Nevena Radonjić, MD, PhD, Norton College of Medicine at SUNY Upstate Medical University
Sabahath Shaik, MD, NP, Norton College of Medicine at SUNY Upstate Medical University
Rebecca Shields, DO, Norton College of Medicine at SUNY Upstate Medical University
Sunita Singh, MD, Norton College of Medicine at SUNY Upstate Medical University
Amanda Stallone, MD, Norton College of Medicine at SUNY Upstate Medical University
Charles Welch, MD, University of Missouri School of Medicine
Mark Wiener, MD, Weill Cornell School of Medicine

List of icons

 Pre- and post-test self-assessment question; question

 Patient evaluation on intake; patient evaluation on initial visit

 Psychiatric history

 Social and personal history

 Medical history

 Family history

 Medication history

 Current medications

 Psychotherapy history; psychotherapy moment

 Mechanism of action moment

Attending physician's mental notes

 Further investigation

 Case outcome; use of outcome measures

 Case debrief

 Take-home points

 Performance in practice: confessions of a psychopharmacologist

 Tips and pearls

 Two-minute tutorial

Abbreviations

5-HT	serotonin	BB	beta blocker
5-HT$_{1A}$/$_{2A}$, etc.	serotonin (receptors)	BDNF	brain-derived neurotrophic factor
α_1A	alpha 1A receptor	BED	binge eating disorder
α_1B	alpha 1B receptor	BIF	borderline intellectual functioning
α_2	alpha 2 receptor	BMI	body mass index
α_2A	alpha 2A receptor	BN	bulimia nervosa
σ_1	sigma 1 receptor	BP	bipolar disorder
AA	Alcoholics Anonymous	BP1	bipolar I disorder
ACC	anterior cingulate cortex	BP2	bipolar II disorder
ACE	angiotensin-converting enzyme	BPD	borderline personality disorder
ACh	acetylcholine	BZ	benzodiazepine
AChR	acetycholine receptors	BZRA	benzodiazepine receptor agonist
ACTH	adrenocorticotropic hormone	CAD	coronary artery disease
ADHD	Attention-Deficit/Hyperactivity Disorder	CAGE	cut down, annoyed, guilty, and eye opener
AIMS	Abnormal Involuntary Movement Scale	CAM	complementary and alternative medicine
AMPA	alpha-amino-3-hydroxy-5-methyl-4-isoxazole-propionic acid	CBC	complete blood count
		CBT	cognitive behavioral therapy
AMPAR	alpha-amino-3-hydroxy-5-methyl-4-isoxazole-propionic acid receptor	CD	covert dyskinesia
		CIWA	Clinical Institute Withdrawal Assessment
AMRS	Altman Mania Rating Scale	CKD	chronic kidney disease
ANA	antinuclear antibodies	CMP	comprehensive metabolic panel
ANC	absolute neutrophil count	CNS	central nervous system
ASD	autism spectrum disorder	COWS	Clinical Opiate Withdrawal Scale
ASRS	Adult ADHD Self-Report Scale	CPG	clinical practice guideline
aTL	anterior temporal lobe	CPT	cold pressor time
AUD	alcohol use disorder	CR	controlled release
BARS	Barnes Akathisia Rating Scale	Cre	creatinine

CRF	corticotropin-releasing factor	EPS	extrapyramidal symptom/s
CRPS	complex regional pain syndrome	ER	emergency room; extended release
CSTC	cortico-striatal-thalamo-cortical circuit	ERP	exposure and response prevention
CUD	cannabis use disorder	ERs	estrogen receptors
CVS	cerebrovascular system	ESR	erythrocyte sedimentation rate
CYP450	cytochrome P450	FBG	fasting blood glucose
D_2	dopamine-2 receptor	FDA	US Food and Drug Administration
D_3	dopamine-3 receptor	FM	fibromyalgia
DA	dopamine	FSH	follicle-stimulating hormone
dACC	dorsal anterior cingulate cortex		
DAT	dopamine transporter	fT4	free thyroxine
DBS	deep brain stimulation	GABA	gamma-aminobutyric acid
DBT	dialectical behavioral therapy	GAD	generalized anxiety disorder
DDP	dynamic deconstructive psychotherapy	GAD7	Generalized Anxiety Disorder Questionnaire
DID	dissociative identity disorder	GED	general educational development
DLPFC	dorsolateral prefrontal cortex	GERD	gastroesophageal reflux disease
DM2	diabetes mellitus type 2	GFR	glomerular filtration rate
DORA	dual orexin receptor antagonist	GHB	γ-hydroxybutyrate
DSM-5	*Diagnostic and Statistical Manual of Mental Disorders*, 5th edn.	GI	gastrointestinal
		GluR 1–4	glutamate receptor 1–4
dTMS	deep transcranial magnetic stimulation	GlyT	glycine transporter
		GPER1	G-protein coupled ER1
ECT	electroconvulsive therapy	GWAS	genome-wide association studies
ED	erectile dysfunction	H1	histamine 1 receptor
EEG	electroencephalogram	HbA1c	hemoglobin A1c
EKG	electrocardiogram	HIV	human immunodeficiency virus
EMDR	eye movement desensitization and reprocessing	HLD	hyperlipidemia
		HPA	hypothalamic–pituitary–adrenal
ENDS	electronic nicotine delivery system	HPL	hyperprolactinemia
EPDS	Edinburgh Postnatal Depression Scale	HRT	hormone replacement therapy

HSDD	hypoactive sexual desire disorder	NaSSA	norepinephrine antagonist / selective serotonin antagonist
HTN	hypertension		
IBS	irritable bowel syndrome	NDRI	norepinephrine–dopamine reuptake inhibitor
ICU	intensive care unit		
ID	intellectual disability		
IM	intramuscular	NE	norepinephrine
IPT	interpersonal psychotherapy	NET	norepinephrine transporter
IR	immediate release	NMDA	N-methyl-D-aspartate
IUD	intrauterine device	NMDAR	N-methyl-D-aspartate receptor
IV	intravenous		
LAI	long-acting injectable	NMJ	neuromuscular junction
LC	locus coeruleus	NMS	neuroleptic malignant syndrome
LD	learning disability		
LDL	low-density lipoproteins	NNH	number needed to harm
LFT	liver function testing	NR1	NMDA receptor subunit 1
LH	luteinizing hormone		
LMWH	low-molecular-weight heparin	NR2	NMDA receptor subunit 2
LSD	lysergic acid diethylamide	NR3	NMDA receptor subunit 3
M1/M3/M5	muscarinic receptor 1/3/5	NRI	norepinephrine reuptake inhibitor
MAOI	monoamine oxidase inhibitor	NRT	nicotine replacement therapy
MC	myasthenic crisis		
MDD	major depressive disorder	NSAIDs	nonsteroidal anti-inflammatory drugs
MDE	major depressive episode	OC	oculogyric crisis
MDMA	methylenedioxymethamphetamine	OCD	obsessive–compulsive disorder
MDQ	Mood Disorders Questionnaire	OCI-R	Obsessive–Compulsive Inventory – revised
MG	myasthenia gravis	OCP	oral contraceptive pill
mPFC	medial prefrontal cortex	OCPD	obsessive–compulsive personality disorder
MRI	magnetic resonance imaging	ODD	oppositional defiant disorder
MS	multiple sclerosis	ODT	oral dissolving tablet
mTOR	mammalian/mechanistic target of rapamycin	OFC	orbital frontal cortex
		OSA	obstructive sleep apnea
NA	nucleus accumbens	OTC	over-the-counter
NAC	N-acetylcysteine	OUD	opioid use disorder

PAHs	polycyclic aromatic hydrocarbons	SAMe	S-adenosyl-methionine
PAM	positive allosteric modulator	SARI	serotonin antagonist / reuptake inhibitor
PC12	pheochromocytoma cell line	SCARED	Screen for Child Anxiety-Related Disorders
PCC	primary care clinician	SERT	serotonin transporter
PCL 5	PTSD Checklist for DSM-5	SIADH	syndrome of inappropriate antidiuretic hormone
PCP	phencyclidine	SIB	self-injurious behavior
PD	panic disorder	SLC6	solute carrier gene family
PDD	pervasive developmental disorders	SMM	serotonin multimodal
PDP	psychodynamic psychotherapy	SNRI	serotonin–norepinephrine reuptake inhibitor
PFC	prefrontal cortex	SP	schizophrenia
PHQ-9	Patient Health Questionnaire	SPARI	serotonin partial agonist / reuptake inhibitor
PLLR	Pregnancy And Lactation Labeling Rule	SRI	serotonin reuptake inhibitor
PMADs	perinatal mood and anxiety disorders	SSRI	selective serotonin reuptake inhibitor
PMC	prefrontal motor cortex	SSS	Symptom Severity Score
POCS	Perinatal Obsessive Compulsive Scale	STEPPS	systems training for emotional predictability and problem-solving
POMC	pro-opiomelanocortin		
PPD	pack per day		
PRN	pro re nata (as needed)	SUD	substance use disorder
PT/INR	prothrombin time / international normalized ratio	TCA	tricyclic antidepressant
		TD	tardive dyskinesia
PTSD	post-traumatic stress disorder	TEAs	treatment-emergent activations
QTc	QT corrected for heart rate	TFP	transference-focused therapy
RCT	randomized controlled trial	TGA	triglycerides
		Tmax	peak plasma time
REM	rapid eye movement	TMN	tuberomammillary nucleus
REMS	risk evaluation and mitigation strategy	TMS	transcranial magnetic stimulation
RID	relative infant dose		
RMS	Rapid Mood Screener	TPJ	temporo-parietal junction
SAD	seasonal affective disorder		

TRD	treatment-resistant depression	VMAT2	vesicular monoamine transporter 2
TRS	treatment-resistant schizophrenia	VMPFC	ventromedial prefrontal cortex
TSH	thyroid-stimulating hormone	VMS	vasomotor symptoms
		VNS	vagal nerve stimulation
UDS	urine drug screen	VPA	valproic acid
UTI	urinary tract infection	VTA	ventral tegmental area
VA	Veterans Affairs	WHO	World Health Organization
VEGF	vascular endothelial growth factor	WNL	within normal limits
VLPO	ventrolateral preoptic area	Y-BOCS	Yale–Brown Obsessive Compulsive Scale

Case 1: Usage of esketamine spray for treatment-resistant major depressive disorder (MDD)

The Question: What is the therapeutic dose and duration of treatment for esketamine (Spravato) nasal spray in depression?

The Psychopharmacological Dilemma: Finding an effective treatment regimen utilizing esketamine (Spravato) spray for treatment-resistant depression (TRD)

Sunita Singh

Pretest self-assessment question

How are the antidepressant effects of esketamine (Spravato) pharmacodynamically mediated?
A. N-methyl-D-aspartate receptor (NMDAR) antagonism
B. Increases brain-derived neurotrophic factor (BDNF) and mammalian target of rapamycin (mTOR) activity
C. Alpha-amino-3-hydroxy-5-methyl-4-isoxazole-propionic acid receptor (AMPAR) antagonism
D. Dopamine-2 receptor (D_2) agonism
E. A and B
F. All of the above

Patient evaluation on intake

- A 42-year-old woman with a chief complaint of being "depressed, hanging on barely"
- Chronically depressed with comorbid panic disorder (PD), uses polypharmacy and vagal nerve stimulation (VNS), all of which seem to be failing over last several weeks
- Presents for first esketamine (Spravato) spray treatment today
- Recurrent MDD now in recurrence with extensive treatment failures
- Panic disorder is remitted though
- Currently exhibits anhedonia, dysphoric mood and constricted congruent affect which are affecting her performance at work
- MDD symptoms escalating with occasional passive suicidal ideation which is worrisome
- Compliant with previous medication management
- Reports no side effects on current regimen
- No contraindications to esketamine (Spravato) nasal spray treatment, has prior authorization, and has read the patient guide regarding treatment

Psychiatric history

- Long history of MDD with some resultant anxiety, with fear of others' judgments, and also suffers from PD with mild agoraphobic symptoms
- Previously endorsed symptoms of fatigue, hypersomnia, social isolation, low motivation, appetite disturbance, feelings of guilt and low self-worth, and negative self-thinking
- VNS implanted in 2007 with adequate response for several years, but response now fading
- Prior to today, failed 30+ medications (including electroconvulsive therapy [ECT], VNS, IV ketamine [weekly dosing], and psychotherapy)

Social and personal history

- Former smoker, quit several years ago
  - Recently restarted smoking with onset of recurrent MDD symptoms
  - Prior history of light daily cigarette-smoking
- Rare alcohol use
- No recreational drug use
- Single parent with grown son
- Works as a nurse per diem

Medical history

- Osteoarthritis
- Gastroesophageal reflux disease (GERD)
- Kidney stones
- Raynaud phenomenon

Family history

- History of depression and anxiety, but extent is unknown
- Patient's family places emphasis on appearances and impressions, which causes her to fear making mistakes and looking foolish
- Anxiety disorder in her paternal aunt and grandmother

Medication history

Previous therapeutic failures:

- SSRIs: selective serotonin reuptake inhibitors
  - Fluoxetine (Prozac)
  - Sertraline (Zoloft)
- SNRIs: serotonin–norepinephrine reuptake inhibitors
  - Venlafaxine (Effexor XR)

- ○ Duloxetine (Cymbalta)
- SARIs: serotonin antagonist / reuptake inhibitors
  - ○ Trazodone (Desyrel)
  - ○ Nefazodone (Serzone)
- NDRI: norepinephrine–dopamine reuptake inhibitor
  - ○ Bupropion (Wellbutrin XL)
- NaSSA: norepinephrine antagonist / selective serotonin antagonist
  - ○ Mirtazapine (Remeron)
- TCAs: tricyclic antidepressants
  - ○ Doxepin (Adapin)
  - ○ Desipramine (Norpramin)
  - ○ Amitriptyline (Elavil)
  - ○ Clomipramine (Anafranil)
- MAOIs: monoamine oxidase inhibitors
  - ○ Selegiline (Emsam)
  - ○ Tranylcypromine (Parnate)
- SPARIs: serotonin partial agonist / reuptake inhibitors
  - ○ Vilazodone (Viibryd)
- Augmentations
  - ○ Benzodiazepines (BZs)
    - Lorazepam (Ativan)
    - Diazepam (Valium)
    - Clonazepam (Klonopin)
    - Estazolam (Prosom)
    - Zolpidem (Ambien)
- Atypical antipsychotics
  - ○ Quetiapine (Seroquel)
  - ○ Aripiprazole (Abilify)
  - ○ Olanzapine (Zyprexa)
- Anticonvulsant
  - ○ Divalproex (Depakote)
  - ○ Lamotrigine (Lamictal)
- Stimulant
  - ○ Dextroamphetamine (Dexadrine)
  - ○ d/l-amphetamine (Adderall)
  - ○ Methylphenidate (Ritalin)
  - ○ Dexmethylphenidate (Focalin)
  - ○ Modafinil (Provigil)
  - ○ Armodafinil (Nuvigil)
- Nutraceutical
  - ○ N-acetylcysteine (NAC)
  - ○ L-methylfolate (Deplin)

- D_2/D_3 partial agonist
  - Pramipexole (Mirapex)
- Others
  - Buspirone (Buspar), a serotonin 1A (5-HT_{1A}) partial receptor agonist
  - Lithium (Eskalith), a calcium modulating mood stabilizer
  - Liothyronine (Cytomel), a thyroid augmentation
  - Atomoxetine (Strattera), a norepinephrine reuptake inhibitor (NRI)
- Interventional
  - VNS
  - ECT
  - Ketamine (Ketalar) IV failed (6 sessions, 0.5 mg/kg once weekly)

Psychotherapy history

- Limited success in weekly psychotherapy
- Admits that she has given up quickly with psychotherapy when she feels uncomfortable
- Not currently in psychotherapy

Current medications

- Vortioxetine (Trintellix) 20 mg/d (SPARI)
- Alprazolam (Xanax) 0.75 mg/d, a BZ
- Cariprazine (Vraylar) 0.75 mg/d, an atypical antipsychotic
- Lisdexamfetamine (Vyvanse) 70 mg/d, a stimulant
- L-methylfolate (Deplin) 15 mg/d, a nutraceutical one carbon cycle enhancer
- Vagus nerve stimulator

Question

Considering the patient's multiple failed treatments, including previous failure of ketamine IV, do you think it is likely that the esketamine (Spravato) intranasal spray treatment will be effective?

- Yes: as the ketamine (Ketalar) IV was given weekly, and esketamine (Spravato) will use a loading dose with multiple sessions within the first few weeks
- No: as ketamine (Ketalar) IV is absorbed more efficiently than intranasal esketamine (Spravato), it is unlikely that intranasal esketamine (Spravato) will be effective at this time

Attending physician's mental notes: initial psychiatric evaluation

- Although intranasal absorption of a drug is much less compared to IV administration, esketamine has four-fold more potency for NMDAR antagonism compared to racemic ketamine
- Given the ease of intranasal administration compared to IV treatments, it is worth evaluating intranasal esketamine spray as a treatment option for TRD even if ketamine (Ketalar) IV failed
- Additionally, her ketamine (Ketalar) IV treatments did not use a loading dose. Therefore, it was possibly subtherapeutic. A loading dose will be used for the esketamine (Spravato) treatments
- Patient with chronic MDD and anxiety is on polypharmacy and VNS, but now has recurrence of a new MDD episode without many new options or new treatments available in the current pipeline
- Esketamine (Spravato) is newly available and likely worth a trial, even if palliative

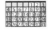

Case outcome: first esketamine (Spravato) treatment

- Patient was prepped and dosed with the usual starting 56 mg esketamine (Spravato) spray over several minutes and tolerated administration well with initial blood pressure of 126/78
- 40 minutes after administration, patient reported mild sedation and some "loopy" feelings for several minutes but was not sedated nor dissociative, with a blood pressure of 110/70
  - Interestingly, blood pressure lowered here when there are regulatory warnings for likely increases during treatment sessions
- 2 hours after administration, patient reported no side effects and was ready to go home, with a final blood pressure of 112/68
  - Patients are obligated to have someone else drive them home after sessions

Question

What adverse effects are common and should be monitored for after esketamine (Spravato) spray administration?

Blood pressure elevation?
Bradycardia?
Wheezing?
Sedation?
Dissociation?
Nausea?
Respiratory suppression?

Attending physician's mental notes: first psychiatric follow-up visit

- Effects of esketamine (Spravato) and ketamine (Ketalar) are primarily mediated by its antagonistic NMDAR activity, causing its anesthetic and analgesic effects
- Esketamine/ketamine also can have antagonistic activity at monoaminergic, muscarinic, and nicotinic receptors, causing a range of adverse effects that should be monitored for after administration
- Patient tolerated first esketamine (Spravato) spray well and had minimal issues with the usual side effects of sedation, nausea, hypertension, and dissociation
- Due to recurrent MDD, we agreed to continue current medications and increase dosing of esketamine (Spravato) sprays to the higher available 84 mg/d dose and continue them twice weekly
- Reported feelings of anxiety are stable and only situational; panic has not worsened due to nasal sprays

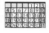

Case outcome: weeks 2 through 8

- Over the next 4 weeks, patient received seven more esketamine (Spravato) 84 mg spray treatments, where the usual is to receive twice a week for the first month and then once weekly for the second month
- For the following 4 weeks, patient received four esketamine (Spravato) spray treatments of 84 mg each, completing the US Food and Drug Administration (FDA) approved protocol
- During this course, patient continued her previous oral medication regimen as well:
  - Vortioxetine (Trintellix) 20 mg/d
  - Cariprazine (Vraylar) 0.75 mg/d
  - Lisdexamfetamine (Vyvanse) 70 mg/d
  - L-methylfolate (Deplin) 15 mg/d
- Patient MDD symptoms went into full remission
- However, once esketamine (Spravato) spray was discontinued at the end of 8 weeks, patient had return of MDD symptoms at 12 days without ongoing nasal sprays

Question

What options exist for patients who relapse when esketamine (Spravato) sessions end?

- Start new 12-dose course of esketamine (Spravato)
- Start maintenance treatments with esketamine (Spravato) every 7–10 days
- Increase dose of esketamine (Spravato) above regulatory limits

Attending physician's mental notes (weeks 2 through 8)

- The approved dosing guidelines for esketamine (Spravato) spray are an induction spray twice weekly for 4 weeks
- Based on patient's response and tolerability, this dose can be increased from 56 mg to 84 mg
- After evaluating its therapeutic benefit for 4 weeks, the established dose (56 mg or 84 mg) can be continued weekly as maintenance therapy up to 8 weeks
- Maintenance therapy for MDD with IV ketamine (Ketalar) is well established, providing support to the use of esketamine (Spravato) spray off label for maintenance therapy, which has not been well delineated or FDA approved
- Since our patient had remission of MDD symptoms with esketamine (Spravato) spray, likely is best to continue ongoing maintenance treatments every 7–10 days

Case outcome: follow-up visit at 2 months

- Patient re-started weekly 84 mg dosing of esketamine (Spravato) spray and MDD symptoms remitted again
- Patient reported that esketamine (Spravato) spray would alleviate depressive symptoms for 7–10 days, but then would lose effectiveness and depressive symptoms would return before next scheduled dose
  - Reports sadness, amotivation, fatigue, and inability to get out of bed when the esketamine (Spravato) spray effect diminishes
- Otherwise tolerating esketamine (Spravato) spray treatment well with no side effects

Attending physician's mental notes: second interim follow-up visit (month 2)

- Because of her intermittent return of symptoms, her current oral medication regimen seems to be inadequate despite ongoing esketamine (Spravato) use
- Need to consider novel treatments of off-label therapies with a similar mechanism of action to esketamine (Spravato) spray, which may help ultimately to taper off esketamine (Spravato) spray

Question

How would you alter her medication regimen to alleviate her return of MDD symptoms between esketamine (Spravato) doses?

- Decrease length of time between esketamine (Spravato) spray treatments and continue its use indefinitely

- Add dextromethorphan / quinidine sulfate (Nuedexta) as it manipulates glutamate activity as well
- Recommend new trial of psychotherapy
- Recommend new trial of ketamine IV (Ketalar)
- Recommend new series of ECT

Attending physician's mental notes: second interim follow-up visit (month 2) (continued)

- Patient likely cannot afford indefinite weekly treatments of esketamine (Spravato) spray and declines psychotherapy. She also declines ECT as it would interfere with her work
- As esketamine (Spravato) spray is helping to decrease her MDD symptoms, another glutamate medication may mimic the effects of esketamine (Spravato) spray and allow increased time between nasal spray sessions
- Decided to add dextromethorphan / quinidine sulfate (Nuedexta) as it will weakly antagonize NMDA receptors (NMDARs), somewhat similar to the effect of esketamine (Spravato) spray
  ○ This agent is approved for use in treating pseudobulbar affect
- Will keep esketamine (Spravato) spray weekly, but patient will take dextromethorphan / quinidine sulfate (Nuedexta) only on days 5/6 when depressive symptoms start appearing again, hopefully avoiding MDD relapse

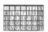

Case outcome: follow-up visit at 3 months

- Reports depressive symptoms are recurrent between sessions, but mild and possibly improving with esketamine (Spravato) spray plus dextromethorphan / quinidine sulfate (Nuedexta) treatment augmentation
- Patient expressed concern about affording esketamine (Spravato) spray treatment long term and is worried about having to stop treatment abruptly
- Chooses to increase length between sessions to 2 weeks as she feels she can only afford 20 more sessions

Attending physician's mental notes: follow-up visit (month 3)

- Esketamine (Spravato) spray every 2 weeks still allows MDD relapses to occur
- Dextromethorphan / quinidine sulfate (Nuedexta) now increased to daily use without side effects
- Still difficult to wean off esketamine (Spravato) spray without MDD relapse

Question

What would you do next?

- Stop dextromethorphan / quinidine sulfate (Nuedexta) and try to find another novel glutamate-based treatment
- Review chart and remove current non-effective medications and restart medications that seemed to help in the past

Case outcome: follow-up at 3 months

- Dextromethorphan / quinidine sulfate (Nuedexta) has not been able to replace esketamine (Spravato) and was discontinued as it was ineffective
- Cariprazine (Vraylar) removed as it was ineffective
- L-methylfolate (Deplin) removed as it was ineffective
- Confirmed alprazolam (Xanax) was not being taken, as some accounts suggest benzodiazepine use may lower ketamine/ esketamine effectiveness
- Main residual MDD symptoms are increased fatigue and amotivation and she has failed multiple stimulant treatments; will try medications that will increase norepinephrine activity perhaps instead of dopamine
- She has never taken the more highly noradrenergic SNRI levomilnacipran (Fetzima), so will titrate that next

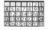

Case outcome: follow-up at 6 months

- With levomilnacipran (Fetzima) 120 mg/d treatment, she only requires esketamine (Spravato) spray now every 30–45 days
- Maintenance began with nasal sprays every 7 days, then 10 days, then 15 days, and so on until 45+ days was achieved
- Nasal sprays continue to be spaced farther apart in this manner
- Lisdexamfetamine (Vyvanse) effectively lowered from 70 mg/d down to 20 mg/d
- Vortioxetine (Trintellix) lowered to 10 mg/d to avoid serotonin toxicity when combining with newer levomilnacipran (Fetzima)
- Current medications now include:
  - Vortioxetine (Trintellix) 10 mg/d
  - Lisdexamfetamine (Vyvanse) 20 mg/d
  - Levomilnacipran (Fetzima) 120 mg/d
  - Esketamine (Spravato) 84 mg every 2 months
- Vagal nerve stimulator battery depleted and not replaced due to its ineffectiveness

Case debrief

- This patient has clear TRD and had failed practically every treatment available, including psychotherapy, polypharmacy, and intervention with ECT, VNS, and ketamine (Ketalar) IV
- Interestingly, nasal esketamine (Spravato) helped to gain temporary remission from MDD when the IV racemic ketamine treatment failed previously
  - Assume this is due to the fact that the nasal spray used an induction or loading strategy with multiple treatments per week, whereas the IV used an older once-weekly protocol
- Patients often do not remit in a sustained or durable fashion from their depression symptoms after acute IV treatment, nor do they from the nasal sprays
- In this case, ineffective medications were streamlined and taken away (l-methylfolate [Deplin], cariprazine [Vraylar]) or lowered (vortioxetine [Trintellix], lisdexamfetamine [Vyvanse]), and new medications (dextromethorphan/quinidine [Nuedexta] and levomilnacipran [Fetzima]) were tried to gain a more durable response to allow a tapering off of esketamine (Spravato) nasal sprays, seemingly with good effectiveness
- This approach allowed for minimizing esketamine (Spravato) nasal spray treatments, to occur every 3 months instead of every week

Take-home points

- Incidence of TRD is common, 30% or greater prevalence
- Some definitions suggest this is a failure to respond to two different antidepressants from different classes
- Many patients are actually more treatment resistant than this, as this case illustrates
- It is unclear when patients become truly refractory, but the goal of treatment regardless should be to keep trying for symptom remission prior to assuming a more palliative psychiatric approach
- Interestingly, nasal esketamine (Spravato) can work even if IV ketamine has previously failed
- Finally, many patients who use esketamine (Spravato) will likely need maintenance treatment, whereas the most recent 4-year data suggests that about 70% of patients who respond will durably maintain their responses

Performance in practice: confessions of a psychopharmacologist

What could have been done better here?

- Perhaps continuing esketamine (Spravato) in a weekly maintenance fashion for those patients with clearly recurrent TRD is warranted instead of stopping at 8 weeks per indication, as TRD patients are known to relapse and have recurrences at a greater rate than others with alternative antidepressant treatments

What are possible action items for improvement in practice?

- Review the literature on maintenance IV ketamine (Ketalar) use for TRD
- Review similar for esketamine (Spravato)
- Review literature and texts to determine whether there are other oral medications with similar mechanism of action to ketamine and esketamine for possible cross-titration
  - Dextromethorphan/quinidine (Nuplazid) for pseudobulbar affect
  - Dextromethorphan/bupropion (Auvelity) for MDD

Mechanism of action moment

- Ketamine:
  - Acts to blockade excitatory synaptic glutamate activity, due to its antagonistic effects on NMDA glutamate receptors (NMDARs) (Figure 1.1)

Site of action of PCP and ketamine: bind to open channel at PCP site to block NMDA R

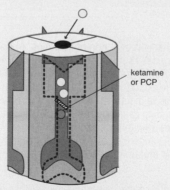

ketamine or PCP

Figure 1.1 Site of action of ketamine. Ketamine binds to the open channel conformation of the NMDAR. Specifically, it binds to a site within the calcium channel of this receptor, which is often termed the PCP site because it is also where phencyclidine (PCP) binds. Blockade of NMDARs may prevent the excitatory actions of glutamate, which is postulated to be a therapeutic mechanism for treating depression.

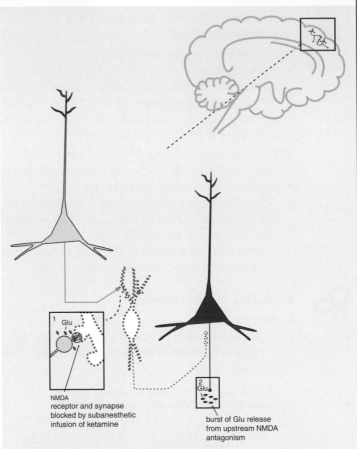

NMDA
receptor and synapse
blocked by subanesthetic
infusion of ketamine

burst of Glu release
from upstream NMDA
antagonism

Figure 1.2 Mechanism of action of ketamine. Shown here are two cortical glutamatergic pyramidal neurons and a GABAergic interneuron. (1) If an NMDAR on a GABAergic interneuron is blocked by ketamine, this prevents the excitatory actions of glutamate (Glu) there. Thus, the GABA neuron is inactivated and does not release GABA (indicated by the dotted outline of the neuron). (2) GABA binding at the second cortical glutamatergic pyramidal neuron normally inhibits glutamate release: thus, the absence of GABA there means that the neuron is disinhibited, and glutamate release is increased.

- At higher doses is responsible for loss of alertness/ responsiveness when used for anesthesia
- At moderate to higher doses is responsible for feelings of dissociation and delirium
- Lower doses may cause an increase in glutamate cycling and extracellular glutamate availability as NMDARs are blocked,

allowing more activity downstream, with now greater binding at glutamate AMPAR sites.

- As stated above, NMDAR antagonism increases secondary activation of AMPA (alpha-amino-3-hydroxy-5-methyl-4-isoxazole-propionic acid) glutamate receptors
- This increased AMPA binding activity may lead to activation of improved neuroplasticity-related signaling pathways that utilize mechanistic target of rapamycin (mTOR) and BDNF, causing increased synaptogenesis (Figure 1.3)
  - Increased synaptogenesis likely combats the prolonged stress model of depression, which describes MDD as being associated with neuronal atrophy and synaptic depression in the prefrontal cortex and hippocampus
  - In this manner, use of ketamine may allow improvement in neurophysiologic communication and adaptive changes within the depressed brain to improve CNS functioning and hinder phenotypic depressive symptoms from manifesting
- Ketamine additionally acts as:
  - A Sigma-1 (σ_1) receptor agonist, potentiating nerve growth factor-induced neurite outgrowth in PC12 cells
    - This suggests that Sigma receptor mediated neuronal modeling contributes to antidepressant effects
- A norepinephrine transporter (NET), serotonin transporter (SERT)
  - Ketamine inhibits NET and SERT function, increasing the amount of norepinephrine and serotonin at the synapse, contributing to antidepressant effects, and can lead to μ-opioid receptor activation (Figure 1.4)
  - likely also contributes to antidepressant effects

- Esketamine: S-enantiomer of ketamine
  ○ It is four times more potent for antagonizing the NMDA receptor compared to ketamine
    - Provides option of administering lower dose of esketamine, which would reduce the dose-dependent dissociative side effects associated with ketamine use
  ○ A systematic review of 24 different trials concluded that IV ketamine demonstrated a more significant overall response and remission rate compared to placebo
    - However, due to the esketamine treatment being a fairly new option, more research is needed to investigate this compared to ketamine IV

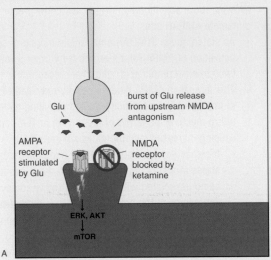

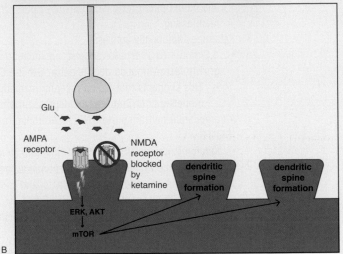

Figure 1.3 Ketamine, AMPA receptors, and mTOR. Glutamate activity heavily modulates synaptic potentiation; this is specifically modulated through NMDA and AMPARs. Ketamine is an NMDAR antagonist; however, its rapid antidepressant effects may also be related to indirect excitatory effects on AMPA receptor signaling and the mTOR pathway. (A) It may be that blockade of the NMDA receptor leads to rapid activation of AMPA and mTOR signaling pathways. (B) This in turn would lead to rapid AMPA-mediated synaptic potentiation. Traditional antidepressants also cause synaptic potentiation; however, they do so via downstream changes in intracellular signaling. This may therefore explain the difference in onset of antidepressant action between ketamine and traditional antidepressants.

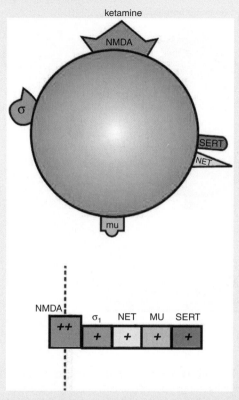

Figure 1.4 Ketamine. Ketamine is an NMDAR antagonist, with additional weak actions at σ_1 receptors, NET, μ-opioid receptors, and SERT.

- Dextromethorphan/bupropion (Auvelity):
  - ○ Dextromethorphan has activity at the same NMDARs as ketamine, supporting that it may have a similar effect
    - · It is a weaker NMDA receptor antagonist, however
    - · Inhibits SERT/NET:
      - • Increasing amounts of serotonin and norepinephrine at the synapse, providing antidepressant effects via reuptake inhibition
    - · σ_1 agonist:
      - • Neuroprotective actions and antidepressant effects
    - · μ-opioid receptors:
      - • Although structurally similar to other opioid agonists, dextromethorphan does not have relevant activity at opioid receptors

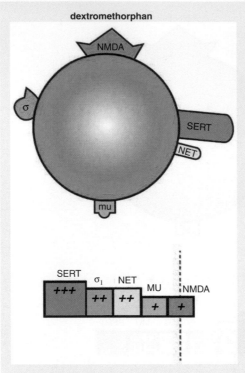

dextromethorphan

Figure 1.5 Dextromethorphan. Dextromethorphan is a weak NMDAR antagonist, with stronger binding affinity for SERT, σ_1 receptors, and NET. It also has some affinity for μ-opioid receptors. Dextromethorphan (in combination with quinidine, which increases its bioavailability) may have therapeutic utility in depression as well, especially in patients that respond well to ketamine, as dextromethorphan and ketamine have similar mechanisms of action.

- ○ Dextromethorphan (Figure 1.5) is combined with bupropion for MDD so it cannot be easily metabolized into its cough suppressing metabolite, thus increasing its plasma concentrations and bioavailability
  - ▪ Bupropion is an inhibitor of the CYP450 2D6 enzyme used to metabolize dextromethorphan
  - ▪ A similar agent combines dextromethorphan and quinidine (Nuedexta) for pseudobulbular affect
    - • Here, also quinidine inhibits CYP450 2D6 and adds an NDRI antidepressant combination component

Tips and pearls

What does each esketamine (Spravato) spray 2-hour session involve?

- To avoid nausea, patient should not eat at least 2 hours prior to esketamine (Spravato) spray administration and avoid liquids 30 minutes prior
- If patient requires a nasal corticosteroid or decongestant, allow this at least 1 hour prior to esketamine administration
- Assess blood pressure prior to administration
  - If elevated (> 140/90) consider risks/benefits of short-term elevation of blood pressure (10–40 mm) with an esketamine (Spravato) spray
  - Sometimes patients are asked to avoid use of stimulants the day of treatment
  - Sometimes patients are asked to taper off or lower dosing of opioids and benzodiazepine sedatives as they may lower effectiveness of the nasal sprays and cause respiratory suppression
- Patient should gently blow nose prior to administration of first device
- Patient should recline at 45-degree angle and close opposite nostril when lightly breathing in dose
- Each nasal spray device has two sprays (one for each nostril)
  - Both sprays are metered and deliver total of 28 mg
  - Use two devices for 56 mg total dose, or three devices for 84 mg total dose
  - A 5-minute rest between using each device to allow adequate absorption is suggested
- 40 minutes after dosing, reassess blood pressure (timing corresponds to peak plasma concentration) and respiration
- Monitor patient for 2 hours after administration for signs of sedation, dissociation, or other significant adverse effects
- If blood pressure is decreasing and patient is stable 2 hours after administration, may discharge patient with someone else driving
- There is a Risk Evaluation and Mitigation Strategy (REMS) monitoring program that requires the treating clinician to register the patient in the REMS system prior to the start of treatment and then during each session to capture the information above on an individual worksheet that must be submitted to the coordination center

Two-minute tutorial

What is palliative psychiatry?

- Palliative psychiatry: an approach that improves the quality of life of patients and their families in facing the problems associated with severe persistent mental illness when a remission of symptoms in the future is unlikely
  - Emphasizes prevention and relief of suffering and treatment of associated physical, mental, social, and spiritual needs
- Focuses on harm reduction and on avoidance of burdensome psychiatric interventions with questionable impact especially where remarkable side effect burdens may result
- Difficult situations that might benefit from palliative psychiatry:
  - Treatment-refractory depression, schizophrenia, post-traumatic stress disorder (PTSD)
  - Severe anorexia in which patients have repeat hospitalizations with involuntary feeding
- Patients who cycle through different treatment options without any improvement of symptoms can feel demoralized, as they feel they are caught in a cycle of false hope
- Palliative psychiatry suggests that in patients with treatment-resistant chronic mental illness, shifting the focus from finding a "cure" to acceptance of chronicity and refocusing on improving quality of life may be more beneficial
  - Focusing on improving patient's quality of life improves therapeutic alliance between patient and practitioner
  - Palliative psychiatry is not withholding treatment – instead redefining goals, such as maintaining meaningful relationships with family and others in the patient's interpersonal environment
  - In this case, there were very few if any treatments that had not been tried in the seeking of remission. Esketamine (Spravato) was released and deemed to be novel so it was utilized with good effectiveness so far
  - In the absence of a novel treatment, the clinician in this case likely may have switched to a more palliative, coping strategy approach

Post-test question

How are the antidepressant effects of esketamine (Spravato) pharmacodynamically mediated?

A. N-methyl-D-aspartate receptor (NMDAR) antagonism
B. Increases brain-derived neurotrophic factor (BDNF) and mammalian target of rapamycin (mTOR) activity

C. Alpha-amino-3-hydroxy-5-methyl-4-isoxazole-propionic acid receptor (AMPAR) agonism
D. Dopamine-2 receptor (D_2) agonism
E. A and B
F. All of the above

Answer: E

The most theorized mechanism of action of esketamine suggests that initial antagonism of NMDA leads to agonism of AMPA receptors. There seems to be downstream increased activity of mTOR and BDNF, suggesting this agent is improving synaptic plasticity and neuroanatomic circuitry communication across a variety of brain areas.

References

1. Abdallah, CG, Adams, TG, Kelmendi, B, et al. Ketamine's mechanism of action: a path to rapid-acting antidepressants. *Depress Anxiety* 2016; 33:689–97
2. Bahji, A, Vazquez, GH, Zarate, CA, Jr. Comparative efficacy of racemic ketamine and esketamine for depression: a systematic review and meta-analysis. *J Affect Disord* 2021; 278:542–55
3. Berk, M, Singh, A, Kapczinski, F. When illness does not get better: do we need a palliative psychiatry? *Acta Neuropsychiatr* 2008; 20:165–6
4. Lauterbach, EC. An extension of hypotheses regarding rapid-acting, treatment-refractory, and conventional antidepressant activity of dextromethorphan and dextrorphan. *Med Hypotheses* 2012; 78:693–702
5. Pai, A, Heining, M. Ketamine. *BJA Educ* 2007; 7:59–63
6. Phillips, JL, Norris, S, Talbot, J, et al. Single, repeated, and maintenance ketamine infusions for treatment-resistant depression: a randomized controlled trial. *Am J Psychiatry* 2019; 176:401–9
7. Popova, V, Daly, EJ, Trivedi, M, et al. Efficacy and safety of flexibly dosed esketamine nasal spray combined with a newly initiated oral antidepressant in treatment-resistant depression: a randomized double-blind active-controlled study. *Am J Psychiatry* 2019; 176:428–38
8. Sial, OK, Parise, EM, Parise, LF, et al. Ketamine: the final frontier or another depressing end? *Behav Brain Res* 2020; 383:112508
9. Singh, JB, Fedgchin, M, Daly, EJ, et al. A double-blind, randomized, placebo-controlled, dose-frequency study of intravenous ketamine in patients with treatment-resistant depression. *Am J Psychiatry* 2016; 173:816–26

10. Sleigh, J, Harvey, M, Voss, L, et al. Ketamine – more mechanisms of action than just NMDA blockade. *Curr Anaesth Crit Care* 2014; 4:76–81

11. Stahl, SM. Treatments for mood disorders: so-called "antidepressants" and "mood stabilizers. In *Stahl's Essential Psychopharmacology: Neuroscientific Basis and Practical Applications*, 5. Cambridge: Cambridge University Press, 2021, 283–358

12. Taylor, CP, Traynelis, SF, Siffert, J, et al. Pharmacology of dextromethorphan: relevance to dextromethorphan/quinidine (Nuedexta®) clinical use. *Pharmacol Ther* 2016; 164:170–82

13. Trachsel, M, Irwin, SA, Biller-Andorno, N, et al. Palliative psychiatry for severe persistent mental illness as a new approach to psychiatry? Definition, scope, benefits, and risks. *BMC Psychiatry* 2016; 16:260

14. Williams, NR, Heifets, BD, Bentzley, BS, et al. Attenuation of antidepressant and antisuicidal effects of ketamine by opioid receptor antagonism. *Mol Psychiatry* 2019; 24:1779–86

15. Yuen, EY, Wei, J, Liu, W, et al. Repeated stress causes cognitive impairment by suppressing glutamate receptor expression and function in prefrontal cortex. *Neuron* 2012; 73:962–77

16. Zhao, Y, Sun, L. Antidepressants modulate the in vitro inhibitory effects of propofol and ketamine on norepinephrine and serotonin transporter function. *J Clin Neurosci* 2008; 15:1264–9

Case 2: The man who is confused about his identity

The Question: What to do when comorbid anxiety disorders are resistant to polypharmacy treatment?

The Psychopharmacological Dilemma: NMDAR antagonists on top of standard-of-care treatment achieve quick remission for major depressive disorder (MDD) – however, may be less effective for comorbid anxiety disorders?

Shiyu Chen

Pretest self-assessment question

Does ketamine or esketamine worsen dissociation in patients with post-traumatic stress disorder (PTSD)?
A. Yes, this is seen clinically much of the time
B. At the low doses typically used, this is infrequent
C. Typically, this is not seen at all clinically
D. Literature is limited but suggests minimal at worst
E. B and D

Patient evaluation on intake

- 31-year-old man with a chief complaint of being "chronically depressed since his teenage years"

Psychiatric history

- Father was American, and mother is a Chinese national
- Well-adjusted childhood up until relocating to China at age 10 after his parents' divorce
- Had a hard time adjusting to Chinese culture and language
- Went back to an American high school and had a hard time readjusting to American culture and relearning English
- Confused about his identity as a biracial white/Asian man
- Never felt he "fit in" and was "always bullied"
- Sexually traumatized at the age of 14
- Gradually developed depression, anxiety, and paranoid traits after this series of unfortunate childhood events
- Admits to full chronic major depressive disorder (MDD) symptoms
  - Feeling depressed since his teenage years without any remission
  - Has frequent passive suicidal ideation with occasional active thoughts and plans, but no attempts
  - Has fatigue, low energy, poor concentration, sense of guilt, worthlessness, and sleep problems

- Admits to full generalized anxiety disorder (GAD) symptoms
  - Feels generally anxious, on edge, fatigued
  - Has poor concentration and difficulty making decisions
  - Has extreme muscle tension in neck and shoulders, and tightness in his chest when anxious and agitated
- Admits to mild social anxiety disorder symptoms
  - Feels generally socially anxious most of time around people
  - Reports anticipatory anxiety and fear of being scrutinized, or feeling as though he will not fit in
  - Reports increased chest discomfort, sweating, palpitations with these events
- Admits to moderate PTSD symptoms
  - Reports childhood sexual trauma
  - Was recently physically assaulted
  - Reports intrusive flashbacks, daytime memories, and sleeping difficulties
  - Reports hyperarousal and agitation
- Has some dependent, avoidant, and paranoid traits
  - Likely part of his temperament or personality
  - Shaped through his life experiences and traumas

Social and personal history

- Has a stable engineering job; however, relies on others for some instrumental activity support such as driving
- Has a significant girlfriend of several years
- Attended college
- Estranged from his biological mother, stepfather passed away, biological father was never part of his life
- Drinks about 500 mg of caffeine per day, usually energy drinks
- Used to smoke about half a pack of cigarettes per day and switched to vaping
- Does not misuse or overuse current medications or use any other drugs
- Drinks alcohol only occasionally

Medical history

- Irritable bowel syndrome (IBS), constipation predominant
- Hypertension

Family history

- Denies any known mental illness in any family member

Medication history

- Failed to respond to the norepinephrine–dopamine reuptake inhibitor (NDRI) antidepressant bupropion (Wellbutrin XL) 300 mg/d
- Is on his first full-course trial of selective serotonin reuptake inhibitor (SSRI), now in combination with his NDRI above
  - ○ Taking the maximum dose of the SSRI sertraline (Zoloft) 200 mg/d
  - ○ Augmented with the sedative anxiolytic benzodiazepine (BZ) alprazolam (Xanax) 1.5 mg/d, and the benzodiazepine receptor agonist (BZRA) hypnotic zolpidem (Ambien) 5 mg/d
- Reports minor benefit with depression and irritable bowel symptoms on current regimen

Current medications

- Bupropion (Wellbutrin XL) 300 mg/d
- Sertraline (Zoloft) 200 mg/d
- Alprazolam (Xanax) 1.5 mg/d
- Zolpidem (Ambien) 5 mg/d

Psychotherapy history

- Has never had weekly psychotherapy sessions
- Attended monthly dialectical behavioral therapy (DBT) group sessions occasionally in the past

Patient evaluation on initial visit

- Chronic depressive and anxiety symptoms associated with unfortunate series of negative life events
- Had to move between two countries and adjust to two cultures and is biracial
- Felt like he never fit in into either American or Asian culture
- Likely did not have the opportunity to create own identity in teenage years and now has existential dilemma. This might be the root cause for most of his psychiatric symptoms
- Also has moderate PTSD symptoms from being abused and being bullied
- Currently has frequent passive suicidal ideation – however, had active thoughts and plans in the past but never acted on them
- Seems very depressed, despondent with flat affect
- Has risks of harming himself but has been resilient and able to maintain not acting on suicidal impulses

- However, currently guarded about committing to his safety plan
- Suggests possible need for inpatient stay
- Reports no current side effects besides slight decrease of libido

Question

In your clinical experience, would you expect a patient such as this to recover?

- Yes, he has good social support and is functional at work
- No, his depression and anxiety with comorbid PTSD are likely chronic and unremitting

Attending physician's mental notes: initial psychiatric evaluation

- This patient currently has moderate to severe chronic MDD, moderate GAD, and moderate PTSD. They are likely generated by his long-term stressors and early negative life events
- The traits and defense mechanisms he developed over the years have made him relatively resilient, and he can maintain a demanding job and a significant relationship with his girlfriend
- He has been somewhat undertreated; only has had a full course of two antidepressant trials
- He is at risk of harming himself now, based on his current presentation
- His prognosis is fair to good if we can generate reasonable, appropriate, and aggressive psychotherapy, pharmacotherapy, and possibly neuromodulation interventions
- Likely needs an inpatient stay or a faster-acting treatment with increased outpatient monitoring

Question

Which of the following would be your next step?

- Increase zolpidem (Ambien) and alprazolam (Xanax) to a higher dose for his insomnia and anxiety disorders
- Augment the current medications with psychotherapy to consolidate treatment results
- Augment the current medications with 5-HT1A receptor partial agonist anxiolytic buspirone (BuSpar)
- Augment the current medications with an atypical antipsychotic
- Refer for inpatient electroconvulsive therapy (ECT)
- Refer for outpatient esketamine (Spravato) nasal spray treatment
- Do nothing additionally outside of wait for current medication regimen effectiveness to occur

Attending physician's mental notes: initial psychiatric evaluation (continued)

- Patient was recently started on a standard-of-care treatment for his MDD with comorbid anxiety disorders using sertraline (Zoloft) and bupropion (Wellbutrin XL)
  - This is likely not adequate as he has had a minimal response and he may need more aggressive treatment now
  - His MDD presentation is of profound despair with increased suicidal thinking
- Does meet criteria now for severe MDD, moderate GAD, and moderate PTSD
- Zolpidem (Ambien) and alprazolam (Xanax) can be continued for now
- Starting buspirone (BuSpar) or aripiprazole (Abilify) to augment sertraline (Zoloft) makes sense, but delayed response time likely
- While one of these is being considered, will attempt to obtain esketamine (Spravato) prior authorization from his insurance company

Further investigation

Is there anything else that you would like to know about the patient?

What about details concerning current medication regimen?

- Currently on the maximum dose of sertraline (Zoloft) at 200 mg/d
  - Has had some minor benefit for his MDD and IBS
  - Tolerates the drug well but has decreased libido
- Currently taking bupropion (Wellbutrin XL) 300 mg/d
  - Tolerates well
  - Could be increased further
- Currently taking zolpidem (Ambien) and alprazolam (Xanax)
  - Improves his sleep and agitation somewhat
  - Both have been generally less and less effective over the years

Attending physician's mental notes: interim follow-up through 8 weeks

- This patient has continuing symptoms and we can be more aggressive with the current medications
- Also could consider rational polypharmacy, given the patient has had enough time on current drugs to see that they are not fully helping to reduce his symptoms

Case outcome: interim follow-up at 8 weeks

- Buspirone (BuSpar) 30 mg/d was gradually added to his bupropion (Wellbutrin XL) and sertraline (Zoloft) regimen by his primary care provider after the initial intake
  - This rational polypharmacy approach adds 5-HT$_{1A}$ receptor partial agonism as a unique mechanism to treat his symptoms better
- Patient has had more therapeutic time on the well-dosed SSRI and NDRI products
- Still reports same severe MDD symptoms as 8 weeks ago
- Specifically calls to request to start esketamine (Spravato) nasal spray treatment for his resistant MDD and suicidal thoughts

Question

How would you change his medication regimen?

- Continue everything as is
- Continue current medication regimen at higher doses, except for sertraline (Zoloft) since it is already at maximum dose
- Start esketamine (Spravato) nasal spray 56–84 mg twice weekly treatment and continue his current medication regimen
- Start esketamine (Spravato) nasal spray 56–84 mg twice weekly treatment, but discontinue all previous psychotropics as none was effective

Case outcome: interim follow-up visit at 12 weeks

- Patient started and has had seven consecutive esketamine (Spravato) treatment sessions in the past 4 weeks
  - He took 56 mg/d for his first two sessions, which he tolerated well, but showed no improvement
  - He now takes 84 mg/d routinely twice weekly
  - During treatments, he experienced mild sedation only
- Depression symptoms seemingly improving per the Patient Health Questionnaire (PHQ-9)
  - PHQ-9 rating scale scores decreased from 22 4 weeks ago to 13 now
- Reports remarkably less GAD and PTSD agitation
- Now uses alprazolam (Xanax) and zolpidem (Ambien) only sparingly
- No PTSD symptom improvement outside of hyperarousal, but also no exacerbation

Question

Would you expect PTSD symptoms to worsen with esketamine (Spravato)?

- Yes, esketamine (Spravato) treatment is known to cause dissociation which is a hallmark symptom of PTSD
- Yes, only to a minor degree, but the gains for alleviating his depression and suicidality would be worth it
- No adverse effects for his PTSD are expected

Case outcome: third interim follow-up visit at 16 weeks

- Continues sertraline (Zoloft), alprazolam (Xanax), zolpidem (Ambien), buspirone (Buspar), and bupropion XL (Wellbutrin XL)
- The NDRI bupropion XL (Wellbutrin XL) now increased to 450 mg/d, to maximal dosing, as full remission not yet gained from esketamine (Spravato) use
- Has had 13 esketamine (Spravato) intranasal spray treatment sessions in the past 2 months
- Adjusted frequency and dosage of esketamine (Spravato) as needed
  - 56 mg twice weekly for 1 week
  - 84 mg twice weekly for 3 weeks
  - 84 mg once weekly thereafter
- After this course, opted to spread out his dosing schedule to every 2 weeks, 4 weeks, then 6 weeks, etc., to try to wean off this treatment
- Blood pressure has been increasing, with diastolic hovering around 90 mmHg, which may be his new normal
  - Possibly due to noradrenergic drive from the increased bupropion (Wellbutrin XL) vs. the beginning of idiopathic essential hypertension
  - Unlikely due to esketamine (Spravato) as this drug now washes out between his treatment sessions
  - Interestingly, his pressure lowers 10 points during esketamine (Spravato) treatment sessions, where esketamine (Spravato) is supposed to escalate blood pressure 10 points, per regulatory agencies, during a session
- Patient is asking about further treatment options for PTSD
  - Still complains of some insomnia and intrusive thoughts

Attending physician's mental notes: third interim follow-up visit (month 8)

- Patient's MDD symptoms are remitted
  - He has better range of affect, is psychomotor normal, no longer despondent nor suicidal

- ○ Esketamine (Spravato) intranasal spray can eventually be tapered off
- ○ He can continue SSRI/SNRI and buspirone (BuSpar) as his maintenance augmentation treatment
- ○ Is not using any sedative/hypnotic agents now
- PTSD and generalized anxiety symptoms persist
  - ○ His PTSD hyperarousal symptoms did respond to esketamine (Spravato) intranasal spray treatment sessions; however, his remaining reliving and avoidance PTSD symptoms continue
  - ○ No increases in dissociative PTSD symptoms noted
  - ○ Can see whether he has had specialized psychotherapy for his trauma vs. more complex polypharmacy for his residual PTSD symptoms may be needed

Question

What would you do next?

- As his PTSD symptoms persist, refer him to eye movement desensitization and reprocessing (EMDR) therapy for his persisting PTSD symptoms
- As his PTSD symptoms persist, add another psychotropic agent for PTSD, such as an atypical antipsychotic or noradrenergic-dampening blood pressure lowering agent
- Continue to wait on the current regimen for full effectiveness to occur as he doesn't have severe side effects

Case outcome: fourth interim follow-up visit at 20 weeks

- As his PTSD symptoms persisted, he was referred for EMDR therapy
- He continued all oral medications
- He continued to have esketamine (Spravato) sessions spread further apart while maintaining good effectiveness

Case debrief

- This patient had unfortunate early life experiences
- This likely contributed to his chronic MDD, PTSD, social anxiety disorder, and GAD since his teenage years
- His symptoms were relatively undertreated, until there was maximization of his SSRI and NDRI antidepressants
- Despite this, plus a buspirone (BuSpar) augmentation, his symptoms persisted
- Given his remarkable depression and increased suicidal thoughts, his insurance company allowed him to start weekly esketamine

(Spravato) nasal spray treatment, which likely helped to avoid an inpatient stay
- MDD symptoms drastically improved during his several-month esketamine (Spravato) intranasal spray trial, with some frequency and dosage adjustments in between
- GAD symptoms also improved but not as significant as the improvement of his MDD symptoms
- PTSD symptoms did not exacerbate and actually mildly improved
- In practice, this patient plans to continue to spread out the esketamine (Spravato) treatments and eventually taper off
- He asked to try EMDR therapy for his PTSD

Take-home points

- The Food and Drug Administration (FDA) and other guidelines suggest a few drugs and devices be used for treatment-resistant depression (TRD) or MDD augmentation
  - Olanzapine–fluoxetine combination (Symbyax)
  - Aripiprazole (Abilify)
  - Quetiapine (Seroquel)
  - Brexpiprazole (Rexulti)
  - Cariprazine (Vraylar)
  - ECT
  - Transcranial magnetic stimulation (TMS)
  - Vagal nerve stimulation (VNS)
- Most antidepressants can take weeks before starting to alleviate MDD
- Ketamine is a non-competitive antagonist of glutamate receptors of the N-methyl-D-aspartate (NMDA) type and has compelling off-label data for use in TRD
- Esketamine (Spravato) is the S-enantiomer of ketamine that has stronger affinity to antagonize NMDARs, which was recently approved by the FDA for TRD
  - Intranasal esketamine (Spravato) given in conjunction with standard-of-care antidepressant treatment may result in rapid improvement in MDD symptoms compared to standard-of-care treatment alone and is considered an augmentation strategy
  - Esketamine (Spravato) can also lower suicidal thinking from MDD according to the FDA
- PTSD has a prevalence of 8.7% in the United States and is often treatment resistant
- Individuals with PTSD are 80% more likely than those without PTSD to be diagnosed with at least one other psychiatric disorder, commonly including MDD, substance use disorders (SUDs), and anxiety disorders

- SSRIs are the only psychotropic class approved for treating PTSD – however, many patients tend not to achieve full remission with SSRI therapy
- There is some evidence that ketamine IV infusion can lead to rapid reduction in symptom severity in patients with chronic PTSD, albeit with slight increased risk of dissociation
- In our case, the patient's resistant MDD symptoms achieved remission gradually after a 2-month initial trial of esketamine (Spravato). However, his PTSD definitely did not worsen
- Interestingly his hyperarousal remarkably improved

Performance in practice: confessions of a psychopharmacologist

What could have been done better here?

- Should more psychotherapy (CBT, psychodynamic, or EMDR) have been given sooner?
  ○ This may have alleviated the MDD, GAD, and PTSD symptoms if started in conjunction with the esketamine (Spravato) intranasal spray
  ○ However, it was felt that his level of MDD and PTSD may have actually interfered with the provision of and benefit from psychotherapy
- Should more aggressive medications be prescribed for his insomnia, GAD, and PTSD?
  ○ Insomnia is a stand-alone risk factor that increases suicide risk
- Should failure of the SSRI and NDRI warrant a trial on other FDA-approved medication for TRD before starting esketamine (Spravato)?
  ○ This is unclear. He has not tried tricyclic antidepressants (TCAs) or monoamine oxidase inhibitor (MAOI) antidepressants
  ○ Some may argue that these agents are riskier in overdose and carry a higher side-effect burden than the regimen used in this case

What are possible action items for improvement in practice?

- Research information available for treatment guidelines regarding TRD with comorbid PTSD and GAD
- Research data or clinical trials on effectiveness of esketamine (Spravato) for treatment-resistant PTSD
- Further exploration on other future indications for esketamine (Spravato), such as bipolar depression
- Research information on potential side effects of esketamine (Spravato) when combined with other medications

- ○ This patient had a mildly elevated systolic and diastolic blood pressure while taking esketamine (Spravato) trial plus an increased dose of bupropion XL (Wellbutrin XL)

Tips and pearls

- About one-third of patients with MDD do not respond to available antidepressants and suffer from TRD
- Current treatment options for TRD are limited
- Intranasal esketamine (Spravato) has rapid antidepressant effects within 4 hours to 1 day after a single dose, and the response rates are ultimately comparable to 8-week trials of monoaminergic-based antidepressants
- Esketamine (Spravato) plus oral antidepressant is more effective than oral antidepressants alone per regulatory trials
- Most common side effects include nausea, headache, sedation, and sometimes mild dissociation
- Abuse and misuse of esketamine (Spravato) is a concern of this newly approved medication but it is held and dispensed by the provider, so addiction and diversion in reality are quite negligible
- Esketamine (Spravato) can also transiently increase patient's blood pressure, with some occasionally increasing more than 40 mmHg, while the average is 10 mmHg, and it may lower breathing rate
  - ○ The blood pressure increase usually peaks around 40 minutes after administration
- A Risk Evaluation and Mitigation Strategy (REMS) was implemented by the FDA for esketamine to ensure safe use
- PTSD can often be treatment resistant and SSRIs have limited efficiency
- Ketamine and esketamine (Spravato) might be a novel treatment for PTSD; however, more data is needed
- Clinicians should likely supplement PTSD pharmacologic treatment with psychotherapy

Mechanism of action moment

Why might NMDA antagonists potentially be able to treat both depression and anxiety disorders?

- Glutamate is an important excitatory neurotransmitter in the brain
  - Glutamatergic system dysfunction is likely related to the pathophysiology of multiple psychiatric disorders, such as MDD, GAD, PTSD, and schizophrenia (SP)
  - Reduced glutamate levels in the prefrontal cortex have been associated with failed antidepressant treatment
- N-methyl-D-aspartate receptors (NMDARs) are ionotropic glutamate receptors
  - Allow calcium ions to enter the cell from extracellular space
    - Calcium influx through the NMDARs leads to long-term potentiation and synaptic plasticity
  - Composed of subunits NR1, NR2 (NR2A–NR2D), and NR3 (NR3A and NR3B)
    - NR1 binds glycine and NR2 binds glutamate
  - Ketamine is a non-competitive NMDA antagonist and decreases the opening frequency of NMDARs
  - NMDAR blockade allows downstream disinhibition of glutamate signaling of alpha-amino-3-hydroxy-5-methyl-4-isoxazole-propionic acid receptors (AMPARs) as well
  - Increased downstream glutamate activity may increase neuronal dendritic growth, synaptogenesis, brain-derived neurotrophic factor (BDNF) availability, vascular endothelial growth factor (VEGF), and mTOR signaling, all of which seem to be biomarkers of good antidepressant activity
- Alpha-amino-3-hydroxy-5-methyl-4-isoazolepropionic acid receptors (AMPARs) are ionotropic glutamate receptors
  - Composed of subunits GluR 1–4
  - Ketamine rapidly increases downstream glutamate activity in the medial prefrontal cortex (mPFC), leading to increased synaptic transmission of AMPARs in the mPFC
  - Ketamine can also upregulate AMPAR subunit (GluR1 and GluR2) expression, and increase synaptogenesis and connectivity in the prefrontal cortex (PFC) and hippocampus through activating BDNF and mTOR pathways
  - This reverses stress- and depression-induced loss of connectivity between the PFC and other structures in the limbic system, which may also explain the antidepressant action of ketamine

- Esketamine is the S(+)-enantiomer of ketamine and has greater affinity and anesthetic potency than R-ketamine, and therefore also seems to rapidly resolve MDD symptoms
- GAD and PTSD symptoms are also linked to NMDAR overactivity
  - Impaired connection in glutamatergic synapses in corticolimbic circuits can lead to hypothalamic–pituitary–adrenal (HPA) axis dysfunction, which is implicated in development of PTSD and other anxiety disorders
  - BDNF then may decrease while under social stress which may lead to anxiety symptoms when there's loss of top-down cortical control over limbic structures which are felt to control fight or flight responses in mammals
  - Treatment with some antidepressants, CBT, ECT, VNS, and NMDA antagonists can increase BDNF expression, ideally reversing this process
  - This may explain the potential for NMDA antagonists such as esketamine (Spravato) to be effective for anxiety disorders
  - This potential mechanism still needs to be further investigated with translational and clinical trials

Two-minute tutorial

Treatment for PTSD

- SSRIs are the first-line recommendation for patients with PTSD
  - There is great phenotypic symptom overlap between DSM-5-diagnosed MDD and PTSD and GAD (Figure 2.1)
  - Among all the SSRIs, only sertraline (Zoloft), paroxetine (Paxil), and fluoxetine (Prozac) were recommended based on evidence for efficiency by the 2017 Veterans' Affairs / Department of Defense Clinical Practice Guideline (CPG)
  - Only sertraline (Zoloft) and paroxetine (Paxil) are approved for PTSD treatment by the FDA
  - All other medications, including the ones mentioned below, are used "off label" with practice guideline support only
  - Maximum benefit from SSRI treatment depends on adequate dosages, duration of treatment, and treatment adherence
- Other antidepressant options for PTSD
  - Venlafaxine, an SNRI, is a promising medication with both serotonergic and noradrenergic characteristics that balances serotonergic and noradrenergic neurotransmission via dual monoaminergic reuptake inhibition

- Nefazodone may also be effective
  - Blocks serotonin-2A receptors and serotonin reuptake
  - Not utilized much due to liver toxicity and unavailability
- TCAs can be beneficial too since some are serotonergic/noradrenergic-balanced as well
  - A potential alternative only if a patient fails to respond to SSRI/SNRI
  - Must observe EKG for QT prolongation, check plasma levels, and watch for remarkable anticholinergic effects
- MAOIs can be effective, because they increase serotonin, dopamine, and norepinephrine simultaneously
  - Requires dietary restriction
  - Interaction with other serotonergic agents can be fatal
- Beta blockers (BBs) (noradrenergic β_1 and β_2 receptor antagonists)
  - May be used for comorbid conditions with PTSD, such as performance anxiety or social anxiety disorder
  - Tends to improve hyperautonomic symptoms (palpitations) and tremulousness
  - Not supported by evidence in treating core PTSD symptoms
- Alpha blockers (noradrenergic α_1 receptor antagonists)
  - Specifically studied and utilized for nightmares associated with PTSD
  - Not supported by evidence in treating core PTSD symptoms
- BZs
  - Studies have not shown that they are effective overall in treating core PTSD symptoms
  - Concerns including falls, addiction, danger in driving, having trouble integrating the traumatic experience, and withdrawal are well noted in the literature
  - PTSD outcome may worsen with BZs and unfortunately increase overall mortality
  - Interestingly, some reports suggest that their use may lower the effectiveness of ketamine and esketamine treatment in MDD

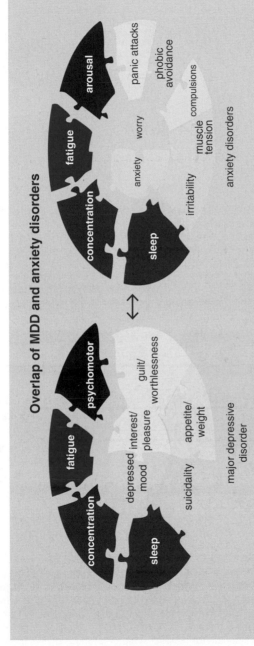

Figure 2.1 Overlap of MDD and anxiety disorders. Although the core symptoms of anxiety disorders (anxiety and worry) differ from the core symptoms of major depression (loss of interest and depressed mood), there is considerable overlap among the rest of the symptoms associated with these disorders (compare the "anxiety disorders" puzzle on the right to the "MDD" puzzle on the left). For example, fatigue, sleep difficulties, and concentration difficulties are common to both types of disorders. If certain SSRI antidepressants are able to alleviate both depression and anxiety symptoms, it makes intuitive sense that ketamine and esketamine may also share in an ability to treat both disorders. In this case, for example, we saw a remarkable reduction in psychomotor agitation and insomnia.

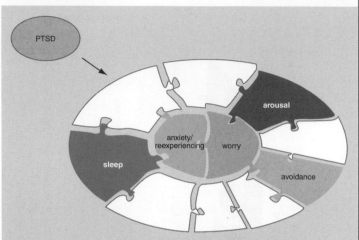

Figure 2.2 PTSD. The characteristic symptoms of PTSD are shown here. These include the core symptoms of anxiety while the traumatic event is being re-experienced as well as worry about having the other symptoms of PTSD, such as increased arousal and startle responses, sleep difficulties including nightmares, and avoidance behaviors. It would be interesting to see whether future research into esketamine use for PTSD will show an ability to treat all PTSD symptom clusters or just the hyperarousal components as seen in this case.

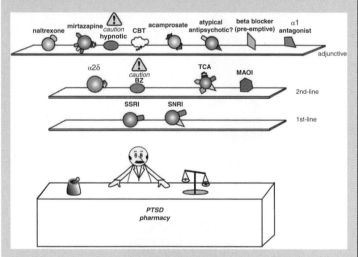

Figure 2.3 PTSD pharmacy. First-line pharmacological options for PTSD are SSRIs and SNRIs. In PTSD, unlike other anxiety disorders, BZs have not been shown to be as helpful, although they may be considered with caution as a second-line option. Other second-line treatments include α_2 ligands, TCAs, and MAOIs. Several medications may be used as adjuncts for residual symptoms, and cognitive behavioral therapy (CBT) is typically recommended as well.

Post-test question

Does ketamine or esketamine worsen dissociation in patients with post-traumatic stress disorder (PTSD)?
A. Yes, this is seen clinically much of the time
B. At the low doses typically used, this is infrequent
C. Typically, this is not seen at all clinically
D. Literature is limited but suggests minimal at worst
E. B and D

Answer: E

The data for use in PTSD is limited but, given that doses are kept low to avoid dissociative effects, there has not been much worsening of PTSD noted so far in trials.

References

1. Albott, CS, Lim, KO, Forbes, MK, et al. Efficacy, safety, and durability of repeated ketamine infusions for comorbid posttraumatic stress disorder and treatment-resistant depression. *J Clin Psychiatry* 2018; 79:17m11634
2. Aleksandrova, LR, Phillips, AG, Wang, YT. Antidepressant effects of ketamine and the roles of AMPA glutamate receptors and other mechanisms beyond NMDA receptor antagonism. *J Psychiatry Neurosci* 2017; 42:222–9
3. Browne, CA, Lucki, I. Antidepressant effects of ketamine: mechanisms underlying fast-acting novel antidepressants. *Front Pharmacol* 2013; 4:161
4. Canuso, CM, Singh, JB, Fedgchin, M, et al. Efficacy and safety of intranasal esketamine for the rapid reduction of symptoms of depression and suicidality in patients at imminent risk for suicide: results of a double-blind, randomized, placebo-controlled study. *Am J Psychiatry* 2018; 175:620–30
5. Collins, A, Rutter, S, Feder, A. Development of ketamine administration as a treatment for chronic PTSD. *Psychiatric Annals* 2020; 50:68–76
6. Feder, A, Parides, MK, Murrough, JW, et al. Efficacy of intravenous ketamine for treatment of chronic posttraumatic stress disorder: a randomized clinical trial. *JAMA Psychiatry* 2014; 71:681–8
7. Henter, ID, de Sousa, RT, Zarate, CA, Jr. Glutamatergic modulators in depression. *Harv Rev Psychiatry* 2018; 26:307–19
8. Hidalgo, R, Hertzberg, MA, Mellman, T, et al. Nefazodone in post-traumatic stress disorder: results from six open-label trials. *Int Clin Psychopharmacol* 1999; 14:61–8

9. Kew, JN, Kemp, JA. Ionotropic and metabotropic glutamate receptor structure and pharmacology. *Psychopharmacology (Berl)* 2005; 179:4–29

10. Kim, J, Farchione, T, Potter, A, et al. Esketamine for treatment-resistant depression – first FDA-approved antidepressant in a new class. *N Engl J Med* 2019; 381:1–4

11. Liriano, F, Hatten, C, Schwartz, TL. Ketamine as treatment for post-traumatic stress disorder: a review. *Drugs Context* 2019; 8:212–305

12. Murrough, JW, Perez, AM, Pillemer, S, et al. Rapid and longer-term antidepressant effects of repeated ketamine infusions in treatment-resistant major depression. *Biol Psychiatry* 2013; 74:250–6

13. Rasmussen, KG. Ketamine for posttraumatic stress disorder. *JAMA Psychiatry* 2015; 72:94–5

14. Sartori, SB, Singewald, N. Novel pharmacological targets in drug development for the treatment of anxiety and anxiety-related disorders. *Pharmacol Ther* 2019; 204:107402

15. Sattar, Y, Wilson, J, Khan, AM, et al. A review of the mechanism of antagonism of N-methyl-D-aspartate receptor by ketamine in treatment-resistant depression. *Cureus* 2018; 10:e2652

16. Stahl, SM. *Stahl's Essential Psychopharmacology: Neuroscientific Basis and Practical Applications*, 5. Cambridge: Cambridge University Press, 2021

17. *VA/DoD Clinical Practice Guideline for the Management of Posttraumatic Stress Disorder and Acute Stress Disorder.* Washington, DC: Veterans' Association, 2017

Case 3: Propane, shattered glass, and parasites

The Question: How do you avoid psychiatric readmission?

The Psychopharmacological Dilemma: Non-compliance in schizophrenia care leads to great risk and readmission

Charles Welch

Pretest self-assessment question

Some atypical antipsychotics exert their antipsychotic and antidepressant effects via partial agonism of the dopamine-2 receptor (D_2). The inhibition of which hepatic cytochrome P450 (CYP450) enzyme would have the most prominent effect on a patient's serum concentration of this class of atypical antipsychotic drugs (sometimes called the PIPS and the RIPS …)?
A. CYP3A4
B. CYP2D6
C. CYP1A2
D. CYP2C9
E. A and B
F. All of the above

Patient evaluation on intake

- A 24-year-old man presents to the emergency room on a hold placed by police due to perceived dangerousness to the community
- Found along a major highway, picking up trash, darting back and forth dodging cars
- Told police he had consumed 750 mL of alcohol 1 day prior
- Ruminates about telling officers he "cannot touch certain metals" and is also "a study subject for a medication experiment"

Psychiatric history

- Diagnosed with Attention-Deficit/Hyperactivity Disorder (ADHD) as a 14-year-old
- Moved from the Midwest to Pennsylvania 3 years ago
- Shortly after moving, the patient started accusing his family of poisoning his water when he visited
- Believed he was infected with tape worms and looked through his feces in the toilet for evidence of this incessantly
- Six months after his move, he was found wandering downtown by his brother after his family could not contact him
- Taken to psychiatric hospital and admitted for 1 week

- ○ Discharged on an atypical antipsychotic, but immediately threw the medication away
- Moved back to the Midwest to be with parents and finish college 1½ years ago
- Parents believe that the patient "has maintained" since he moved back, but now has progressively become more paranoid and is acting more bizarre over the last 6 months
- Highest level of concern when patient was recently seen via video-doorbell on the front porch attempting to set a propane tank on fire with no reason given for this behavior

Social and personal history

- Straight-A student during high school, full scholarship to college
- Heavy marijuana usage during first semester of college along with illicit prescription stimulant usage
- Graduated from college with major in physics, applied but was rejected for job at major engineering company

Medical history

- No significant medical history reported
- Has been on multiple antibiotic/antifungal regimens over the last year for what patient believes are various infections, all of which appear to be psychosomatic in nature and seem unfounded

Family history

- Mother and sister both have major depressive disorder (MDD)
- Grandfather died by suicide

Medication History

- Dextroamphetamine (Dexedrine) prescribed as teenager for ADHD; illicitly obtained and used during college to excess as well
- Discharged from inpatient psychiatric stay taking risperidone (Risperdal) 4 mg/d

Current medications

- Patient denies any current medications and he no longer takes risperidone (Risperdal)

Psychotherapy history

- None. Patient was scheduled to see a psychiatrist and a therapist
  - ○ Followed up with psychiatrist once
  - ○ Never showed for other appointments with either

PATIENT FILE

Patient evaluation on initial visit

- Initial drug screen negative for stimulants or cannabis
- During his interview, answers all questions with loose associations that relate to chemistry and maintains a flat affect throughout the conversation
- He speaks rapidly, though collateral sources later reveal that this has been baseline since he was a young child; speech quality is otherwise of normal volume and enunciation, and he does not display a flight of ideas
- Frequently looks over the provider's shoulder and at the air conditioning vent during interview, appearing to react to internal stimuli, indicating hallucinations
- Ruminates about having an adverse reaction to the handcuffs that he wore while en route to the hospital, which he believes were comprised of nickel or chromium
- Poor insight, unable to state that the police brought him to the hospital for using a propane tank dangerously, dodging cars and disrupting traffic, etc.
- Patient able to provide little meaningful information about his history, and most of this is obtained from his parents via telephone secondarily
- Endorses past non-compliance, and frequently states that risperidone (Risperdal) is a "benzisoxazole derivative"

Question

Given the patient's current presentation, is his mental state likely to stabilize as it is now or continue to worsen without medical intervention?

- Given that what he is experiencing is likely related to stressors of late adolescence and early adulthood, he will most likely stabilize as he emotionally matures
- If he stops using cannabis and stimulants he will get better
- Most likely his function will continue to progress negatively without treatment over time

Attending physician's mental notes: initial psychiatric evaluation

- This patient has displayed a marked pattern of psychotic disorganized thoughts and behaviors, clear somatic and paranoid delusions, a flat affect, and hallucinations in apparent absentia of recent substance use, a concurrent mood disorder, or other medical comorbidities

○ This appears to be a primary psychosis, meeting DSM-5 criteria for schizophrenia

• The signs and symptoms in the context of his history, as well as his poor progression over this time period, is also convincing for schizophrenia

• His first psychotic break correlates to a period of high stress in early adulthood

• His high intellectual (pre-illness) functioning, initially rapid onset of symptoms which occurred within months of leaving for college, and prominence of positive symptoms are indicative usually of a more positive prognosis

• His sex, lack of mood symptoms, non-compliance, unmitigated symptoms, and age of first onset are factors that are indicative of a more negative prognosis

• Illegal use of stimulants and cannabis were risky and may have triggered the onset of schizophrenia; it is good for his long-term prognosis that he is sober now and has good family support

Question

Which of the following would be your next step?

• Admit and only monitor the patient, and observe to confirm the diagnosis for several days in the hospital before taking further steps to make sure this is not all drug-induced psychosis

• Discharge him from the emergency room only after coordinating with social work to ensure he has established outpatient follow-up and if parents agree to assist

• Prescribe an atypical antipsychotic and discharge the patient after outpatient follow-up has been established

• Prescribe a typical antipsychotic and discharge the patient after outpatient follow-up has been established

• Prescribe an atypical antipsychotic and observe the patient while continuing his inpatient admission as he is too psychotic and dangerous to discharge at present

Attending physicians' mental notes: initial evaluation (continued)

• Unmitigated and ongoing psychosis predicts the poorest outcomes

• "Past performance is indicative of future results"

  ○ Non-compliance during this hospitalization or at discharge is likely, given previous encounters

  ○ Very poor insight drives this and worsens his prognosis

- He was brought in on an initial hold placed by the police; that allows several inpatient days to attempt medication management to improve his symptoms
- If he is compliant and improves, it is less likely that a court will grant a lengthened hospital stay
- Hallucinations will improve most quickly, followed by an improvement in marked thought disorder; delusions may likely persist longer and negative symptoms may not improve
- Family members will need to be counseled about a possible new "baseline," as many patients with schizophrenia get worse with each psychotic episode

Further investigation

What else would assist in the guidance of pharmacologic treatment?

- What dose of risperidone (Risperdal) had the patient been taking in the hospital prior, and what sort of improvements and side effects were seen during that hospitalization?
  - Dose upon discharge was 4 mg/d, which is an average dose
  - Documentation was unfortunately sparse from his hospitalization; the only information gleaned was that his reactivity to his hallucinations had improved
  - Patient states he did not want to take this medication because it made him "fat," but otherwise no other side effects were noted

Case outcome: from admission to inpatient day 4

- Patient was started on aripiprazole (Abilify) 5 mg/d, then increased to 10 mg/d on day 3
  - Does not believe this medication is needed or will work for him
  - He is nevertheless compliant and no adverse effects are noted on this subtherapeutic dose
- Observed on the inpatient ward as pharmacotherapy was initiated for a total of 4 days until the expiration of his commitment status
- Has not been observed reacting to subjective stimuli while on the ward
- Has not needed restraints, and has been behaviorally appropriate
- Continues to endorse delusions and has intermittent loose associations, but these seem to be improving too

Question

What would be your next course of action?

- Continue his admission by filing a petition for a court-ordered extension of his involuntary hold as he is still quite symptomatic with poor insight

- Release patient on current low dose of aripiprazole (Abilify) with planned outpatient follow-up soon after discharge
- Release patient, but increase his aripiprazole (Abilify) prior to discharge to 15 mg/d, which is felt to be a fully therapeutic dose
- Discharge patient, but switch to olanzapine (Zyprexa) as he has not impoved sufficiently while taking aripiprazole (Abilify)
- Discharge patient, but start him on a long-acting injectable (LAI) atypical antipsychotic to improve compliance after discharge

Attending physician's mental notes: from admission to inpatient day 4

- Given the laws of the state in which he has been hospitalized, it is highly unlikely that the court will grant a continued involuntary admission
  - Though a continued hospitalization would be ideal, the treatment team will likely need to release the patient
- Will need to continue upward titration of aripiprazole (Abilify) for this patient as he seems to be responding initially to the lower dose
- Follow-up will be especially critical to monitor patient for potential non-compliance and acute extrapyramidal symptoms (EPS)
- Need to contact the outpatient team to arrange a warm hand-off
- Need to consider an LAI antipsychotic

Case outcome: return to the hospital and a second admission

- Patient was discharged after the short hospital stay during first admission above
- Patient is brought to the hospital again 11 days later on another hold placed by the police
  - Multiple calls were made by the patient to the police about spiders and gasoline being in the patient's house
  - Broken items and shattered glass surrounded the patient's front porch upon police arrival
- Patient oddly removed all "flammable" items from his home before vacuuming, upset his roommate
- Believes that his arrival to the hospital is a "big misunderstanding"
- Tangential on interview, frequently interjects with "fun facts"
- Very poor insight, endorses medication compliance for "3–4 days only after discharge"

Further investigation

What elements of this patient's history since last discharge would you inquire about?

- Was this patient actually compliant with his antipsychotic?
  - ○ Patient's father states they learned that patient immediately flushed his medication down the toilet the evening after discharge
- Did this patient make it to his follow-up appointment?
  - ○ Clinic informs that the patient did not show for his appointment either
- Was patient initially stable upon discharge from the hospital?
  - ○ Roommate states that the patient appeared to be "sort of normal" for roughly 3 days, then began to "act strange again"
- Did the patient remain sober?
  - ○ Urine drug screen collected in the emergency department is negative

Question

The patient has been admitted to the inpatient unit again. What would be your next step in regard to pharmacotherapy?

- Restart aripiprazole (Abilify) 10 mg/d and maintain at this dose
- Restart aripiprazole (Abilify) but increase to 15 mg/d
- Initiate oral risperidone (Risperdal), as the patient has been on this in the past
- Initiate oral olanzapine (Zyprexa), as the patient has not yet been tried on this medication
- Initiate oral paliperidone (Invega) as it has an LAI form to convert to later
- Start paliperidone palmitate IM (Invega Sustenna) LAI right away
- Start a weight-neutral atypical antipsychotic such as ziprasidone (Geodon), lurasidone (Latuda), or lumateperone (Caplyta) given his fear of weight gain

Further investigation (continued)

- Were there any other items to note in regard to medications?

  - ○ Medication reconciliation reveals the patient had been on fluconazole (Diflucan) 400 mg/d for tinea capitis for several weeks leading up to last admission, which he resumed immediately following discharge

Attending physician's mental notes: second hospitalization day 1

- Improvement during last visit (albeit mild) on low-dose aripiprazole (Abilify) indicates it might be effective at a higher dose
- Medication non-compliance with subsequent decompensation 3 days after last dose roughly correlates with mean half-life of his medication (30–146 hours dependent on rapid or poor metabolism)
- Resumption of fluconazole (Diflucan) at discharge slowed the elimination of aripiprazole (Abilify), likely increasing its expected half-life, however
  - Fluconazole (Diflucan) inhibits CYP3A4, a key enzyme in the metabolism of aripiprazole (Abilify)
- Throughout his treatment with aripiprazole (Abilify), it had been well tolerated
- He is a good candidate for an LAI, possibly aripiprazole monohydrate (Abilify Maintena) or aripiprazole lauroxil (Aristada)
  - It makes sense to use the same oral and LAI product whenever possible
- Potentially can use aripiprazole (Abilify Mycite), which, when taken, has a built-in sensor that alerts the clinician each time this aripiprazole product is swallowed

Case outcome: second hospitalization

- Patient is restarted on his aripiprazole (Abilify) 10 mg/d
- Risks, benefits, and alternatives to different LAIs were discussed
  - Though initially hesitant due to the injection, he agrees to this later
- On day 3 of second hospitalization, he is given:
  - Aripiprazole (Abilify) 30 mg once orally
  - Aripiprazole lauroxil (Aristada Initio) 675 mg IM once
  - Aripiprazole lauroxil (Aristada) 1024 mg IM once
  - This dosing regimen ensures no supplemental oral aripiprazole (Abilify) is needed to achieve therapeutic serum concentrations after the day of injection
- Over next several days, patient's hallucinations, loose associations, and disorganization improve
- Follow-up is again planned, parents agree to allow patient to return to their home to stay with them instead of with roommate
- Patient voices the need to be compliant with his medications
- Odd behavior such as eating his food exclusively while being seated on the ground is observed, but otherwise improved from admission
- No adverse reactions from LAI are seen

- Patient is discharged home on hospital day 6
- Unfortunately, patient does not return to clinic for follow-up and his long-term course is uncertain; he has not been seen within the same hospital system since the second discharge
- Attempts need to be made to reach the patient prior to the LAI effectiveness wearing off

Case debrief

- This patient was diagnosed with schizophrenia based on his pattern of delusions, hallucinations, disorganized behavior, and disorganized speech that negatively progressed over a period of multiple years
- He was indeed responsive to antipsychotics whenever he was actually receiving them consistently
- His past non-compliance and his concern over weight gain led the treatment team to pick a more weight-neutral medication, aripiprazole (Abilify)
- Initial response was positive, and the team gave the patient the opportunity for medication compliance on his own accord
- This failed, and the patient decompensated over the course of several days following cessation of aripiprazole (Abilify) after his first hospital stay
- During second hospitalization, the cytochrome P450 (CYP3A4) inhibitor fluconazole (Diflucan) was discovered and removed from his home medication list to maintain appropriate plasma levels and efficacy of aripiprazole (Abilify)
- Due to non-compliance with oral agents, this patient was a clear candidate for an LAI, and the dose he was given would maintain him at a serum level roughly equivalent to 15 mg/d orally of aripiprazole (Abilify) for up to 2 months

Take-home points

- Medication non-compliance is a persistent issue in all fields of medicine, including behavioral health where rates of non-compliance in those with primary psychosis are extremely high
  - Several large literature reviews have demonstrated compliance rates of only 41.2% to 58%
  - One VA study of over 34,000 veterans with schizophrenia showed that 61% of patients had at least one year of poor compliance
- Relapse rates for psychosis after medication discontinuation are very high, even after only a single episode

- One literature review from 2013 demonstrated recurrence rates of nearly 80% during the first 12 months following the first episode of psychosis
- Some theorize a "kindling effect" or "downward drift" with psychosis, meaning that with each relapse the disease will progress faster with increasing severity, and the patient's baseline of psychosocial functioning will decline over time
- Advancements in LAIs ensure patients can have a steady dose of antipsychotics in their system for weeks to months, and likely should be used more often

Pharmacokinetic moment

- One consideration for initiation of atypical antipsychotics is to consider drug–drug interactions, as many schizophrenia patients have comorbid medical conditions
- Diabetes, hyperlipidemia, and coronary artery disease are often seen within this population
  - Often associated with the very medications taken to control their psychosis
  - Some patients are placed on extensive medication regimens as sequelae of these comorbid conditions, many of which possess pharmacokinetic interactions
  - Not limited to medications, as even smoking induces CYP1A2, which can be associated with reduced efficacy of olanzapine (Zyprexa) or clozapine (Clozaril)
- Aripiprazole (Abilify), cariprazine (Vraylar), and brexpiprazole (Rexulti) are all partial D_2 and D_3 receptor agonists metabolized by CYP3A4 and CYP2D6
  - Common inhibitors of CYP3A4 include most macrolide antibiotics, diltiazem (Cardizem), azole-class antifungals, ritonavir (Norvir), verapamil (Verelan), and grapefruit, which increase these antipsychotics' plasma levels to some degree
  - Common inducers of CYP3A4 include phenobarbital (Luminal), carbamazepine (Tegretol), rifampicin (Rifadin), phenytoin (Dilantin), St. John's Wort, as well as glucocorticoids. These will lower plasma levels
  - Common inhibitors of CYP2D6 include bupropion (Wellbutrin), fluoxetine (Prozac), metoclopramide (Reglan), paroxetine (Paxil), duloxetine (Cymbalta), and terbinafine (Lamisil). These will remarkably increase plasma levels
  - Common inducers of CYP2D6 include tocilizumab (Actemra) and tumor necrosis factor inhibitors. These will lower plasma levels

Pharmacokinetic moment: hepatic metabolism and the antipsychotics

In Table 3.1, we see the differences between the atypical antipsychotics. One of the most common enzymatic pathways that the liver uses to detoxify and rid our patients of their prescribed antipsychotics seems to be 2D6 (Figure 3.1). Therefore, any concomitant medication that inhibits 2D6 may remarkably increase plasma levels of the antipsychotics. Typically, in these cases, we worry about an increase in extrapyramidal symptoms (EPS) such as dystonia or akathisia. Some patients are genetically poor metabolizers as they have inherited genes from their parents which make the 2D6 enzyme less aggressive, allowing medication levels to build up more quickly, and again this is associated typically with a greater side-effect burden. In this case, the patient was taking an antifungal which actually inhibited 3A4 enzymes and, according to the table above, likely increased his aripiprazole plasma levels. This actually may have been helpful in this case, allowing for more drug availability to help lower his acute psychotic symptoms.

Table 3.1 The hepatic enzymes involved in the metabolism of 17 antipsychotics

Drug	Metabolized by
Clozapine	CYP450 1A2, 3A4, 2D6
Risperidone	CYP450 2D6
Paliperidone	Is only weakly metabolized
Olanzapine	CYP450 1A2
Quetiapine	CYP450 3A4, 2D6
Ziprasidone	Not affected by CYP450 enzymes
Aripiprazole	CYP450 3A4, 2D6
Zotepine	CYP450 1A2, 3A4
Perospirone	CYP450 3A4
Sertindole	CYP450 3A4, 2D6
Loxapine	Unknown
Cyamemazine	Unknown
Amisulpride	Is only weakly metabolized
Sulpiride	Is only weakly metabolized
Bifeprunox	CYP450 2C9, 3A4, only little 2D6
Iloperidone	CYP450 3A4, 2D6
Asenapine	CYP450 1A2, 3A4

Source: Stahl's Essential Psychopharmacology, 4th edn.

1 = family
A = subtype
1 = gene product

Figure 3.1 The cytochrome P450 system encompasses a large number of enzymes. These are classified according to family, subtype, and gene product, using the following nomenclature: 1 = family, A = subtype, and 1 = gene product. Thus, as depicted in the figure, the five most common and relevant systems are CYP450 1A2, 2D6, 2C9, 2C19, and 3A4. The atypical antipsychotics differ as to which of these degradative metabolic pathways are utilized to lower drug plasma levels within our patients. There are genetic polymorphisms for each, which may allow a patient's liver to metabolize a drug away faster or really inhibit and slow down catabolism, sometimes allowing for toxicity and side effects to occur more robustly.

Two-minute tutorial

Long-acting injectables (LAIs)

- Long-acting injectables have been developed for many atypical antipsychotics
- Typically, oral antipsychotics may provide reasonable plasma levels for a few days to a few weeks, depending on the drug's half-life
- LAIs use intramuscular slow-release preparations which can allow for adequate plasma levels for weeks to months, depending on the LAI

Table 3.2 below lists the available LAIs and their typical dosing regimen. The latest approval is for paliperidone (Invega Hayfera), which can be used now every 6 months. Note that older typical antipsychotic decanoate injections are used sparingly – haloperidol (Haldol) and fluphenazine (Prolixin).

- Another option for monitoring patient compliance is a novel formulation of aripiprazole tablets with a sensor (Abilify Mycite)
  - Includes an ingestible event marker sensor, a patch (wearable sensor), a smartphone app for the patient, and a web-based portal for the provider

Table 3.2

Generic name	Brand name	Available formulation	Common dosing schedule
Aripiprazole monohydrate	Abilify Maintena	300 or 400 mg prefilled syringes 720 or 960 mg prefilled syringes	Monthly Every 2 months
Aripiprazole lauroxil	Aristada	441, 662, 882, 1064 mg prefilled syringes (675 mg Initio option)	Monthly (441/662 mg) Every 6 weeks (882 mg) Every 2 months (1064 mg)
Risperidone microspheres	Risperdal Consta	12.5, 25, 37.5, 50 mg vials	Every 2 weeks
Paliperidone palmitate	Invega Sustenna	39, 78, 117, 156, or 234 mg prefilled syringes	Monthly
Paliperidone palmitate	Invega Trinza	273, 410, 546, 819 mg prefilled syringes	Every 3 months
Olanzapine pamoate	Zyprexa Relprevv	210, 300, 405 mg vials	Every 2 weeks (150–300 mg) Monthly (405 mg)

- ◦ Digitally tracks whether patients have been compliant with their oral aripiprazole dosing
- ◦ This formulation of aripiprazole utilizes a silicon chip with a logic circuit as well as a piece of copper and magnesium
- ◦ Whenever the mechanism makes contact with the gastric acid of the stomach, it generates a small current that powers the chip to send a signal to the sensor

Post-test question

Some atypical antipsychotics exert their antipsychotic and antidepressant effects via partial agonism of the dopamine-2 receptor (D$_2$). The inhibition of which hepatic cytochrome P450 (CYP450) enzyme would have the most prominent effect on a patient's serum concentration of this class of atypical antipsychotic drugs (sometimes called the PIPS and the RIPS …)?

A. CYP3A4

B. CYP2D6

C. CYP1A2

D. CYP2C9

E. A and B

F. All of the above

Answer: E

The atypical antipsychotics aripiprazole (Abilify), cariprazine (Vraylar), and brexpiprazole (Rexulti) are all metabolized to a great extent by these two enzymes. Therefore, concurrent administration of a medication which inhibits these enzymes would cause a remarkable increase in serum levels of these antipsychotics.

References

1. Bak, M, Fransen, A, Janssen, J, et al. Almost all antipsychotics result in weight gain: a meta-analysis. *PLoS One* 2014; 9:e94112

2. Cochran, JM, Fang, H, Le Gallo, C, et al. Participant engagement and symptom improvement: aripiprazole tablets with sensor for the treatment of schizophrenia. *Patient Prefer Adherence* 2022; 16:1805–17

3. Doane, MJ, Bessonova, L, Friedler, HS, et al. Weight gain and comorbidities associated with oral second-generation antipsychotics: analysis of real-world data for patients with schizophrenia or bipolar I disorder. *BMC Psychiatry* 2022; 22:114

4. Higashi, K, Medic, G, Littlewood, KJ, et al. Medication adherence in schizophrenia: factors influencing adherence and consequences of nonadherence, a systematic literature review. *Ther Adv Psychopharmacol* 2013; 3:200–18

5. Lian, L, Kim, DD, Procyshyn, RM, et al. Long-acting injectable antipsychotics for early psychosis: a comprehensive systematic review. *PLoS One* 2022; 17:e0267808

6. Reymann, S, Schoretsanitis, G, Egger, ST, et al. Use of long-acting injectable antipsychotics in inpatients with schizophrenia spectrum disorder in an academic psychiatric hospital in Switzerland. *J Pers Med* 2022; 12:441

7. Stahl, SM. *Stahl's Essential Psychopharmacology: Neuroscientific Basis and Practical Applications*, 5. Cambridge: Cambridge University Press, 2021

Case 4: Hit by a car

The Question: Why do patients not respond to medications?

The Psychopharmacological Dilemma: What medication to try first, second, third …

Cecilia Albers

Pretest self-assessment question

What is not a potential complication of using antipsychotics in a patient with agitation when there is no available history?

A. Could worsen hyperactive catatonia
B. Could cause respiratory complications in patients who previously received IM lorazepam (Ativan)
C. Could worsen delirium
D. Could cause cardiac complications due to QTc prolongation
E. Could cause allergic reactions

Patient evaluation on intake

- A 22-year-old man brought to the hospital involuntarily after having run into the street screaming that he was "being chased" and being ultimately hit by a car
- Given lorazepam (Ativan) 1 mg IV and 2 mg midazolam (Versed) IV in the emergency room (ER) because he was screaming and fighting with staff on arrival
- Friend reported that he had been acting erratically, quit going to work and broke up with his long-term girlfriend recently
- Initially, nursing reports he has been difficult to care for and would not speak to them
- On examination, he responded to his name, but when asked any questions would blankly respond "I don't know," then would stare toward the wall and TV
- He would flip the channel every 45 seconds to a minute and did not appear to be engaged with what was on the TV
- Police stated the patient claimed at the scene that he was "being shot at"
- Since patient could not provide history, it was obtained from his mother, father, and a sister

Psychiatric history

- Family reported that the patient had never been diagnosed with a mental illness, but they had been worried about him for the last 4 months

- Mother reports that patient was "feeling anxious" since an incident where he was robbed at gun-point in his home at about that time
- Mother reported that he seemed more depressed than usual
- No previous suicide attempts or hospitalizations for psychiatric symptoms
- No previous medication trials
- Urine Drug Screen (UDS) was positive for methamphetamines
- Roommate reports that he was using methamphetamines daily in the 4 weeks prior to admission
- Also reported that the patient had not slept for a week prior to admission

Social and personal history

- Did well in high school and college
- Recently broke up with his long-term partner
- Was gainfully employed working as a paralegal
- Family reported no history of drug use, but UDS was positive for methamphetamines and also cannabis

Medical history

- Fracture of left leg from being hit by the car
- No chronic medical concerns
- Patient is negative for Clinical Institute Withdrawal Assessment (CIWA) or Clinical Opiate Withdrawal Scale (COWS) for withdrawal

Family history

- Uncle had episodes of sadness in which he would not get out of bed for days and episodes of fast talking and excessive spending, but had refused any care and had no formal diagnosis
- No other known family history of mental illness

Medication history

- No previous medication trials for any psychiatric reason

Current medications

- None

Psychotherapy history

- A few sessions of family therapy during his parents' divorce when he was a child, but none since then

Patient evaluation on initial visit

- New onset of anxiety 4 months after being robbed
- New onset of paranoid delusions one week prior to admission
- Police suggest that he was having visual hallucinations
- UDS was positive for methamphetamines and cannabis
- Patient is unable to participate in evaluation and does not have decision-making capacity at this time; parents are the surrogate decision-makers

Question

Should delirium be considered a possible diagnosis in this patient?

- No, this is a healthy 26-year-old male with no previous medical conditions
- Yes, despite otherwise being low risk, his drug use and recently being hit by a car is enough to cause a medical delirium
- No, delirium unlikely, but may be stimulant and cannabis intoxication
- No, the drug use unmasked a psychiatric diagnosis such as schizophrenia

Attending physician's mental notes: initial psychiatric evaluation

- This patient is in the age range for new onset of psychotic psychiatric conditions
- He can provide us with very little information, his family lives out of state, and after initial conversation roommate stopped returning our phone calls
- While patients who are withdrawing from methamphetamines may refuse to participate in care, they are usually asleep and have increased appetite while in a "crash" withdrawal; he is presenting differently
- He is lucid and does not show a waxing or waning of consciousness, nor confusion associated with a delirium
- While the exact time of last drug use was unknown, he was taken into police custody more than 24 hours ago, which makes acute intoxication very unlikely and he does not appear to be in a withdrawal state now
- Busch-Francis is a scale that evaluates the common symptoms of catatonia, where greater than two symptoms is considered concerning for catatonia and the total score reflects severity (Table 4.1)
  - Score was 10 with symptoms of mutism, withdrawal, staring, and immobility, which suggests catatonia

Table 4.1

Busch-Francis Catatonia Rating Scale

1. Immobility/stupor: extreme hypoactivity, immobile, minimally responsive to stimuli

   0 – Absent
   1 – Sits abnormally still, may interact briefly
   2 – Virtually no interaction with external world
   3 – Stuporous, non-reactive to painful stimuli

2. Mutism: verbally unresponsive or minimally responsive

   0 = Absent
   1 = Verbally unresponsive to majority of questions; incomprehensible whisper
   2 = Speaks less than 20 words / 5mins
   3 = No speech

3. Staring: fixed gaze, little or no visual scanning of environment, decreased blinking

   0 = Absent
   1 = Poor eye contact, repeatedly gazes less than 20 sec between shifting of attention; decreased blinking
   2 = Gaze held longer than 20 sec, occasionally shifts attention
   3 = Fixed gaze, non-reactive

4. Posturing/catalepsy: spontaneous maintenance of posture(s), including mundane (e.g., sitting or standing for long periods without reacting)

   0 = Absent
   1 = Less than 1 min
   2 = Greater than 1 min, less than 15 min
   3 = Bizarre posture, or mundane maintained more than 15 min

5. Grimacing: maintenance of odd facial expressions

   0 = Absent
   1 = Less than 10 sec
   2 = Less than 1 min
   3 = Bizarre expression(s) or maintained more than 1 min

6. Echopraxia/echolalia: mimicking of examiner's movements (echopraxia) or speech (echolalia)

   0 = Absent
   1 = Occasional
   2 = Frequent
   3 = Constant

7. Stereotypy: repetitive, non-goal-directed motor activity (e.g., finger-play, repeatedly touching, patting or rubbing self); abnormality not inherent in act but in its frequency

   0 = Absent
   1 = Occasional
   2 = Frequent
   3 = Constant

8. Mannerisms: odd, purposeful movements (hopping or walking tiptoe, saluting passers-by or exaggerated caricatures of mundane movements); abnormality inherent in act itself

   0 = Absent
   1 = Occasional
   2 = Frequent
   3 = Constant

9. Stereotyped & meaningless repetition of words & phrases (verbigeration): repetition of phrases or sentences (like a scratched record)

   0 = Absent
   1 = Occasional
   2 = Frequent, difficult to interrupt
   3 = Constant

10. Rigidity: maintenance of a rigid position despite efforts to be moved (exclude if cog-wheeling or tremor present)

    0 = Absent
    1 = Mild resistance
    2 = Moderate
    3 = Severe, cannot be repostured

11. Negativism: apparently motiveless resistance to instructions or attempts to move/examine patient. Contrary behavior, does exact opposite of instruction.

    0 = Absent
    1 = Mild resistance and/or occasionally contrary
    2 = Moderate resistance and/or frequently contrary
    3 = Severe resistance and/or continually contrary

12. Waxy flexibility: during repositioning of patient, patient offers initial resistance before allowing him/herself to be repositioned, similar to that of a bending candle. (Also defined as slow resistance to movement as the patient allows the examiner to place his/her extremities in unusual positions. The limbs may remain in the position in which they are placed or not)

    0 = Absent
    3 = Present

13. Withdrawal: refusal to eat, drink and/or make eye contact

0 = Absent
1 = Minimal oral intake / interaction for less than 1 day
2 = Minimal oral intake / interaction for more than 1 day
3 = No oral intake / interaction for 1 day or more

14. Excitement: extreme hyperactivity, constant motor unrest which is apparently non-purposeful. Not to be attributed to akathisia or goal-directed agitation

1 = Excessive motion, intermittent
2 = Constant motion, hyperkinetic without rest periods
3 = Full-blown catatonic excitement, endless frenzied motor activity

15. Impulsivity: patient suddenly engages in inappropriate behavior (e.g., runs down hallway, starts screaming, or takes off clothes) without provocation. Afterwards can give no, or only a facile, explanation

0 = Absent
1 = Occasional
2 = Frequent
3 = Constant or not redirectable

16. Automatic obedience: exaggerated cooperation with examiner's request or spontaneous continuation of movement requested

0 = Absent
1 = Occasional
2 = Frequent
3 = Constant

17. Passive obedience (mitgehen): patient raises arm in response to light pressure of finger, despite instructions to the contrary

0 = Absent
3 = Present

18. Muscle resistance (gegenhalten): involuntary resistance to passive movement of a limb to a new position. Resistance increases with the speed of the movement

0 = Absent
3 = Present

19. Motorically stuck (ambitendency): patient appears stuck in indecisive, hesitant motor movements

0 = Absent
3 = Present

20. Grasp reflex: striking the patient's open palm with two extended fingers of the examiner's hand results in automatic closure of patient's hand

0 = Absent
3 = Present

21. Perseveration: repeatedly returns to same topic or persists with the same movements

0 = Absent
3 = Present

22. Combativeness: belligerence or aggression. Usually in an undirected manner, without explanation

0 = Absent
1 = Occasionally strikes out, low potential for injury
2 = Frequently strikes out, moderate potential for injury
3 = Serious danger to others

23. Autonomic abnormality: abnormality of body temperature (fever), blood pressure, pulse, respiratory rate, inappropriate sweating, flushing

0 = Absent
1 = Abnormality of one parameter (exclude pre-existing hypertension)
2 = Abnormality of two parameters
3 = Abnormality of three or more parameters

- Patient has several possible diagnoses, but some treatments will be contraindicated
- If patient has hypoactive delirium, lorazepam (Ativan) could worsen his condition; if patient has catatonia, then antipsychotics could worsen his condition
- Treatment must proceed based on what diagnosis is most likely and what can be the most dangerous if treated incorrectly

Question

Which of the following would be your next step for this patient?

- Start a typical antipsychotic, haloperidol (Haldol) 1 mg/d for treatment of delirium
- Start an atypical antipsychotic, olanzapine (Zyprexa) 5 mg q6h for treatment of agitation due to psychosis
- Give a sedative anxiolytic benzodiazepine (BZ), lorazepam (Ativan) 1–2 mg IV and observe for 1 hour for improvement of catatonia

Attending physician's mental notes: lorazepam (Ativan) challenge

- This BZ challenge should be definitive in helping us to decide the level of catatonia present

Case outcome: lorazepam (Ativan) challenge

- Patient was given 2 mg of IV lorazepam (Ativan) and 60 minutes later was observed to be very sedated, but much more verbally responsive
- Could not repeat Busch-Francis scale due to level of sedation; patient would only speak a few sentences before drifting off to sleep
- Asked nurse to observe him over the next few hours
  - Reported that he was not speaking spontaneously, but would more easily respond to direct questions and was able to eat lunch 2–3 hours later

Attending physician's mental notes: lorazepam (Ativan) challenge

- This BZ challenge seems definitive and helped us to see that some catatonia was present
- May need to continue this BZ treatment for a few days

Question

Was this an adequate response to a lorazepam (Ativan) catatonia challenge?

- Yes, the patient showed improvement in key symptoms of catatonia, such as reversal of mutism and fixed staring
- No, patient was too sedated to perform a full Busch-Francis Scale so the challenge should be repeated before making the diagnosis of catatonia

Case outcome: lorazepam (Ativan) challenge continued

- Mutism and withdrawal symptoms in this case have resolved
- Some of ongoing symptomatology is secondary, and complicated due to the sedation from using 2 mg IV as the initial lorazepam (Ativan) dose

Attending physician's mental notes: lorazepam (Ativan) challenge outcome

- This BZ challenge seems definitive and helped us to see that some catatonia was present
- May need to continue this BZ treatment for a few days

Case outcome: hospital day 3

- Patient was started on oral lorazepam (Ativan) 1 mg twice daily in a divided dose to ideally reduce sedation, but yield ongoing anti-catatonia clinical effectiveness
- Significant speech latency continued, but patient was able to participate in interview process
- Reports now that he has some depression, but is vague
- When pressed empathically to elaborate further on answers he would lapse into long staring spells

Question

What would be the next most reasonable medication step for this patient?

- No further medications, as patient's symptoms are likely due to resolving catatonia which will be further treated with ongoing oral lorazepam (Ativan)
- Start an atypical antipsychotic, aripiprazole (Abilify), as speech latency could be due to new-onset psychotic disorder that is causing the catatonia
- Start an antidepressant such as fluoxetine (Prozac) to address patient's reported depression and mother's report of his anxiety
- Start a mood stabilizer such as lithium (Eskalith) as the patient's initial symptoms of poor sleep and paranoia are more consistent with mania

Attending physician's mental notes: hospital day 3

- Good that the catatonia is better treated, but the patient is still a poor historian
- May need to continue this BZ treatment for a few days, but we will need a better history to obtain a more conclusive sense of what has caused the catatonia

Case outcome: hospital day 4

- Deemed medically stable as the patient was eating and drinking now and was transferred from the medical floor to the inpatient psychiatric floor
- On initial evaluation by inpatient team, he again reported that he was depressed
- Reported having recently quit his job, but could not provide details
- Reported that he did run into the street and was hit by the car, but could not say why
- It was noticed that he had some echopraxia and mimicking of the clinician's motions
- Collateral history was obtained from the mother which stated that the patient had
  - Stopped cleaning up after himself
  - Made a phone call 1 month ago in which he was speaking so fast she could not understand him
  - That "his whole world fell apart" when he quit his job
- Given his reported history of periods of sleep loss, rapid speech, with disorganized and hyperactive behaviors prior, it was felt that he most likely experienced a manic event
  - Not all mood elevation events were concurrent with methamphetamine use
- Started on lithium (Eskalith) 600 mg/d after baseline labs obtained, with a new working diagnosis of bipolar I disorder (BP1), now with catatonia

Attending physician's mental notes: hospital day 4

- After gaining more history from the patient and outside sources, it seems that his catatonia may be driven by a bipolar disorder (BP)
- Will need to make sure we strive for optimal mood stabilization medications to prevent a return of catatonia

Case outcome: hospital days 5–7

- Continued to deny paranoia and stated that running out in front of the car was "something that happened"
- Tolerated the lithium (Eskalith) with no side effects
- On hospital day 7, lithium (Eskalith) level was 0.5 mEq/L
- Denied hallucinations but was still observed to be responding to unseen stimuli while on the unit
- He reported that his mood was "good" though and was observed to be interacting socially and normally on the unit without current catatonia symptoms

- Busch-Francis score was normalizing gradually
- On hospital day 7, it was felt that he had received the maximum benefit from inpatient hospitalization and, with the right supports and psychiatric follow-up plan, he could safely transition to outpatient care
- On the day of discharge, there was still some concern that he was hallucinating, but he was consistently denying hallucinations and did not appear to be impaired to the level that he was a danger to himself or others to warrant further involuntary hospitalization
    - The outpatient team was apprised of his improving, albeit residual, symptoms

Case debrief

- In young adults with no previous diagnosis, there can be many possible causes of catatonia
    - Drug use, depression, or psychosis-induced
- The most likely disorders associated with catatonia are mood disorders, particularly bipolar disorder (BP) and sometimes major depressive disorder (MDD)
- Although this patient had a history of recent stimulant use, his behaviors were much better explained by BP once collateral and corroborative history was obtained
    - Strong risk factors were noted for BP because of a first-degree relative with similar symptoms
    - Mother reports a previous history of depressive episodes and possibly one mania for this patient
    - Symptoms of paranoia did not improve once stimulant acute intoxication resolved
    - BP is much more likely to cause catatonia than stimulant or cannabis use disorder
        - However, there are many case reports of the high-potency synthetic cannabinoids, such as "Spike," causing catatonic states in some patients
    - Patient most likely presented in a BP depressive state with psychosis and catatonia
- Any patient who presents with new-onset catatonia should have a work up for medical conditions that can be the possible cause of catatonia, such as dystonias, HIV encephalopathy, progressive multifocal leukoencephalopathy, encephalitis, and renal failure, as well
- Both BZ and clozapine (Clozaril) withdrawal are associated with catatonia and can be considered as possible causes

- Patients whose catatonia symptoms do not respond to BZ therapy or who have autonomic dysregulation should be considered for ECT treatment
- Catatonia can be considered a medical emergency if the patient is failing to thrive, especially if they have no oral intake of fluids due to their symptoms
- This case shows classically how BZs can be used to stop catatonia and how to use lithium (Eskalith) to treat underlying BP to ultimately maintain the patient out of a catatonic state

Take-home points

- It is often not possible at the initial time of presentation to know the totality of the patient's diagnosis, prior to starting medication treatment in the emergency setting
  ○ We must always strive to obtain collateral history, which was a key element of this case
- In these cases, it makes sense to focus on the most urgent concerns and treat using the most likely diagnosis
- Patients may experience sedation during a BZ catatonia challenge and still respond to it for treatment of their catatonia
- Catatonia can look like other diagnoses, particularly psychosis and delirium
  ○ With medical causes ruled out, delirium becomes less likely
- Dopamine-2 receptor (D_2) antagonizing antipsychotics used for treatment of psychosis and delirium can actually worsen catatonia; likewise the BZ used to treat catatonia can worsen delirium
- Therefore, patients should be thoroughly evaluated to determine whether delirium or catatonia is the most likely diagnosis

Performance in practice: confessions of a psychopharmacologist

What could have been done better here?

What are possible action items for improvement in practice?

- Use more effective lorazepam (Ativan) challenges
  ○ The typical range of dosing for a lorazepam (Ativan) challenge is 1–2 mg IV
  ○ While 2 mg IV is not an unreasonable dose for a lorazepam (Ativan) challenge, 1 mg should have been administered first and, if the patient did not respond, then an additional 1 mg dose could have been given
  ○ This dose would have caused less sedation and would have made interpretation easier

- ○ The IV preparation has double the bioavailability of oral lorazepam
- ○ Factors to consider when deciding on initial dose are severity of symptoms, past history of treatment response, weight, age, medication interactions, and prior history of BZ use
- Should an atypical antipsychotic have been considered for treatment of this patient's bipolar disorder?
  - ○ Perhaps earlier use of an antipsychotic, paired with the lorazepam (Ativan), may have helped his hallucinations to resolve faster
- Should more have been done to address the patient's prior methamphetamine use prior to discharge?
  - ○ Continued methamphetamine use will significantly worsen the patient's long-term prognosis and cause future manic episodes
  - ○ However, in the acute setting, in a patient who is on the pre-contemplative level of change, intervention is difficult and unlikely to be effective
  - ○ Also, cannabis use can foster onset of schizophrenia and other psychotic symptoms and destabilize affect in those patients with known mood disorders
  - ○ His substance use complicated this case and increased the complexity of his differential diagnosis
  - ○ His catatonia symptoms lasted well past the time expected for symptoms of acute stimulant withdrawal

What are possible action items for improvement in practice?

- Research information on the treatment options for BP with catatonia
- Research available US and international guidelines regarding treatment of methamphetamine use disorder
- Create a standardized procedure for performing the lorazepam (Ativan) challenge, including what criteria would need to be met for a higher or lower initial dose

Tips and pearls

- The evaluation of catatonia is complicated by the fact that many symptoms of catatonia are similar to those of delirium (e.g., waxing and waning of symptoms) and they can have similar causes
- The DSM-5 criteria for delirium are
  - ○ A disturbance in attention and awareness
  - ○ A disturbance in cognition, such as memory, orientation, or language
  - ○ This disturbance is an acute sudden change from the baseline and is usually short in duration, lasting a few hours to days

- ◦ The disturbance is the direct consequence of an underlying physiological condition, substance, toxin, or withdrawal
- There are several drugs of abuse that are associated with catatonia and whose acute intoxication may mimic some symptoms of catatonia (hyperactivity, withdrawal, and negativism), such as phencyclidine (PCP), cannabis, mescaline, lysergic acid diethylamide (LSD), cocaine, and methylenedioxymethamphetamine (MDMA)
- A patient can still have catatonia even if they do not respond to a single dose of a BZ challenge; if there is no response, consider retrying in 3 hours
- Patients with underlying schizophrenia or longer-standing catatonia are less likely to respond to BZs, unfortunately
- If the evidence for catatonia is strong, but the patient is only partially responding to lorazepam (Ativan), consider higher dosing or consider referral for ECT
- The patient's entire medication list should be evaluated for potential iatrogenic medication causes of catatonia
- The withdrawal of clozapine (Clozaril) and BZs are another potentially overlooked cause of delirium and catatonia
- Typical antipsychotics are generally contraindicated in catatonia, but atypical antipsychotics are a possible treatment option when a primary psychotic disorder is the suspected cause after initial BZ treatment of the catatonia
- Consider use of an antipsychotic with lower D_2 affinity, such as quetiapine (Seroquel), or with D_2 partial agonism, such as aripiprazole (Abilify), brexpiprazole (Rexulti), cariprazine (Vraylar), or lumateperone (Caplyta)
- Catatonia can become a medical emergency when there is severe autonomic instability, prolonged refusal of oral intake, or complications of prolonged immobility, such as embolism, stasis ulcers, and aspiration pneumonia

Mechanism of Action Moment

How do benzodiazepines (BZs) work to treat catatonia?

- The exact mechanism of action of the treatment of catatonia is not fully understood, because the pathophysiology of this condition is not fully understood
- However, there are two prominent theories about how BZs may work:
  - ◦ Catatonia as an anxiety process
    - ▪ Suggests that catatonia may be an extreme version of the fight or flight response causing tonic immobility, and sometimes it is called "fight, flight, or freeze" response

- Patients with catatonia in some studies have shown hyperactivation in the orbital frontal cortex (OFC) and ventromedial prefrontal cortex (VMPFC), which is similar to processing of negative (anxious) emotion
- BZs primarily bind with GABA-A receptors to act as a positive allosteric modulator (PAM) on the BZ-sensitive GABA-A receptors
- Once bound, they cause an increase in the frequency of chloride channel opening, which increases the level of inhibition for neurons in these hyperfunctioning brain areas

○ Catatonia as a motor disorder

- Patients with catatonia show some overlap symptoms with Parkinson's Disease patients
- Patients with catatonia have also shown decreased activity in the dorsolateral prefrontal cortex (DLPFC), and altered orbitofrontal cortex (OFC), prefrontal cortex (PFC), parietal cortex, and motor cortical regions
- Many of these regions are regulated by GABAergic projections of the basal ganglia
- Lorazepam (Ativan) and other BZs may help to increase the effectiveness of GABA-A receptors via PAM and facilitate improved neurotransmission in these hypothetically affected neuro-circuits as well

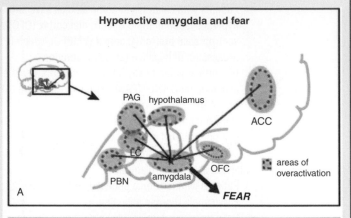

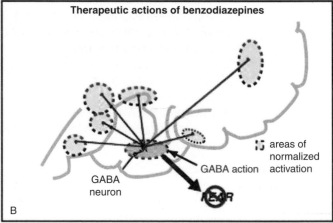

Figure 4.1 As noted here, GABA neurons are involved and tend to dampen central nervous system (CNS) hyperactivity in several brain areas that seem to be hyperactive based upon functional neuroimaging studies involving catatonia patients. Theoretically, use of BZs can normalize the activity in these abnormally functioning areas. (PAG – periaqueductal gray; PBN – parabrachial nucleus; LC – locus coeruleus; OFC – orbitofrontal cortex; ACC – anterior cingulate cortex)

Two-minute tutorial

Treatment of catatonia

Benzodiazepines (BZs)

- Although there is limited research regarding the treatment of catatonia, BZs are considered the first line of treatment for rapid resolution of symptoms in most guidelines
- A rapid response to a BZ is considered a diagnostic sign of catatonia

- Lorazepam (Ativan) is the most common to be used because it comes in PO, IM, and IV formulations, meaning that it can be used in patients who refuse all oral intake
- A BZ trial for a patient with suspected catatonia is usually done by giving 1–2 mg of IM or IV lorazepam (Ativan) and observing the patient for 30 minutes to an hour for resolution of symptoms
  - If symptoms do not resolve, then one or two more similar trials may be given at 3-hour intervals
  - A patient can be considered responsive if there is a 50% reduction of catatonia symptoms after these administrations
- Lorazepam (Ativan) is not the treatment of choice in patients with symptoms of profound autonomic dysfunction, also referred to as malignant catatonia, because these symptoms can be fatal and ECT can bring about more rapid resolution
- Higher doses of lorazepam (Ativan) may have notable side effects of sedation, cognitive impairment, dizziness, ataxia, hypotension, respiratory suppression, and, in addition, physiological dependence
  - It is also relatively contraindicated in patients with pulmonary compromise (such as obstructive sleep apnea and chronic obstructive pulmonary disease [COPD]) and narrow angle glaucoma as it can worsen these conditions

Benzodiazepine receptor agonists

- Zolpidem (Ambien) is a PAM and typically used as a hypnotic agent
- It is thought to work by selectively binding to α_1 isoform subunits of the BZ receptors which are located on GABA-A receptors, which are clustered mostly in sleep-promoting centers of the brain, such as the ventrolateral preoptic area (VLPO)
  - This binding at the same time as a GABA molecule binds allows for a higher frequency of chloride channel openings, allowing greater neuronal inhibition
- Zolpidem (Ambien) is thought to have possibly less cognitive blunting when compared to true BZ use
- It only comes in an oral formulation and therefore is not appropriate for patients who are refusing oral intake
- It can be used in place of lorazepam (Ativan) for a challenge, using a single 10 mg initial dose and observing for 15 minutes to an hour later
- Important psychiatric side effects include hallucinations, anterograde amnesia, and complex sleep behaviors such as sleep walking, eating, and driving
- Other notable, albeit rare, side effects include respiratory depression and angioedema

Glutamate antagonists

- Amantadine (Symmetrel) 100–500 mg three times a day, and memantine (Namenda) 5–20 mg/d, have both been used off label for treatment of catatonia
- Both are thought to have their proposed effect in catatonia due to their glutamate N-methyl-D-aspartate acid receptor (NMDAR) antagonist properties
- This is a treatment option with limited available research so far, but may be an option when first-line treatments have failed, because of its unique mechanism of action
- Notably could lead to worsening of psychiatric symptoms
- Other possible side effects include seizures, dizziness, and constipation

Mood stabilizers

- Mood stabilizers are typically not used as an initial treatment for catatonia, but are often used as an adjuvant in treatment-resistant cases
- DIvalproex (Depakote), carbamazepine (Tegretol), and topiramate (Topamax) have all been used in cases of treatment-resistant catatonia
- Lithium (Eskalith) may be considered for prevention of reoccurrence of catatonia
- Given the relationship between mania and catatonia, this may be a consideration in selecting a mood stabilizer for patients with BP

Electroconvulsive therapy (ECT)

- ECT is a treatment option for patients who do not respond to BZ or other medication options, or if a rapid response is required because life-threatening symptoms – such as, in malignant catatonia, dehydration – are present
- This treatment option can be complicated by the fact that the majority who require ECT for catatonia are also unable to provide informed consent, requiring the need for surrogate decision-makers
- Potential complications directly related to ECT are prolonged seizures and associated hypoxia, arrhythmias, damage to teeth and mouth, and cardiac events / hypertension
- Other concerns are related to retrograde amnesia that is often associated with this treatment, especially if being used for maintenance

Transcranial magnetic stimulation (TMS)

- TMS is not FDA approved for the treatment of catatonia, and the possible mechanism of action is not fully understood; however,

some case reports and small studies have shown improvements in catatonic symptoms when TMS is utilized
- The most common placement is over the left DLPFC
- This treatment option has the advantage of not requiring anesthesia, therefore reducing associated complicated risk. This makes it a potential treatment option for patients who are not candidates for ECT due to safety concerns
- The difficulty is that the patient must sit still for 20–30 minutes each session. This is generally all right with catatonic stupor, but not if there are bouts of catatonic excitement

Antipsychotics
- Many patients with catatonia will have an underlying psychotic disorder or BP, which can be treated with typical or atypical antipsychotics
- There is some evidence that aggressive D_2 blockade of the nigrostriatal pathway could worsen the motor symptoms of catatonia, which suggests generally avoiding the typical antipsychotics
- Patients with catatonia may be at increased risk of developing neuroleptic malignant syndrome (NMS) when on antipsychotic medications
- The treatment of catatonia must be balanced with the treatment of the underlying psychiatric condition, so treating the catatonia first and then treating the underlying condition second via starting an atypical antipsychotic with lower antagonistic affinity for the D_2 is clinically warranted and justified

Post-test question

What is not a potential complication of using antipsychotics in a patient with agitation when there is no available history?

A. Could worsen hyperactive catatonia
B. Could cause respiratory complications in patients who previously received IM lorazepam (Ativan)
C. Could worsen delirium
D. Could cause cardiac complications due to QTc prolongation
E. Could cause allergic reactions

Answer: C

Antipsychotics are unlikely to worsen delirium, although there is questionable evidence if they actually improve delirium, despite being commonly used in its treatment. Using IM olanzapine (Zyprexa) in combination with IM lorazepam (Ativan), however, can cause respiratory complications. Most antipsychotics can cause QTc prolongation to some degree, which can be particularly hazardous when combined with other QTc-prolonging drugs or in patients with hereditary prolonged QT Syndrome. On initial presentation, the symptoms of hyperactive catatonia are very similar to those of agitation due to psychosis, and use of high-potency antipsychotics can worsen catatonia. Without a thorough history, clinicians are not aware of the patient's previous allergies and the risk of provoking an unknown allergic reaction must be weighed against the benefits of managing severe and acute agitation.

References

1. Cristancho, MA, Cristancho, P, O'Reardon, JP. Other therapeutic psychiatric uses of superficial brain stimulation. *Handb Clin Neurol* 2013; 116:415–22

2. Ellul, P, Choucha, W. Neurobiological approach of catatonia and treatment perspectives. *Front Psychiatry* 2015; 6:182

3. Grisaru, N, Chudakov, B, Yaroslavsky, Y, et al. Catatonia treated with transcranial magnetic stimulation. *Am J Psychiatry* 1998; 155:1630

4. McKeown, NJ, Bryan, JH, Horowitz, BZ. Catatonia associated with initiating paliperidone treatment. *West J Emerg Med* 2010; 11:186–8

5. Pelzer, AC, van der Heijden, FM, den Boer, E. Systematic review of catatonia treatment. *Neuropsychiatr Dis Treat* 2018; 14:317–26

6. Penland, HR, Weder, N, Tampi, RR. The catatonic dilemma expanded. *Ann Gen Psychiatry* 2006; 5:14

7. Rasmussen, SA, Mazurek, MF, Rosebush, PI. Catatonia: our current understanding of its diagnosis, treatment and pathophysiology. *World J Psychiatry* 2016; 6:391–8

8. Sienaert, P, Dhossche, DM, Vancampfort, D, et al. A clinical review of the treatment of catatonia. *Front Psychiatry* 2014; 5:181

9. Stahl, SM. *Stahl's Essential Psychopharmacology: Neuroscientific Basis and Practical Applications*, 4. Cambridge: Cambridge University Press, 2015

10. Stahl, SM. *Stahl's Essential Psychopharmacology: Neuroscientific Basis and Practical Applications*, 6. Cambridge: Cambridge University Press, 2018

11. Stip, E, Blain-Juste, ME, Farmer, O, et al. Catatonia with schizophrenia: from ECT to rTMS. *Encephale* 2018; 44:183–7

Case 5: Caring for the whole person

The Question: Are medications effective in dissociative identity disorder (DID)?

The Psychopharmacological Dilemma: Is poor response due to medication non-compliance, misdiagnosis, or a condition not treatable with medication?

Nekpen Sharon Ekure

Pretest self-assessment question

Which of the following medications is FDA-approved for dissociative identity disorder (DID)?

A. Risperidone (Risperdal)
B. Aripiprazole (Abilify)
C. Divalproex (Depakote)
D. Fluoxetine (Prozac)
E. Both A and B
F. None of the above

Patient evaluation on intake

- A 48-year-old woman seen in outpatient setting for major depressive disorder (MDD) with recurrent suicidal ideation
- Recent inpatient hospitalization one week prior for self-harming behavior (cutting) and suicidal thinking
- Treated with electroconvulsive therapy (ECT) and discharged on a mood stabilizer, lamotrigine (Lamictal), and a tricyclic antidepressant (TCA), amitriptyline (Elavil)
- Now reports mild depressive symptoms: depressed mood, anhedonia, poor concentration, guilt feelings, and chronic passive suicide thinking without intent or plan to hurt self, despite the upcoming anniversary of the death of her mother
- Fixated upon the idea that she was lied to by her family regarding the circumstances surrounding her mother's death
- Moderate generalized anxiety disorder (GAD) symptoms have been comorbid with her MDD
- Mild post-traumatic stress disorder (PTSD) symptoms that are also comorbid
- Will also have occasional panic attacks that seem adjustment-based and related to social or stressful circumstances
- Frustrated that medications have not been helpful so far
- Frankly appears unwilling to consider any treatment recommendation at times

Psychiatric history

- PTSD, borderline personality disorder (BPD), bipolar disorder (BP), and learning disability (LD) were some of the several psychiatric diagnoses discussed with the patient
- The first contact with mental health providers dated to her preteen years when she had behavioral issues that made her parents send her off to a long-term residential treatment center
- Diagnosed with DID at the center
- Psychiatrically hospitalized at least 50 times since
- Several previous suicide attempts, one of which was by overdose on acetaminophen (Tylenol) and carbamazepine (Equetro)
- Has taken many psychotropic medications with no sustainable responses
- Some response in early antidepressant trials; however, effects wore off quickly
- Similar response with antipsychotics and mood stabilizers, unfortunately

Social and personal history

- The patient is the middle of three children with a history of sexual abuse by her uncle
- Unable to complete high school due to LD
- Strained relationship with siblings
- Obtained her GED certificate and worked in retail businesses for a brief period. However, she has been predominantly unemployed in the past two decades
- Currently on disability and lives in supportive housing
- Never married and has no children
- Has had romantic relationships, some of which were emotionally and verbally abusive
- Denies alcohol or recreational drug use

Medical history

- Hypertension, prediabetes, hyperlipidemia, vertigo, sleep apnea
- ECT treatment was halted due to pericardial effusion during one of the inpatient hospitalizations
- Surgeries – cholecystectomy

Family history

- Significant for maternal aunt with MDD, sister with self-harming behavior, and paternal relative with alcohol use disorder (AUD)
- Family history of suicide attempts in a cousin

Medication history

- Medication trials include but not limited to
  - Antipsychotics: clozapine (Clozaril), quetiapine (Seroquel), aripiprazole (Abilify), olanzapine (Zyprexa), perphenazine (Trilafon), lurasidone (Latuda)
  - Antidepressants: amitriptyline (Elavil), sertraline (Zoloft), paroxetine (Paxil), fluoxetine (Prozac), venlafaxine (Effexor XR), duloxetine (Cymbalta)
  - Mood stabilizers: lithium (Eskalith), divalproex (Depakote), lamotrigine (Lamictal)
- History of non-compliance with many of these medications
- Hydroxyzine (Vistaril) was prescribed at the last outpatient visit for anxiety and insomnia; refused to take, and accused the provider of "setting her up" for suicide by giving her so many pills at once
  - Hydroxyzine (Vistaril), as needed for anxiety and sleep, re-started after therapeutic intervention and safety planning
- Sertraline (Zoloft) was started again on the last inpatient admission and continued at outpatient follow-up for a short period
- Inpatient ECT was partially effective after several treatments at lowering MDD and suicidal thinking. Unfortunately, she chose to discontinue outpatient maintenance ECT due to a previous cardiovascular complication which had resolved without issue

Current medications

- Sertraline (Zoloft) 100 mg/d, a selective serotonin reuptake inhibitor (SSRI) antidepressant
- Prazosin (Minipress) 2 mg nightly, an α-1 receptor agonist used to treat nightmares or insomnia
- Melatonin 5 mg nightly, an MT1/MT2 receptor agonist

Psychotherapy history

- Individual supportive outpatient psychotherapy once monthly
- Benefited previously from group therapy in an inpatient setting during her stay in long-term treatment centers
- Has not had a bona fide course of dialectical behavioral therapy (DBT), nor psychodynamic psychotherapy (PDP)

Patient evaluation on the initial visit

- Endorses sleep disturbance with difficulty initiating and maintaining sleep
- Has recurrent nightmares that interfere with sleep
  - Mood is frequently depressed with situational anxiety, and especially with reminders of traumatic experience
  - Avoids places and events that remind her of abuser or trauma
- Harbors recurrent thoughts of dying or wishing to be dead with occasional self-harm behavior by cutting
- Frequently has inappropriate giggles with isolation of affect
- She perseverates on the loss of her family members, which usually triggers low mood and suicidal ideation
- Vehemently denies auditory or visual hallucinations or any psychotic symptoms
- There is no history of sustained (hypo)mania
- Previously reports having "eight persons in her head"; however, in recent encounters, identifies only three "Alters" aged 6, 11, and 13
  - 6-year-old thinks "she did something bad"
  - 11-year-old is "shy and does not talk much"
  - 13-year-old is the one that "constantly wishes to die"
- It is unclear whether she loses time when in an altered state as she frequently responds with "I don't know"
- Family members think she is "weird" – will rarely have contact with her only brother in the city
- Other providers have noticed that her affect is incongruent with her speech with constant giggles
- Symptoms of BPD include affective and emotional instability, recurrent suicidal ideation, unstable sense of self, a pattern of unstable and intense interpersonal relationships marked by switching between extremes of idealization and devaluation, chronic feelings of emptiness, as well as frequent outbursts of rage

Question

Do you think the patient's non-response to treatment (medications and ECT) could be due to misdiagnosis?

- Possibly, but it seems there has been a solid ruling in support of a BP and schizophrenia (SP) spectrum disorder, and no addictive issues have been noted

- Unlikely, as she seems to have comorbid MDD, PTSD, GAD, BPD, and has a traumatic upbringing, making her prognosis and response to medications poor overall
- No, she has DID, and there are no FDA-approved medications to help this condition

Attending physician's mental notes: initial evaluation

- The patient seems to have DID, but this could be due to dissociation from BPD
- Unfortunately, has MDD, PTSD, G and GAD, too
- Thankfully, there are no addiction-related symptoms
- She has a poor support system in place
- Psychotropic medications often are used secondarily to intensive psychotherapy protocols for DID. However, they can play a role in reducing anxiety, depressive symptoms, and stabilization of mood lability using a target symptom approach
- There are reports of success in small clinical trials with SSRIs, TCAs, and monoamine oxidase inhibitor (MAOI) antidepressants in addition to antihypertensives ($\beta_{1/2}$ receptor antagonists, α_2 receptor agonists, anticonvulsant mood stabilizers, and benzodiazepines [BZs]) in reducing hyperarousal, intrusive symptoms, and anxiety in patients with DID
- Clinical research suggests nightmares may respond to prazosin (Minipress), a norepinephrine α_1 receptor antagonist which is approved to lower blood pressure
- ECT for some patients can be helpful to alleviate refractory mood disorders without worsening dissociative memory issues
- Unfortunately, the patient is relatively non-compliant with care

Further investigation

Is there anything else that you would like to know about the patient?

- Has psychological or other testing been completed with this patient?
- What are her most troubling symptoms, in her opinion?

Question

What would be the next most appropriate course of action?

- Stop all medications and re-evaluate her symptoms over several days or weeks to delineate her diagnosis better with an extended drug-free evaluation period
- Titrate sertraline (Zoloft) upward

- Try to continue ECT
- Add a mood stabilizer
- Refer for intensive psychotherapy recommended for BPD
- Refer for specialized integrative therapy for DID

Case outcome: first interim follow-up visits through 4 weeks

- Sertraline (Zoloft) was increased to 75 mg/d to improve mood and anxiety symptoms
- Melatonin 5 mg at bedtime for sleep continued
- Hydroxyzine (Vistaril) 75 mg/d as needed for anxiety exacerbation was increased
- Goal is to maximize current medications before adding even more medications
  - Must try to avoid irrational polypharmacy
- ECT was not re-started per the patient's choice
- Attempted to refer for specific psychotherapy
- Symptoms continued to be poorly controlled

Attending physician's mental notes: first interim follow-up visits through 4 weeks

- Likely to be an uphill battle clinically
- Try to motivate for psychotherapy as a critical initiative specifically for her ongoing symptoms and her medication non-compliance in the past
- Escalate and use the safest medications given her lethality and self-injury patterns would be ideal

Case outcome: 1 month through 4 months

- The patient presented to emergency room for a severe headache and elevated blood pressure
  - Discharged same day with negative medical work-up
- Continued on sertraline (Zoloft) and hydroxyzine (Vistaril)
  - Voiced ambivalence about continuing sertraline (Zoloft) as she thought it was responsible for her medical issues
- Sleep disturbance is still her major concern
- The patient stopped her melatonin as she felt it was ineffective for her insomnia
- No psychological testing is done in the period of working with her because she was unavailable with frequent emergency room visits and inpatient hospitalizations
  - This would have been helpful to delineate whether any psychotic processes are underlying her symptoms

Question

What else can be done to increase compliance?

- Prescribe medications as patient wishes, regardless of indication or side-effect burden
- Minimize medications used and refer for psychotherapy
- Use motivational techniques to work with the patient directly on compliance

Case outcome: interim follow-up visit at 4 months

- No-showed for a previously scheduled visit because she was hospitalized on an inpatient unit for suicidal ideation for 3 days
- She thought she was a "burden to society, not contributing meaningfully"
- Sertraline (Zoloft) increased to 100 mg/d for depressive symptoms that included depressed mood, anhedonia, guilt related to feelings of inadequacy, poor concentration, sleep disturbance, and recurrent suicidal ideation
- She refused to acknowledge any benefit from sertraline (Zoloft); however, willing to continue with upward titration

Question

What would you do next?

- Continue to titrate sertraline (Zoloft) upward despite no reported response
- Combine now with a sedating antidepressant such as mirtazapine (Remeron) to target sleep disturbance and residual depressive symptoms
- Stop all medications and focus on psychotherapy
- Re-evaluate diagnoses

Further investigation

Is there anything else that you would like to know about the patient?

- Was she screened for BPD?
  - Yes, the patient's symptoms suggestive of BPD are emotional instability, affective lability, recurrent suicidal ideation, a sense of self that is unstable, including a pattern of intense interpersonal relationships typically characterized by switching between extremes of idealization and devaluation, chronic feelings of emptiness, and frequent displays of temper

- Does she meet formal criteria for DID?
  - Yes, having presented with at least three personality states / identities accompanied by changes in behavior, memory, and thinking observed by others and reported by the patient. These are not part of her culture or religious practices and have interfered with two areas of functioning – the ability to relate to others and to hold a consistent job
  - These do not appear to be psychotic in nature
- Does she meet criteria for PTSD?
  - Yes, she has a history of sexual abuse in childhood with ongoing associated intrusion symptoms (dissociative reactions outside of her alters and marked physiological reactions to internal and external cues that symbolize or resemble the traumatic event), avoidance (avoidance of external reminders, e.g., people, places, etc.), altered mood (persistent negative emotional state and ongoing and exaggerated negative beliefs about herself), altered reactivity (sleep disturbance, problems concentrating, reckless or self-destructive behavior), all lasting more than 1 month and causing clinically significant distress

Attending physician's mental notes: follow-up visit (month 4)

- Diagnosis is confusing and likely multifactorial
- Patient may not be able to care for self
- Medication non-compliance likely thwarting our outcome as well

Case outcome: interim follow-up visit at 5 and 6 months

- The patient requested a long-term inpatient hospitalization as symptoms of depression persisted
- Worked with a case manager and her local housing agency to get on a wait-list for a long-term inpatient admission
- Taking sertraline (Zoloft); however, unsure if she is taking it as prescribed
- Takes hydroxyzine (Vistaril) for anxiety only occasionally because of complaint that it makes her "tired all day"
- The patient became suicidal and was acutely hospitalized again
- Sertraline (Zoloft) was switched to another SSRI, fluoxetine (Prozac), during inpatient hospitalization, at her request
- Hydroxyzine (Vistaril) was continued

Attending physician's mental notes: interim follow-up (month 6)

- Only apparent pattern is that she will have reasons to discontinue both medications
- It may be ideal to transfer her from an acute psychiatric inpatient setting to the longer-term option that was being arranged prior

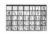

Case outcome: follow-up at 9 months

- Requested to discontinue fluoxetine (Prozac) with complaints of "feeling agitated and not sleeping"
- Re-started on sertraline (Zoloft) at her request
- Improved enough to leave the psychiatric hospital
- Missed her 8-month appointment (4 weeks post-discharge), presented to emergency room for agitation
  - Complained of "having weird thoughts like her mother is not really dead, faked her death to get away from her because she is a burden"
  - Discharged but presented again 2 days later
- This time she was admitted with complaints of "racing thoughts, paranoia and thoughts of harming herself"
  - Discharged after 3 days' stay on prazosin (Minipress) and now an atypical antipsychotic, lurasidone (Latuda)
- Didn't like taking lurasidone (Latuda) 40 mg/d, requested to be off it despite some mood improvement
- She was re-started on sertraline (Zoloft), and prazosin (Minipress) was continued for nightmares per her request

Attending physician's mental notes: interim follow-up (month 9)

- Only apparent pattern is that she will have reasons to discontinue her medications, likely driven by psychotic thought processes and denial
- Need to try for a longer-term inpatient option because attempts to increase rapport, case management, and other ambulatory options are clearly failing

Case outcome: follow-up through 12 months

- Still taking sertraline (Zoloft) and prazosin (Minipress)
- Continued with monthly supportive therapy
- The patient declined DBT skills group referral because she "has tried it in the past" and possibly could not utilize it well due to LD
- Signed a release to try to join an independent living program

Case debrief

- Dissociative symptoms, a hallmark of PTSD, can be very disabling and challenging to treat
- This case was challenging because there are currently no precise existing data or comprehensive guidelines on pharmacological management of DID or dissociation in general
- Regarding BPD, the clinicians involved tried to work with atypical antipsychotics, mood stabilizers, and antidepressants, all of which have shown some effectiveness with different target symptoms of BPD
- However, in this case, non-adherence to both psychotherapy and medication treatment recommendations played a key role in her recurrent relapses and decompensations
- It is difficult to determine whether all of the patient's medications were ineffective as she did not give a good amount of them a full therapeutic trial as far as dosing and duration of drug treatment are concerned
- BPD may have contributed a great deal to her splitting transference with providers, frequent emergency room presentations, and self-harming behavior
- Dynamically, she would probably have done well with highly structured psychotherapy for the development of mature defenses or an integrated, dependable, and positively valued sense of self
- Unfortunately, she reported that she could only afford her 30 minutes of supportive therapy monthly
- Her situation was not helped by frequent changes of providers within the clinic because of her splitting and disruptions due to inpatient hospital stays
  - She could not connect easily with providers as such
  - She would often feel that "no one listens" to her, and she mistrusts almost everyone

Take-home points

- Wow, this was tough
- Poor medication adherence detracts from the number of days on drug
- Improving therapeutic alliance can be tried
- Improving a team-based approach with peer mentoring, case management, etc., can be tried
- Despite best efforts, patients with severe and persisting psychotic-level disorders can repeat this poor adherence and compliance pattern for months to years
- Unfortunately, longer-term psychiatric stays are harder to obtain

Performance in practice: confessions of a psychopharmacologist

What could have been done better here?

- Wait for full psychological testing battery to be completed
  - ○ Probably will not have changed the outcome or made any difference in her behavior in the short term
  - ○ It would help to delineate better whether there is a psychotic process behind her MDD, BPD, DID, to help focus treatment if psychosis present
- Use outpatient ECT for maintenance
  - ○ Likely to improve mood and affective lability as she was thought to be a sustained partial responder while undergoing this treatment
- Obtain pharmacogenomic testing
  - ○ Evidence to support this is not overwhelmingly compelling
  - ○ However, it could have provided clarity regarding medications that could potentially be effective for her while avoiding adverse effects, which had hurt compliance in some situations
  - ○ Despite lacking evidence, sometimes testing can yield increase in medication adherence as a clear reason for choosing and using a medication is assigned, which can increase rapport and confidence in the prescriber
- Reassess her diagnoses earlier in treatment and focus more on safety and establishing therapeutic alliance rather than medication provision
- Referred earlier for DBT or CBT and reinforced this need for her regarding her overall treatment regimen

Tips and pearls

- If you can gain some medication adherence:
  - ○ Try using once-a-day medication as this approach is easier for patients to remember and tolerate
  - ○ Try to use a single medication and, if you have to use multiple medications, try to dose all at the same time of the day
  - ○ Try to use medications with longer half-lives because if the patients tend to miss some doses, it is more likely that some medication will remain in their system between doses

Two-minute tutorial

Biopsychosocial causes of DID and treatment options

- Like other mental health disorders, DID is diagnosed based on DSM-5 criteria, requiring an understanding of the biopsychosocial elements obtained on the psychiatric interview
  - The etiopathology of DID is poorly understood
  - The validity of its diagnosis is questioned because of the lack of reliable diagnostic tools
  - Relies solely on history-taking and the patient's subjective report
- Several clinical studies highlight the neuroanatomical basis of DID, with evidence that patients and healthy controls can potentially be discriminated using patterns of neuroimaging biomarkers
- Some research uses machine learning to distinguish between individuals with DID and healthy control subjects based on their brain morphology, as there seems to be marked differences in the gray and white matter brain on MRI
  - Connectivity studies suggest greater amygdala functional connectivity (synchronization) with prefrontal regions involved in emotion regulation, including the middle and medial frontal gyrus as well as the default mode network, among PTSD individuals with dissociative symptoms
- DID is defined in the fifth edition of the DSM-5 as an identity disruption indicated by the presence of two or more distinct personality states (experienced as possession in some cultures), with discontinuity in the sense of self and agency, and with variations in affect, behavior, consciousness, memory, perception, cognition, or sensory-motor functioning
- It is considered the most severe form of dissociative disorder and of childhood-onset PTSD
- Exposure to trauma is reported to be a common cause of DID, especially when the trauma is severe, chronic, or occurring during critical periods of brain development, when emotional systems are susceptible to a stressful experience
- Dissociative phenomena are considered to be psychological events related to defense mechanisms in managing anxiety related to psychological trauma
- Dissociation has been recognized as a moderator of poorer outcomes for PTSD patients and perhaps this may be extrapolated to DID

- There is sometimes a clinical temptation to use antipsychotic medications for dissociative symptoms as they can appear hallucinatory or delusional in nature
  - Dissociation could reflect a breakdown in reality testing
  - However, we are aware of no formal studies examining the potential efficacy of antipsychotic drugs for dissociative symptoms (or, for that matter, derealization or depersonalization), but in practice they do not often alleviate these symptoms
- Noradrenergic dampening, opioid dampening, and serotonin elevating agents have been studied in small, uncontrolled trials
- Perhaps use of PTSD approaches are most warranted, given their association with dissociative symptoms

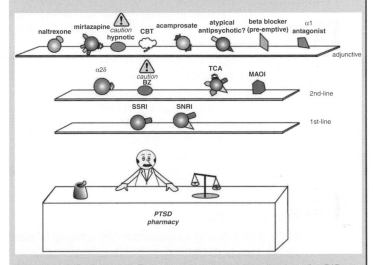

Figure 5.1 DID pharmacy. There are no approved medications for DID, but much of DID's psychogenesis may be created from trauma or neglect. First-line pharmacological options likely are still the selective serotonin reuptake inhibitors (SSRIs) and serotonin–norepinephrine reuptake inhibitors (SNRIs). We suspect that, similar to PTSD, the BZs may not be as helpful. BZs have been shown to worsen dissociation. Perhaps they may be considered with caution as a second- or third-line option. Other second-line treatments include $\alpha_2\delta$ ligands (gabapentin or pregabalin), TCAs, and MAOIs. Several medications may be used as adjuncts for residual symptoms. The atypical antipsychotics can not only treat psychosis, but lower agitation, improve mood, etc., and can be considered a broad-spectrum treatment approach for some, especially if the dissociative symptoms have a more psychotic feel to them after clinical assessment

Rating scales in action moment

- Throughout this case, there has been debate regarding this patient's diagnosis
  - Schizophrenia vs. PTSD vs. BPD vs. DID
- It was suggested at one point that intensive psychological testing with an expert, using methods such as the Thematic Apperception Test or the Rorschach test might help delineate psychosis from the other diagnoses
- Clearly, if this patient was felt to be psychotic instead of dissociative, there may have been a greater drive to use atypical antipsychotics and their long-acting injectables (LAIs) to improve psychotic symptoms and medication compliance
- Another area of concern is the validity of a patient with purported DID in self-reporting about his/her alters. If these symptoms are not psychotic in nature, are they volitional, fabricated, or embellished by the patient, or clearly dissociative?
  - This may occur in BPD patients who are using splitting defenses spread across multiple providers either to obtain the sick role or secondary gain perhaps of acquiring a disability, or to create stress across providers who are trying to help, thus perpetuating feelings that no one can, in fact, help them, or that people will ultimately leave and abandon them (projective identification)
- The Test of Memory Malingering is a bedside test that does not require a psychologist's referral for specific testing but is proprietary and must be purchased for use

Post-test question

Which of the following medications is FDA-approved for dissociative identity disorder (DID)?

A. Risperidone (Risperdal)
B. Aripiprazole (Abilify)
C. Divalproex (Depakote)
D. Fluoxetine (Prozac)
E. Both A and B
F. None of the above

Answer: F

Unfortunately, there are no FDA-approved medications for DID. A literature review suggests that the medications with the greatest effectiveness are paroxetine (Paxil) and naloxone (Narcan). They were found to have modest evidence for controlling depersonalization and dissociative symptoms. However, it is recommended that initial treatment focus be on safety issues, symptom stabilization, and establishment of a therapeutic alliance.

References

1. Blihar, D, Delgado, E, Buryak, M, et al. A systematic review of the neuroanatomy of dissociative identity disorder. *Eur J Trauma Dissociation* 2020; 4:100148

2. Brand, BL, Sar, V, Stavropoulos, P, et al. Separating fact from fiction: an empirical examination of six myths about dissociative identity disorder. *Harv Rev Psychiatry* 2016; 24:257–70

3. Brand, BL, Webermann, AR, Snyder, BL, et al. Detecting clinical and simulated dissociative identity disorder with the Test of Memory Malingering. *Psychol Trauma* 2019; 11:513–20

4. Kalin, NH. Trauma, resilience, anxiety disorders, and PTSD. *Am J Psychiatry* 2021; 178:103–5

5. Lebois, LAM, Li, M, Baker, JT, et al. Large-scale functional brain network architecture changes associated with trauma-related dissociation. *Am J Psychiatry* 2021; 178:165–73

6. Menon, V. Dissociation by network integration. *Am J Psychiatry* 2021; 178:110–12

7. Reinders, A, Marquand, AF, Schlumpf, YR, et al. Aiding the diagnosis of dissociative identity disorder: pattern recognition study of brain biomarkers. *Br J Psychiatry* 2019; 215:536–44

8. Sadock, B, Sadock, V, Ruiz, P. *Synopsis of Psychiatry: Behavioral Sciences/Clinical Psychiatry*. Philadelphia: Lippincott Williams & Wilkins, 2015

9. Stahl, SM. *Stahl's Essential Psychopharmacology: Neuroscientific Basis and Practical Applications*, 5. Cambridge: Cambridge University Press, 2021

10. Sutar, R, Sahu, S. Pharmacotherapy for dissociative disorders: a systematic review. *Psychiatry Res* 2019; 281:112529

Case 6: The man whom clozapine (Clozaril) could not touch

The Question: How do you treat psychosis when increasing the clozapine (Clozaril) dose does not seem to be significantly affecting the plasma level?

The Psychopharmacological Dilemma: Super-dose clozapine (Clozaril) or add other agents?

Rebecca Shields

Pretest self-assessment question

Which of the following is true regarding clozapine (Clozaril) dosing?

A. Start at 12.5 – 25 mg/d
B. Increase by 25 – 50 mg each day as tolerated
C. Usual dosing is 300 – 400 mg/d and FDA maximum dose is 900 mg/d
D. Usual therapeutic plasma clozapine (Clozaril) level is 350 – 1000 ng/mL
E. A, B, and C are true
F. All of the above are true

Patient evaluation on intake (inpatient unit)

- A 27-year-old man, brought in by mother, for reported auditory and visual hallucinations, delusions, and aggressive behavior
- Admitted now to inpatient unit
- According to the patient, "Mom brought me in because I cut my arm on the counter top at home"
- Patient presented as restless
- Denied any suicidal ideation, homicidal ideation, or auditory or visual hallucinations, and did not appear manic
- Patient also stated "medications are destroying my brain" and asked to leave the hospital because he was afraid the medications would "likely kill him"

Psychiatric history

- Diagnosed with schizophrenia at 17 years old
- Now carries a diagnosis of schizoaffective disorder. Unclear whether he has had a true manic episode or a major depressive episode (MDE) in the past as patient and family are poor historians
- Has had multiple psychiatric hospitalizations, including three at 19 years old

- Symptoms fairly consistent throughout the years with religious delusions, auditory hallucinations, intermittent and unpredictable aggression, disorganized speech, disorganized behavior, and negative symptoms including decreased emotional expression, avolition, and monotone voice
- No prior suicide attempts or self-injurious behaviors
- Opposed to medication use and keeping medication outpatient visits overall, with remarkable history of medication non-compliance with subsequent psychotic relapse

Social and personal history

- Graduated high school
- Never employed, on social security income
- Lives at home with mother and two sisters
- No known legal or arrest history
- Smokes 1.5 packs of cigarettes daily
- Denies alcohol use
- Has a remote history of trying cannabis, none currently

Medical history

- Hashimoto's Disease but is euthyroid
- History of recurrent sinus infections
- Tardive dyskinesia (TD) reported in past, none currently

Family history

- Sister has schizophrenia (SP) and intellectual disability (ID)
- Uncle completed suicide
- Grandmother had a "nervous breakdown" and was hospitalized
- Mother has some undiagnosed mental illness with evidence of disorganized behavior

Medication history

- Past medications include olanzapine (Zyprexa), fluphenazine (Prolixin), risperidone (Risperdal), aripiprazole (Abilify), ziprasidone (Geodon), lithium (Eskalith), clonazepam (Klonopin)
- Has a history of medication non-compliance, but reported compliance after admission usually, and during hospitalizations

Current medications

- Fluphenazine (Prolixin) 40 mg/d, a typical antipsychotic
- Olanzapine (Zyprexa) 10 mg/d, an atypical antipsychotic
- Lithium (Eskalith) 1200 mg/d, a mood stabilizer
- Clonazepam (Klonopin) 0.25 mg as needed for agitation, a benzodiazepine (BZ) sedative anxiolytic
- Levothyroxine (Synthroid) 25 mcg/d for hypothyroidism

Psychotherapy history

- Bi-weekly supportive psychotherapy and case management

Patient evaluation on initial visit

- Psychosis is worsening and reaching levels that are concerning
- This seems typical of previous non-adherence-induced relapses of his schizophrenia
- He is likely on no medications at this point
- Poor insight but fair family support
- Worsening aggression, paranoid delusions with religious preoccupation, and responding to unseen and unheard stimuli
  - Talked about hearing the "voice of God," including directing him to "kill the family"
  - In explanation of violence to others, he would say that "God told me to do it"

Question

In your clinical experience, what is more effective, antipsychotic polypharmacy, antipsychotic sequential monotherapies, superdosing of a monotherapy, etc. ... ?

- Polypharmacy with two atypical antipsychotics
- Polypharmacy with an atypical plus a typical one
- Successive monotherapies
- Superdosing of a monotherapy

Attending physician's mental notes: initial psychiatric evaluation

- This patient has severe and persistent recurrent psychotic disorder, most likely schizophrenia as can find no sustained manla events nor depressive episodes, so will issue the working diagnosis of schizophrenia
- He has paranoid, disorganized, and negative symptoms predominantly

- His paranoia, hallucinations, and disorganization lead him to be at high risk of violence toward others, unfortunately. He will need ongoing inpatient care
- If off medications, may need to restart them to regain effectiveness
- If on medications, need to consider the current regimen as ineffective and try something new

Question

Which of the following would be your next step?

- Confirm whether he has in fact been taking the medications, either by family report or by drawing blood levels
- Abandon current medications as they have failed
- Raise the dose of his typical antipsychotic
- Raise the dose of his atypical antipsychotic
- Start a new antipsychotic monotherapy
- Start a new polypharmacy combination

Further investigation

Is there anything else that you would like to know about the patient?

- Does he have a history of hurting others when he is psychotic like this?
  - Luckily, so far he has never acted on his command hallucinations
- Does he have access to firearms?
  - No
- When he has been committed in the past, has he taken medications or needed a court order to be treated?
  - No, he typically will take medications when asked in the hospital

Case outcome: inpatient days 1 through 7

- Becoming more paranoid and agitated
- Punched a nurse in the chest, stating that "God told me to"
  - Received haloperidol (Haldol) 5 mg orally, lorazepam (Ativan) 2 mg orally, and diphenhydramine (Benadryl) 50 mg orally for agitation with good effect on re-evaluation 30 minutes later
- Restarted on usual outpatient psychiatric medications as it was confirmed he had not been taking them
  - Olanzapine (Zyprexa) 10 mg/d, fluphenazine (Prolixin) 40 mg/d, lithium (Eskalith) 1200 mg/d, and clonazepam (Klonopin) 0.25 mg/d prn

- However, fluphenazine (Prolixin) was discontinued due to outpatient psychiatrist's report of increased aggression (possible akathisia) on it, and risperidone (Risperdal) 1 mg/d was started due to family report that it was "helpful for his anxiety" in the past

Attending physician mental notes: inpatient days 1 through 7

- Patient is continuing to display disorganized speech and behavior, with paranoia, hallucinations, and religious preoccupation
  - He has been aggressive while on the unit and remains a risk to others
- Usual medications do not seem to be helping, and addition of risperidone (Risperdal) low dose is not helping yet either
- Further review of outpatient records confirms that patient's psychotic symptoms have never been adequately controlled (possibly ever) on multiple trials of antipsychotics, neither monotherapy nor polypharmacy combinations

Question

What would you do next?

- Increase current medications to maximum tolerated safe dose
- Add another antipsychotic for better control of symptoms
- Switch to clozapine (Clozaril) with the goal of taking as a monotherapy

Case outcome: inpatient days 8 through 28

- The atypical antipsychotic clozapine (Clozaril) is started at 12.5 mg/d after reviewing the case and determining that the patient has been resistant to treatment on multiple previous antipsychotics
  - Tapered off risperidone (Risperdal) and olanzapine (Zyprexa)
  - Goal now is to see whether clozapine (Clozaril) monotherapy will be effective
- Lithium (Eskalith) is to be maintained for now and level is 0.75 mmol/L, felt to be low but reasonable as likely to be discontinued in favor of clozapine (Clozaril) monotherapy later in treatment course
- Clozapine (Clozaril) at 100 mg/d. Levels drawn as follows:
  - Clozapine quantitative: 180 ng/mL
- Blood monitoring for clozapine (Clozaril) needed
  - Baseline and weekly absolute neutrophil count (ANC) levels remain safe throughout the admission
  - Side effects
    - Complains of constipation and dry mouth, and that "medications destroyed his brain and voice"

- Continues to report having < 10 bowel movements a year, despite having regular bowel movements while on the unit
- X-ray abdomen on admission was benign
- Discharged home from hospital back to previous outpatient psychiatric team on day 28
  ○ Clozapine (Clozaril) 200 mg/d, lithium (Eskalith) 1200 mg/d as key interventions
  ○ Speech and behavior were more organized, he was less religiously preoccupied and paranoid, he was medication compliant, and attended some groups on the unit, and he is socially appropriate and no longer aggressive
    - He was felt to be safe and amenable to outpatient care, where ideally the rest of his symptoms will continue to resolve

Attending physician mental notes: inpatient days 8 through 28

- Seems to have had a clinically meaningful response as his religious preoccupations, aggression, and disorganized behaviors have decreased
- He is not complaining of new side effects, which is good
- He will likely require increased clozapine (Clozaril) dosing as he is improving but is not in remission yet
- Will need to monitor for impact of smoking cigarettes on clozapine (Clozaril) levels, as he is being discharged from the hospital and may resume smoking

Case outcome: first interim follow-up outpatient visit at 1 week

- Patient is smoking cigarettes again at one pack per day (PPD)
- Mother reports worsening psychosis, including religiously themed auditory hallucinations and delusions, intermittent agitation, and possible vocal and motor tics
- Patient denies drug or alcohol use
- Patient continues to report that "medications destroyed his brain and vocal cords," as well as giving him dry mouth, polydipsia, decreased cognition, and < 10 bowel movements a year
  ○ Had a bowel movement yesterday according to mother
- Clozapine (Clozaril) is increased from 200 mg/d to 250 mg/d for better control of psychosis

- Labs are ordered, including fasting blood glucose (FBG), complete blood count with differential (CBC w/diff), lipid panel, comprehensive metabolic panel (CMP), thyroid-stimulating hormone (TSH), hemoglobin A1c (HbA1c), lithium (Eskalith) level, and continued weekly ANC per risk evaluation and mitigation strategies (REMS) clozapine (Clozaril) protocol

Attending physician mental notes: first interim follow-up at 1 week

- Patient's symptoms appear worse than when he completed his stay in the hospital
  ○ May be due to smoking cigarettes again, which can lower clozapine (Clozaril) levels
- No new side effects reported
- Want to continue to titrate clozapine (Clozaril) to a therapeutic dose

Case outcome: interim follow-up visit at 1 month

- No noticeable change in symptoms from 1-week visit
  ○ Still religiously preoccupied, hearing voices, and intermittently agitated
  ○ Still smoking one PPD of cigarettes
  ○ Still reporting constipation, dry mouth, polydipsia, vocal cord issues, and decreased cognition
- Mother keeps a list of patient's medications and reports giving them to him as prescribed
- Clozapine (Clozaril) is increased from 250 mg/d to 300 mg/d, and then from 300 mg/d to 400 mg/d 2 weeks after
- Senna glycoside (Senna) is increased from 17.2 mg/d to 25.8 mg/d to help prevent constipation with increasing clozapine (Clozaril)
- Clozapine (Clozaril) levels are ordered

Attending physician mental notes: 1 month

- Patient's psychosis does not seem better with the increased clozapine (Clozaril) dose, but the side effects are also unchanged (not worsening)
  ○ Clozapine (Clozaril) dose in hospital was lower at 200 mg/d but seemed to have a greater effect
    ▪ May be due to cigarette smoking lowering plasma clozapine (Clozaril) levels
    ▪ Need to re-check clozapine (Clozaril) levels to compare to inpatient level on 200 mg
- Need to continue to increase clozapine (Clozaril) dose to a clinically therapeutic level, as long as patient continues to tolerate it

Case outcome: interim follow-up visit at 2 months

- Patient is more sociable and conversational, and tics are less pronounced
- He is still intermittently agitated in public and religiously preoccupied, stating that "Jesus and God started trouble at the mall one day"
- Patient continues to complain of the same side effects including constipation, dry mouth, polydipsia, vocal cord issues, and decreased cognition
- Clozapine (Clozaril) levels are reviewed from when dose was at 300 mg/d (previous levels while inpatient at 100 mg/d in parentheses)
  - Clozapine quantitative: 166 ng/mL (180 ng/mL)
- Clozapine is increased from 400 mg/d to 500 mg/d as clozapine (Clozaril) levels are lower now compared to when the patient was in the hospital on a lower dose of clozapine (Clozaril) (100 mg/d)

Question

Why are the patient's clozapine (Clozaril) levels lower now than when the patient was in the hospital, even with the dose increased from 100 mg/d to 300 mg/d?

- Patient is not taking his clozapine (Clozaril) as prescribed, while outpatient
- The patient started smoking cigarettes again which is causing clozapine levels to drop

Attending physician mental notes: 2 months

- Mother is reporting patient medication compliance and is able to show evidence of a medication administration log
- Patient is smoking at least one PPD of cigarettes, which he was not doing in the hospital
  - Cigarettes are likely interacting with clozapine via inducing CYP1A2, leading to decreased serum clozapine (Clozaril) by way of increased metabolic clearance now
  - Patient does not want to quit smoking and is refusing to take nicotine replacement therapy (NRT)
- Will continue to increase clozapine (Clozaril) dose as symptoms are starting to improve but are not well controlled yet

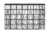

Case outcome: interim follow-up visit at 3 months

- No significant change in presentation compared to last visit
    ◦ Patient is somewhat conversational, but is still religiously preoccupied and intermittently aggressive
- Patient is now smoking 1.5 PPD of cigarettes
- Clozapine (Clozaril) is increased from 500 mg/d to 600 mg/d today, and then from 600 mg/d to 700 mg/d 2 weeks after
- Docusate (Colace) is started at 200 mg/d to help prevent constipation
- Recommend cutting back on smoking, but patient is not interested
    ◦ Patient is aware of risk for clozapine (Clozaril) toxicity if he were to stop smoking suddenly
- Repeat clozapine (Clozaril) levels are ordered

Attending physician mental notes: 3 months

- Patient likely is increasing the amount he is smoking, which may explain why the patient's presentation is remaining psychologically stable despite increased clozapine (Clozaril) dosing
- Patient is not complaining of any new side effects, so will continue to increase clozapine (Clozaril) as tolerated
- Patient is not at high risk for stopping smoking abruptly, which could cause clozapine toxicity, as he does not wish to quit at this time and has been educated about the risk

Case outcome: interim follow-up visit at 4 months

- No major improvement in symptoms or worsening of side effects apart from verbal and motor tics
- Is continuing to smoke and admits to 1.5 PPD of cigarettes
- Labs are reviewed (newest value to oldest from left to right)
    ◦ Clozapine quantitative: 128 ng/mL (166 ng/mL, 180 ng/mL)
    ◦ Li 0.99, TSH 1.76, T4 1.15, ANC 5.5, lipid panel within normal limits (WNL), HbA1c 4.9%, B12 and Vit D WNL
- Clozapine (Clozaril) is increased from 700 mg/d to 800 mg/d, and then from 800 mg/d to 900 mg/d 2 weeks after
- NRT (gum or inhalers) is prescribed to help patient cut down on smoking, as clozapine (Clozaril) levels are not increasing despite escalating doses
- Docusate (Colace) is increased from 200 mg/d to 400 mg/d

Attending physician mental notes: 4 months

- Patient is continuing to have significant psychotic symptoms with intermittent agitation despite escalating doses of clozapine (Clozaril)
- Lab work reveals that clozapine (Clozaril) levels are even lower than they had been in the hospital despite major increases in his daily dose
  - Likely due to cigarette use
  - As doses increase, there should be an increase in side effects
    - In the absence of this, it may suggest subtherapeutic dosing
- To increase plasma clozapine (Clozaril) levels, need to continue to increase clozapine (Clozaril) dose or help patient cut down on smoking
  - Encouraged patient to take NRT to cut down on smoking, but is unlikely he will take NRT as he does not want to quit smoking
  - Increasing clozapine (Clozaril) dose for better control of psychosis likely needed
  - Increasing docusate (Colace) for better control of constipation which can worsen with increasing the clozapine (Clozaril) dose

Case outcome: interim follow-up visit at 5 months

- Clozapine (Clozaril) dose currently at 900 mg/d
- Patient initially appears more calm and conversational during the session but is later heard yelling "F*** you" in the hallway before leaving to smoke more cigarettes
- Mother reports new onset nocturnal enuresis
  - Adult diapers are ordered
  - Nocturnal enuresis treatment is offered, but patient and mother refuse, stating he is already taking too many medications
- Recommend continuing with clozapine (Clozaril) 900 mg/d as it is now at the maximum FDA recommended dose despite the new-onset nocturnal enuresis
- Continue to recommend cutting back on smoking, while also warning about quitting altogether due to risk for clozapine (Clozaril) toxicity
  - NRT has been prescribed and patient is encouraged to try it
- EKG, Li level, CBC w/diff, ANC, CMP, TSH, T4, and plasma clozapine (Clozaril) levels are ordered again

Attending physician mental notes: 5 months

- Continue with clozapine (Clozaril) 900 mg/d instead of increasing the dose as the patient has new-onset nocturnal enuresis, needs a repeat EKG to evaluate for cardiomyopathy, and needs repeat plasma clozapine (Clozaril) level
- Cutting down on smoking would be ideal so clozapine (Clozaril) dose could be lowered. However, patient has not been able to decrease smoking yet. Will continue to encourage for now

Case outcome: interim follow-up visit at 6 months

- Patient is more calm and conversational, perhaps indicating a partial response to clozapine (Clozaril)
  - Lab technician and therapist both report that patient is less agitated during lab draws
- Mother is still skeptical of treatment with medications and says that the patient is "worse than ever." She inquires about inpatient hospitalization
- Patient continues to report dry mouth, constipation, decreased cognition, and nocturnal enuresis
- Labs are reviewed and listed below (newest value to oldest from left to right)
  - Clozapine quantitative: 234 ng/mL (128 ng/mL, 166 ng/mL, 180 ng/mL)
  - Li 0.75, CBC WNL, ANC 3.7, CMP WNL, TSH 3.69, T4 9.6
  - EKG non-actionable; QTc 447 (worth monitoring more often once 450–500 values noted)

Question

What would you do next?

- Superdose clozapine (Clozaril) as patient has a partial response to it so far
- Add another antipsychotic to see whether polypharmacy with clozapine (Clozaril) improves the response without making clozapine-specific side effects worse
- Start fluvoxamine (Luvox) as an adjuvant to help increase plasma clozapine (Clozaril) via known drug–drug interaction, without having to increase the clozapine (Clozaril) dose further
  - Has the potential to lower side effects such as metabolic issues or sedation
- Hospitalize patient so he can be more closely monitored during further medication changes

Attending physician mental notes: 6 months

- Could superdose clozapine (Clozaril) as clozapine (Clozaril) plasma level is still subtherapeutic at 234 ng/mL (< 350 ng/mL)
  - Could worsen side effects, which patient and mother are sensitive to
- Could add another antipsychotic, but he was trialed on different combinations of antipsychotics in the past without success
  - Has never tried clozapine (Clozaril) with another antipsychotic, so could be considered. However, adding another antipsychotic could increase risk for more side effects
- Hospitalizing patient is risky since he would not be allowed to smoke cigarettes, and his clozapine (Clozaril) levels could become toxic
  - This could also mean having to go through the long process of re-titrating once discharged again, but we know target oral doses now needed to gain therapeutic plasma levels
  - Would avoid hospitalization at this point unless patient is an imminent danger to self or others
- Adding fluvoxamine (Luvox), an SSRI, may increase plasma clozapine (Clozaril) levels
  - Fluvoxamine (Luvox) inhibits CYP1A2, whereas cigarettes induce CYP1A2, so fluvoxamine might help counter the negative effect of smoking on clozapine (Clozaril)

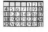

Case outcome: interim follow-up visit at 7 months

- Fluvoxamine (Luvox) 25 mg/d was started at the last visit
- Patient is more conversational, pleasant, and focused in session
  - Mother reports for first time that patient is helping out around the house, is able to concentrate better, is more conversational, is less agitated, and is behaving better outside the house
- For side effects, mother reports improvement in enuresis and constipation, but mildly worse sedation
- Labs are reviewed (newest value to oldest from left to right)
  - Clozapine quantitative: 524 ng/mL (234 ng/mL, 128 ng/mL, 166 ng/mL, 180 ng/mL)
  - CMP WNL, LFTs WNL, TSH 2.4, T4 9, Li 0.77, CBC WNL, ANC 3.5
  - No change in EKG
- Clozapine (Clozaril) is decreased from 900 mg/d to 800 mg/d as clozapine (Clozaril) level increased significantly with the addition of fluvoxamine and may continue to do so over the next couple of weeks

- Repeat clozapine (Clozaril) level is ordered to see whether the level continues to change with the lower dose of clozapine (Clozaril) and addition of fluvoxamine (Luvox)

Attending physician mental notes: 7 months

- The patient looks the best he ever has after the addition of fluvoxamine (Luvox)
  - Improvement may be due to increased clozapine (Clozaril) levels or, less likely, could be due to the effect of fluvoxamine (Luvox) on mood
- The clozapine (Clozaril) levels increased significantly, nearly doubling the quantitative value
  - Since selective serotonin reuptake inhibitors (SSRIs) take 4–6 weeks to clinically exert maximum effect in the brain, but pharmacokinetically should affect plasma level changes within a few days, wondered whether clozapine (Clozaril) levels would continue to rise
    - Decided to lower clozapine (Clozaril) dose to prevent clozapine (Clozaril) from reaching a toxic level
    - Will need to continue to monitor clozapine (Clozaril) levels
    - Lower clozapine (Clozaril) dose could decrease side effects, but also could decrease its efficacy

Case outcome: interim follow-up visit at 8 months

- Patient is clinically worse again with decreased ability to engage in conversation, poorer focus, and reports of worsening aggression and psychosis by mother
- Side effects are unchanged from the last visit with no noticeable improvement in nocturnal enuresis, constipation, or sedation
- Labs are reviewed (newest value to oldest from left to right)
  - Clozapine quantitative: 350 ng/mL (524 ng/mL, 234 ng/mL,128 ng/mL, 166 ng/mL, 180 ng/mL)
    - As seen above, clozapine (Clozaril) levels have decreased significantly with the change from 900 mg/d to 800 mg/d
- Repeat clozapine (Clozaril) levels are ordered to be done in 4 weeks
- Clozapine (Clozaril) is increased back up to 900 mg/d

Attending physician mental notes: 8 months

- Lowering the clozapine (Clozaril) dose from 900 mg/d to 800 mg/d lowered the plasma clozapine (Clozaril) levels significantly and seemed to have led to clinical worsening without improvement in side effects

- ◦ The effect of fluvoxamine (Luvox) on clozapine (Clozaril) level does not need 4–6 weeks to take its full effect, which is the difference between a clinical pharmacodynamic effect and its pharmacokinetic effects which are governed by its half-life
- Clozapine (Clozaril) is increased back up to 900 mg/d to see whether patient's symptoms improve again

Question

Is there anything else to consider in order to optimize this patient's care?

- Recheck clozapine (Clozaril) and eventually decrease to find lowest dose that is safe and effective
- Increase fluvoxamine (Luvox) while decreasing clozapine (Clozaril) and continuing to monitor levels
- Once stable, taper off of lithium (Eskalith) as it was ineffective
- Consider augmenting with electroconvulsive therapy (ECT) if still has residual psychosis
- Pharmacogenetic testing may be considered
- Use varenicline (Chantix) for smoking cessation, and, if successful, would need to lower fluvoxamine (Luvox) and clozapine (Clozaril) as clozapine (Clozaril) plasma levels would rise secondary to varenicline (Chantix) use

Case Debrief

- The patient was started on clozapine (Clozaril) as his psychotic symptoms were not well controlled by > 2 antipsychotics, despite adequate dosing and evidence of reasonable compliance while inpatient
- Serum clozapine (Clozaril) levels initially fell, despite increasing doses of clozapine (Clozaril), which was attributed to increasing cigarette use causing CYP450-1A2 induction while outpatient
- Over the course of 7 months, titrated clozapine (Clozaril) to maximum FDA dose of 900 mg/d with partial improvement, but no remission of symptoms
- Had to decide whether to continue to increase clozapine (Clozaril) past 900 mg/d, to add fluvoxamine (Luvox) to increase serum clozapine by a drug–drug interaction, to augment with aripiprazole (Abilify), or to augment with ECT
  - ◦ Although patient reached 900 mg/d of clozapine (Clozaril), the plasma level was still subtherapeutic at < 350 ng/mL. However, patient was already experiencing significant side effects from

the clozapine (Clozaril), including nocturnal enuresis, so did not want to increase it as sole agent

- ◦ Patient and family were suspicious of all psychiatric care, including medications, often stating that the medications may have caused his psychosis, so did not offer ECT option
- ◦ Adding aripiprazole (Abilify) or another antipsychotic seemed risky as may contribute to increased side effects, and without ever receiving a therapeutic dose (according to serum level) of clozapine (Clozaril)
- ◦ Fluvoxamine (Luvox) had the potential both to increase serum clozapine (Clozaril) and possibly to negate cigarette smoking effects on plasma levels
  - ▪ It increases the clozapine (Clozaril) to norclozapine ratio, which is thought to decrease side effects as norclozapine has more potent serotonin 5-HT_{2A} receptor antagonism which may lower EPS
  - ▪ However, it was also risky as it was not known how much it would increase the clozapine (Clozaril) plasma concentration by and could lead to clozapine (Clozaril) toxicity
- This patient received fluvoxamine (Luvox) 25 mg/d (where its usual dosing range is up to 300 mg/d) in addition to the clozapine (Clozaril) 900 mg/d, which increased serum clozapine (Clozaril) levels by over 200% after 3 weeks
  - ◦ Was associated with a marked improvement in positive symptoms
- Clozapine (Clozaril) was decreased from 900 mg/d to 800 mg/d to prevent further increase in serum clozapine (potential for toxicity) and to see whether the lower dose would have same control of symptoms with fewer side effects
  - ◦ Follow-up labs in 4 weeks showed significant decrease in serum clozapine again with an associated worsening of symptoms
- Clozapine (Clozaril) was increased back up to 900 mg/d, and fluvoxamine (Luvox) 25 mg/d was continued
  - ◦ Repeat plasma clozapine (Clozaril) lab was ordered
  - ◦ This regimen represented the "sweet spot" where adequate blood levels and symptom control seemed to occur
- Of note, patient had a case manager who would do home visits and would take the patient to the lab when needed. If he did not have this support, clozapine (Clozaril) would have been a poor choice for him

Take-home points

- Around 40% of patients with treatment-resistant schizophrenia do not have an adequate response to clozapine (Clozaril)
- Clozapine (Clozaril) non-response could be due to various factors, including cigarette smoking, genetics, non-compliance, medication interactions, or adverse effects
  - Tracking plasma clozapine (Clozaril) levels is a very useful practice and may be more beneficial than tracking the dose itself
- If patient is tolerating clozapine (Clozaril) titration, but serum clozapine (Clozaril) is still low despite being on a high dose:
  - Can add fluvoxamine (Luvox)
  - Can continue to titrate clozapine (Clozaril) as a monotherapy, or even past the maximum dose
  - Can actively treat tobacco use disorder (if present)
- If patient's serum clozapine levels are increasing appropriately, but the patient cannot tolerate increasing the dose further:
  - Can augment with ECT
  - Can augment with aripiprazole (Abilify), a different atypical antipsychotic, or a typical one
  - Can treat side effects to make clozapine (Clozaril) more tolerable, with subsequent dose increases as tolerated
- Beware of transition from inpatient to outpatient and vice versa, as it can dramatically affect the clozapine (Clozaril) levels due to no smoking being allowed while on inpatient units
  - Beware of pharmacokinetic interactions in general as they can both decrease and increase clozapine (Clozaril) levels. Example: cyprofloxacin inhibits CYP 1A2 and could lead to toxic levels of clozapine (Clozaril) if not careful
- Make sure patient has supports in place to be able to comply with taking the clozapine (Clozaril) daily, as well as getting regular blood draws (ANC monitoring)

Performance in practice: confessions of a psychopharmacologist

What could have been done better here?

- Could have more aggressively treated cigarette smoking with varenicline (Chantix) early on
  - Would monitor closely due to older varenicline (Chantix) warnings about possible neuropsychiatric effects including depression, agitation, and suicidality
    - Risks found to be minimal in subsequent FDA-mandated post-approval registries and studies

- Could have augmented with fluvoxamine (Luvox) or aripiprazole (Abilify) sooner, thereby potentially avoiding further side effects with equal or better efficacy
- Could have dosed clozapine (Clozaril) above 900 mg
- Could have pushed for treatment of side effects such as nocturnal enuresis, to make ongoing clozapine (Clozaril) use more likely
- Could have done pharmacogenomic testing to look at the patient's potential enzyme activity, such as CYP 1A2, and how he might have responded to clozapine (Clozaril) and other psychotropic medications

Tips and pearls

- What to try if clozapine (Clozaril) monotherapy fails and is at a therapeutic dose (plasma levels > 350 ng/mL)
  - Augment with electroconvulsive therapy (ECT)
    - Favored over augmenting with medication
  - Augment with an atypical antipsychotic
    - Limited evidence
    - Aripiprazole (Abilify) has been studied the most and may decrease hospitalizations
  - Add a typical antipsychotic
    - Limited evidence
  - Augment with divalproex (Depakote) or lithium (Eskalith)
    - Limited evidence
  - Augment with lamotrigine (Lamictal)
    - Limited evidence, but some support for its use
  - Augment with a BZ sedative anxiolytic
    - Limited evidence
  - Augment with an antidepressant
    - Limited evidence; may help with negative symptoms

Pharmacokinetic moment

How does adding fluvoxamine (Luvox) to clozapine (Clozaril) increase plasma clozapine (Clozaril) levels, while also having the theoretical potential to decrease side effects from clozapine (Clozaril)?

- Clozapine (Clozaril) is predominantly a substrate that is metabolized by the hepatic metabolism enzyme called CYP1A2
  - Fluvoxamine (Luvox) inhibits CYP1A2, leading to increased plasma clozapine (Clozaril) as it can no longer be catabolized normally via this hepatic metabolic pathway

- ○ Smoking (polycyclic hydrocarbons in cigarette or cannabis smoke) induces CYP1A2, leading to decreased serum clozapine (Clozaril) as clozapine (Clozaril) is metabolized faster
    - ▪ Studies suggest that those with at least one gene allele copy of CYP1A2*1F may be more likely to respond poorly to clozapine (Clozaril) therapy while smoking
  - ○ Ingesting the caffeine equivalent of three cups of coffee has been shown to inhibit 1A2 as well, leading to increased serum clozapine (Clozaril)
- Plasma norclozapine, not clozapine (Clozaril), levels are associated with metabolic effects such as weight gain
  - ○ Clozapine (Clozaril) is metabolized to norclozapine by CYP1A2
  - ○ Fluvoxamine (Luvox) is thought to improve the clozapine (Clozaril) to norclozapine ratio, thereby decreasing adverse effects while boosting clozapine (Clozaril) plasma levels for better therapeutic effects
    - ▪ In theory, a clozapine (Clozaril) to norclozapine ratio of > 2 is thought to minimize side effects while having the greatest clinical response

Two-minute tutorial

Hepatic CYP1A2 enzymes and genetic testing
CYP1A2

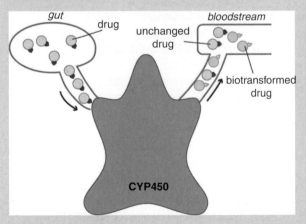

Figure 6.1 Cytochrome P450. The cytochrome P450 (CYP) enzyme system mediates how the body metabolizes many drugs, including antipsychotics such as clozapine (Clozaril). The CYP enzyme in the gut wall or liver converts the drug into a biotransformed product in the bloodstream. After passing through the gut wall and liver (left), the drug will exist partly as unchanged drug and partly as biotransformed drug (right).

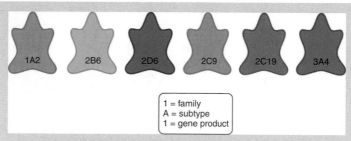

1 = family
A = subtype
1 = gene product

Figure 6.2 Five CYP enzymes. There are many cytochrome P450 (CYP) systems; these are classified according to family, subtype, and gene product. Five of the most important are shown here: CYP1A2, 2D6, 2C9, 2C19, and 3A4. This case focuses on the 1A2 subtype of hepatic enzyme, where the patient presents with either normal, enhanced, or poor enzymatic ability to process clozapine. Pharmacogenetic testing is discussed further below.

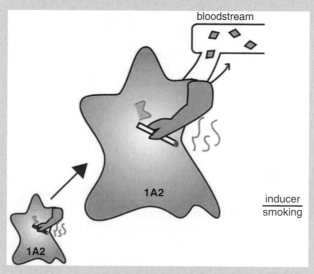

Figure 6.3 CYP1A2 and smoking. Cigarette smoking, quite common among patients with schizophrenia, can induce the enzyme CYP1A2 enzymatic pathway and then lowers the concentration of drugs metabolized by this enzyme, such as olanzapine (Zyprexa) and clozapine (Clozaril), most commonly. Smokers may also require higher doses of these drugs than non-smokers as we have seen in this clozapine (Clozaril) case.

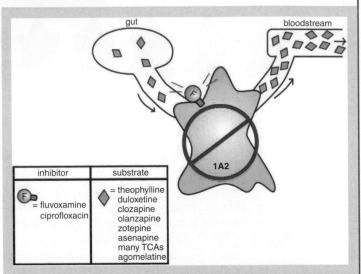

Figure 6.4 Consequences of CYP1A2 inhibition. As seen in this diagram and as utilized in this case, fluvoxamine (Luvox) was added to this patient's regimen and it began blocking his CYP1A2 pathway which allowed clozapine (Clozaril) to be broken down less often and less efficiently so that it was able to build up in the patient's blood stream to more effective levels.

Genetic testing

- Investigates and clarifies a patient's genetic alleles for the CYP450 hepatic enzyme metabolism system
- Pros
  - May help guide treatment
  - May increase medication compliance rate if choosing a likely better-tolerated medication
  - May be another option if several drugs tried are either ineffective or poorly tolerated, before stopping medications altogether
  - May save time in selecting a better-tolerated or effective medication
- Cons
  - Is expensive
  - Has not been shown to necessarily improve clinical outcomes overall across diagnostic patient populations
  - May prevent use of a medication which would have otherwise been the first-line treatment for the condition
- It is unknown for this patient whether he is genetically a normal, excessive, or poor metabolizer. If this type of genetic testing was conducted prior to clozapine (Clozaril) dosing, we might have been able to predict what dose he would need, and to predict how much smoking cigarettes would disrupt his blood levels

Post-test question

Which of the following is true regarding clozapine (Clozaril) dosing?
A. Start at 12.5 – 25 mg/d
B. Increase by 25–50 mg each day as tolerated
C. Usual dosing is 300–400 mg/d and FDA maximum dose is 900 mg/d
D. Usual therapeutic plasma clozapine (Clozaril) level is 350–1000 ng/mL
E. A, B, and C are true
F. All of the above are true

Answer: F

All of the above are true. Clozapine (Clozaril) should be started at 12.5 – 25 mg/d and then increased by 25–50 mg/d as tolerated. Most people achieve a therapeutic response at clozapine (Clozaril) plasma levels > 350 ng/mL, with usual dosing around 300–400 mg/d. Clozapine is most often given in divided doses as the mean half-life of a single dose is 8 hours, while the mean half-life increases to 12 hours with twice-daily dosing. This suggests that the half-life may be concentration dependent. Divided doses may also make clozapine (Clozaril) more tolerable as peak plasma levels tend to stay lower. The maximum FDA-approved dose is 900 mg/d, and is not usually exceeded due to higher risk for seizures. However, keep in mind that dosing above 900 mg/d may be appropriate in cases where the plasma clozapine (Clozaril) levels are still subtherapeutic (< 350 ng/mL).

References

1. Ashton, AK. Aripiprazole augmentation of clozapine: in refractory schizophrenia. *Psychiatry (Edgmont)* 2005; 2:18–19
2. Butler, MG. Pharmacogenetics and psychiatric care: a review and commentary. *J Ment Health Clin Psychol* 2018; 2:17–24
3. Dhillon, N, Heun, R. Nocturnal enuresis is an under-recognised side effect of clozapine: results of a systematic review. *Global Psychiatry* 2019; 2:21–30
4. Ellison, JC, Dufresne, RL. A review of the clinical utility of serum clozapine and norclozapine levels. *Ment Health Clin* 2015; 5:68–73
5. Gee, S, Howes, O. Optimising treatment of schizophrenia: the role of adjunctive fluvoxamine. *Psychopharmacology* 2016; 233:739–40
6. Gray, J, Risch, S. When clozapine is not enough: augment with lamotrigine? *Curr Psychiatry* 2009; 8:40–6

7. Hinze-Selch, D, Deuschle, M, Weber, B, et al. Effect of coadministration of clozapine and fluvoxamine versus clozapine monotherapy on blood cell counts, plasma levels of cytokines and body weight. *Psychopharmacology (Berl)* 2000; 149:163–9

8. Kane, JM, Agid, O, Baldwin, ML, et al. Clinical guidance on the identification and management of treatment-resistant schizophrenia. *J Clin Psychiatry* 2019; 80(2):18com12123

9. Lammers, CH, Deuschle, M, Weigmann, H, et al. Coadministration of clozapine and fluvoxamine in psychotic patients – clinical experience. *Pharmacopsychiatry* 1999; 32:76–7

10. Lu, ML, Lane, HY, Chen, KP, et al. Fluvoxamine reduces the clozapine dosage needed in refractory schizophrenic patients. *J Clin Psychiatry* 2000; 61:594–9

11. Lu, ML, Lane, HY, Lin, SK, et al. Adjunctive fluvoxamine inhibits clozapine-related weight gain and metabolic disturbances. *J Clin Psychiatry* 2004; 65:766–71

12. Meyer, JM, Proctor, G, Cummings, MA, et al. Ciprofloxacin and clozapine: a potentially fatal but underappreciated interaction. *Case Rep Psychiatry* 2016; 2016:5606098

13. Meyer, JM, Stahl, SM. *The Clozapine Handbook*, Cambridge: Cambridge University Press, 2019

14. Olsson, E, Edman, G, Bertilsson, L, et al. Genetic and clinical factors affecting plasma clozapine concentration. *Prim Care Companion CNS Disord* 2015; 17(1):10.4088/PCC.14m01704

15. Polcwiartek, C, Nielsen, J. The clinical potentials of adjunctive fluvoxamine to clozapine treatment: a systematic review. *Psychopharmacology* 2016; 233:741–50

16. Schwartz, D. Interpretation of clozapine levels. *Graylands Hospital Drug Bulletin* 2017; 24:1–8

17. Stahl, SM. *Stahl's Essential Psychopharmacology: Prescriber's Guide*, 5. Cambridge: Cambridge University Press, 2017

18. Stahl, SM. *Transporters, Receptors, and Enzymes as Targets of Psychopharmacological Drug Action*, 5. Cambridge: Cambridge University Press, 2021

19. Stahl, SM, Schwartz, T. *Case Studies: Stahl's Essential Psychopharmacology*. Cambridge: Cambridge University Press, 2016

20. Tanzer, T, Warren, N, McMahon, L, et al. Treatment strategies for clozapine-induced nocturnal enuresis and urinary incontinence: a systematic review. *CNS Spectr* 2022; 28(2):133–44

21. Wigard, ME, van Gool, AR, Schulte, PF. Addition of fluvoxamine to clozapine: theory and practice. *Tijdschr Psychiatr* 2013; 55:113–21

Case 7: Where did her period go?

The Question: Can you reverse antipsychotic-induced hyperprolactinemia?

The Psychopharmacological Dilemma: Finding an effective way to treat psychosis when hindered by amenorrhea

Mark Wiener and Cristiana Mihai

Pretest self-assessment question

Which antipsychotic medications are most commonly associated with causing hyperprolactinemia?

A. Haloperidol (Haldol)
B. Olanzapine (Zyprexa)
C. Quetiapine (Seroquel)
D. Risperidone (Risperdal)
E. A and D
F. A, B, and D
G. All of the above

What is true about antipsychotic-induced hyperprolactinemia?

A. Clinical guidelines recommend treatment of asymptomatic hyperprolactinemia
B. It can be reversed with a partial dopamine-2 receptor (D_2) agonist
C. It does not appear to be dose related
D. There appears to be equal incidence in males and females
E. A and B
F. A, B, and C
G. All of the above

Patient evaluation on intake

- A 26-year-old female with a chief complaint of "auditory hallucinations"

Psychiatric history

- She has experienced symptoms of psychosis since late adolescence
- Started seeing a therapist and psychiatrist after onset of these symptoms
- History of multiple psychiatric hospitalizations for chief complaints that included "hallucinations" and "inability to care for self as a result of psychiatric illness"
- At least one hospitalization followed medication non-compliance which caused worsening of psychotic symptoms
- Denies a history of suicide attempts and self-harm

Social and personal history

- Emigrated from Europe during late adolescence
- Single, with one child, and lost custody of this child due to inability to care for her as a result of psychotic symptoms
- Upset about losing custody of her child to the father
- Lives with her stepfather
- High school graduate, currently working in a part-time minimum-wage retail job
- Engages in social events organized by local community services
- Social drinker, but denies the use of tobacco or recreational drugs

Medical history

- Obese, with a body mass index (BMI) of 33 after past trial with olanzapine (Zyprexa)
- Hypertension (HTN)

Family history

- Mother and maternal aunt were reportedly depressed
- Denies a known family history of substance use
- Denies a known family history of suicide attempts or completions

Medication history

- Past trial with atypical antipsychotic olanzapine (Zyprexa) 15 mg/d for 6 months
  - Generally well tolerated and effective for treatment of her psychotic symptoms
- However, it was ultimately discontinued due to weight gain of 20 lb and because it caused constipation
- Paliperidone (Invega) 6 mg/d was started in its place and was a better-tolerated atypical antipsychotic

Current medications

- Paliperidone (Invega) 6 mg/d, an atypical antipsychotic

Psychotherapy history

- Patient is currently being treated under split treatment model and has been seeing both a therapist and a psychiatrist
  - She is very compliant with visits
- Treatment modalities include both supportive psychotherapy and cognitive-behavioral therapy (CBT)
- Good rapport with her therapist

Patient evaluation on initial visit

- Patient endorses auditory hallucinations which are male, at times multiple voices at once, and content consists of incoherent mumbling
- Evidence of past history of paranoid delusions, but none now
    - She believed she was being poisoned during periods of medication non-compliance
    - She previously thought everyone was conspiring to keep her from her children
- Previous medication trial with a typical antipsychotic, haloperidol (Haldol), was very effective, but was discontinued, interestingly also due to weight gain, which the patient likely erroneously attributed to medication
- Patient has poor insight and does not think she has schizophrenia, reports she lied about hearing voices in the past "for fun," but likes going to therapy and thinks it's helpful
- Pleasant and cooperative, seemingly does not understand the concept of psychosis, but demonstrates fair judgment by agreeing to get help and continue working with therapist and psychiatrist despite lack of insight
- Received the diagnosis schizophrenia (SP) from most past inpatient and outpatient psychiatrists
- She says she would like to lose weight and is agreeable with a referral to a nutritionist for help with weight control

Questions

In your clinical experience, would you expect a patient such as this to be compliant with medication going forward?

- No, because of her history of medication non-compliance and poor insight
- Yes, because she now has a strong support system and is connected to multiple mental health providers

What could you do to increase medication compliance?

- Use drug plasma levels of paliperidone (Invega) as guide to balance efficacy and probability of side effects
- Provide psychoeducation about the importance of medication compliance at each visit
- Ask her family members to regularly encourage and observe for medication compliance

Attending physician's mental notes: initial psychiatric evaluation

- Patient has some strengths including resilience, has a will to live, is agreeable with suggestion to continue counseling and taking medications, has ultimate goal of living more independently
- Prognosis: fair, as she seems to function reasonably well, there is no evidence of dangerous indiscretions, and historically has been able to stay out of hospital as long as compliant with outpatient medication management and psychotherapy
- Her symptoms seem to predate her current stressors
- Despite weight gain and constipation, she reportedly responded to olanzapine (Zyprexa) and haloperidol (Haldol) in the past very well
- She's been taking low therapeutically dosed paliperidone (Invega) 6 mg/d for 3 months, but is still experiencing some auditory hallucinations and paranoid delusions
- Plasma levels of paliperidone (Invega) should be monitored as follows:
  - Therapeutic threshold of 20 ng/mL is used as initial target plasma level for patients who are inadequate responders
  - Point of futility of 90 ng/mL is used as an upper limit, as the benefits of titration beyond this point do not justify the risks because less than 5% of patients will respond to a higher plasma level
- The patient is on a standard approach to treating schizophrenia (SP)
  - Early on, was tried on a typical antipsychotic and responded
  - Switched appropriately to an atypical one and responded
  - Now is on an atypical but has some ongoing psychosis
- Following these trials we can optimize dosing, could consider use of clozapine (Clozaril) for treatment of unremitted psychosis and treatment-resistant schizophrenia (TRS)
- Patient's history of medication non-compliance at times is a poor prognostic factor

Further investigation

Is there anything else that you would like to know about the patient?

What about close-ended questions to screen for side effects of her current medication regimen?

- She denies restlessness, tremors, and abnormal movements
- She has not gained weight recently
- When asked how recent her last menstrual cycle was, she said it has been "at least 2–3 months"

Question

Which of the following would be your next step?

- Obtain a pregnancy test
- Increase the dose of paliperidone (Invega) to 9 mg/d, a higher, potentially more effective dose, to alleviate psychosis
- Switch to an alternative medication, because she has been taking a therapeutic dose long enough for it to be considered an adequate trial
- Check the plasma level of paliperidone (Invega) to ensure it is within the therapeutic range and confirm medication compliance
- Augment the current medications with a second antipsychotic to improve response
- Watchful waiting with current medication regimen

Attending physician's mental notes: initial psychiatric evaluation (continued)

- The typical therapeutic range of paliperidone is 6–12 mg/d, so the dose can be increased
- Although the current medication has a long-acting formulation, no reason yet to switch to this formulation as she has been compliant and we will likely escalate the dose
- Unclear whether there were unforeseen factors in the past that may have increased the likelihood of non-compliance, such as lack of understanding of the medication, lack of insight into her illness, side effect burden, etc.
- Given ongoing symptoms, also spoke with her mother and recommended calling the clinic if symptoms worsened or if there were notable changes in her clinical status
- Will consider checking the plasma level of paliperidone if there is no response

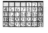

Case outcome: first interim follow-up visit at 2 weeks

- Following a discussion about potential benefits and side effects of increasing the dose of medication, the decision was made to increase the dose to 9 mg/d and follow up in 2 weeks
- Patient reports decrease in the frequency and intensity of auditory hallucinations and there is no current evidence of delusions, paranoia, or thought disorder
- Denies side effects

- Still lacks insight into illness despite denial of recent hallucinations and acknowledgment of past symptoms
- According to her mother, she has been isolating less and has not recently noticed her talking to herself, something which had occurred frequently in the past

Question

Would you continue with oral medication management or transition to a long-acting injectable (LAI)?

- Continue medication management as is, due to its effectiveness and current tolerability, and having a strong support system at present decreases the likelihood of medication non-compliance
- Transition to an LAI due to history of past medication non-compliance, symptom relapse, and multiple psychiatric hospitalizations

Case outcome: follow-up visit at 1 month

- After discussion of risks and benefits of switching to an LAI, an initial dose of 234 mg of paliperidone palmitate IM (Invega Sustenna) was scheduled for 1 week later. This was followed by a maintenance dose of 156 mg of paliperidone palmitate IM (Invega Sustenna) after informed consent, 1 week following
  - ◦ Family felt it was a matter of time, given the patient's poor insight, before she would stop the medication and, as she was nearly psychosis free, all were happy with current outcome and this LAI approach
- Following this maintenance dose of paliperidone palmitate IM (Invega Sustenna), oral dose was decreased to 6 mg/d and patient and her mother were advised to decrease the dose further to 3 mg/d 2 weeks later if symptoms were still in remission

Attending physician's mental notes: follow-up visit (month 1)

- Use of an LAI seems like a good choice to enhance adherence to her medication regimen
- This should increase consecutive days on drug, improve effectiveness, and keep her psychosis away ideally for longer periods of time

Case outcome: interim follow-up visit at 2 months

- Patient still denied auditory hallucinations, her thought process was linear and coherent, and there was no evidence of delusions or thought disorder
- Her mother denies noticing any evidence of ongoing psychotic symptoms and is happy that patient seems more engaging and eager to spend time with her family
- The patient is the best clinically since her SP started

Further investigation

Is there anything else that you would like to know about this patient?

What about closed-ended questions to screen for side effects of her current medication regimen?

- She denies restlessness, tremors, and abnormal movements
- She has not gained weight
- When asked how recent her last menstrual cycle was, she said it has been "at least 4–5 months"
    - She says she has not been sexually active in years
    - Does not recall a history of amenorrhea

Question

How would you proceed, given this information?

- Due to psychotic symptom remission, wait at least 2–3 more months before considering further work-up or switching to an alternative medication, and possibly increase frequency of appointments
- Start cross-titration between paliperidone palmitate IM (Invega Sustenna) and a different more prolactin-sparing atypical antipsychotic medication
- Order prolactin level
- Refer to Obstetrics/Gynecology specialist
- Order MRI of the brain and pituitary gland

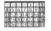

Case outcome: interim follow-up visit at 2½ months

- Patient reports remission of psychotic symptoms with paliperidone palmitate IM (Invega Sustenna)
- Patient said she still has not menstruated, though denies breast tenderness, gynecomastia, galactorrhea, or vaginal dryness
- She again denies sexual activity

Question

How would you proceed, given recent history and elevated prolactin level?

- Start treatment with a D_2 agonist, such as cabergoline (Dostinex) or pramipexole (Mirapex) and continue with monthly paliperidone palmitate IM (Invega Sustenna) injections
- Consider treatment with aripiprazole (Abilify) given its D_2 partial agonism, and continue with monthly paliperidone palmitate IM (Invega Sustenna) injections
    - Use low-dose aripiprazole (Abilify) as an antidote to lower prolactin and add it to the current regimen
    - Use a full dose of aripiprazole (Abilify) and remove paliperidone palmitate IM (Invega Sustenna)
- Stop paliperidone palmitate IM (Invega Sustenna) and restart treatment with oral paliperidone as this seemed to have fewer side effects than the IM formulation
- Lower paliperidone palmitate IM (Invega Sustenna) in hope of controlling psychosis but lowering prolactin

Attending physician's mental notes: interim follow-up visit at 2½ months

- Patient reports remission of psychotic symptoms with paliperidone palmitate IM (Invega Sustenna) and really appears to be her baseline best clinically
- She has a history of psychiatric hospitalizations and poor functioning during periods of medication non-compliance, so really need to keep her on an antipsychotic
- Reports suggest that aripiprazole (Abilify) can reverse antipsychotic-induced hyperprolactinemia

Case outcome: follow-up visits through 7 months

- Patient agreed to start treatment with 5 mg/d aripiprazole (Abilify) and continue her usual medications
- One week after starting treatment, she denied new side effects and dose was increased to 10 mg/d
- A few months after this dose increase, patient said she resumed her normal menstrual cycle

Attending physician's mental notes: interim follow-up (month 7)

- Excluding select cases of treatment-resistant psychosis, there is relative paucity of data suggesting that treatment with more than one antipsychotic is more effective than monotherapy, and continuing to treat her with two antipsychotics may have increased risk-to-benefit ratio due to increased risk of side effects
- Her psychosis, however, is in remission following titration of paliperidone palmitate IM (Invega Sustenna) dose, so discontinuing the medication or even decreasing the dose could come with the risk of worsening symptoms
- In hindsight, should have obtained plasma levels at 9 mg of the oral dose to compare to the current IM LAI dose.
- With such a good response, it's too risky to lower the dose or stop this medication right now
- The patient seems to be in a "win-win" situation where she is on polypharmacy, which can be viewed as a negative, but she is at her positively best clinically now and also has no current amenorrhea

Question

What would you do next?

- Cross-titrate between paliperidone palmitate IM (Invega Sustenna) and aripiprazole (Abilify), with goal of eventually discontinuing paliperidone palmitate IM (Invega Sustenna) entirely
- Continue treatment with both medications concurrently due to effectiveness and resumption of normal menses
    - Paliperidone palmitate IM (Invega Sustenna) is the therapeutic agent
    - Aripiprazole (Abilify) is being used off label as an antidote for hyperprolactinemia
- Discontinue paliperidone palmitate IM (Invega Sustenna) entirely now, increase dose of aripiprazole (Abilify) to 15–30 mg/d, while checking for aripiprazole plasma levels as follows:
    - Therapeutic threshold of 110 ng/mL used as initial target plasma level
    - Point of futility of 500 ng/mL used as an upper limit
    - Could convert to the LAI preparation of aripiprazole called:
        - Aristada – every 4–8 weeks
        - Asimtufii – every 8 weeks
        - Maintena – every 4 weeks

Case outcome: follow-up visits through 16 months

- Decision was made to start cross-titrating between paliperidone palmitate IM (Invega Sustenna) and aripiprazole (Abilify) as she had almost 1.5 years of psychosis remission and improved psychosocial functioning
- Dose of paliperidone palmitate IM (Invega Sustenna) was since decreased to 117 mg/month
- At follow-up, patient still reports that psychotic symptoms are in remission and denies amenorrhea, galactorrhea, and vaginal dryness
- There are no new side effects
- Aripiprazole (Abilify) was increased 15 mg/d while further decreasing paliperidone palmitate IM (Invega Sustenna) over the next few months

Case debrief

- As the patient is a limited historian and some details regarding her remote psychiatric history are scarce, it is unclear whether the patient had other antipsychotic trials besides haloperidol (Haldol), and olanzapine (Zyprexa) was never maximized to 20 mg/d and plasma levels were not checked
- As the patient is obese, and olanzapine (Zyprexa) is considered now to be too metabolically risky, it was deemed a failed trial
- In retrospect, it may have been wise to consider a trial with an antipsychotic with a less significant association with weight gain, dyslipidemia, and glucose intolerance than even paliperidone (Invega)
- Though paliperidone (Invega) is not as strongly associated with metabolic side effects as agents such as olanzapine (Zyprexa), quetiapine (Seroquel), and clozapine (Clozaril), there are other medications, such as aripiprazole (Abilify), ziprasidone (Geodon), lumateperone (Caplyta), and lurasidone (Latuda), that are considered more metabolically neutral or favorable
- Paliperidone (Invega) was initially effective and then switched to its LAI formulation (Invega Sustenna) due to the patient's history of ongoing psychosis with medication non-compliance
- Aripiprazole (Abilify) was started because of its unique prolactin-normalizing capability, not to be used as atypical antipsychotic polypharmacy
- When the patient admitted to loss of menses, laboratory testing confirmed hyperprolactinemia and aripiprazole (Abilify) was

started instead while the dose of paliperidone palmitate IM (Invega Sustenna) was decreased slowly

- Aripiprazole (Abilify) was increased and became the sole treatment ultimately
- If her psychotic symptoms were to remain in remission following completion of a cross-titration between aripiprazole (Abilify) and paliperidone palmitate IM (Invega Sustenna), a long-acting formulation of aripiprazole, such as Abilify Maintena, could be considered next
- In this case, as her symptoms improved, she remained medication compliant with oral aripiprazole (Abilify)

Take-home points

- Hyperprolactinemia (HPL) in individuals taking antipsychotic medication ranges as high as 42% to 89%
- HPL is associated with sexual dysfunction, amenorrhea, gynecomastia, galactorrhea, weight gain, osteoporosis, depression, and anxiety
- Prolactin levels increase in patients treated with risperidone (Risperdal) more than other atypical antipsychotics, and paliperidone (Invega) is its active metabolite and may also cause this side effect, based on numerous case reports in the literature
- Evidence suggests that prolactin levels increase depending upon dosing and this happens more commonly in women at high doses
- The symptoms of HPL can become so severe that adherence to treatment with antipsychotic medications often declines
- Aripiprazole (Abilify) acts as a net antagonist at D_2s in hyperdopaminergic conditions and as a partial agonist in hypodopaminergic conditions, thus not having much adverse effect on serum prolactin levels, and it may actually improve prolactin levels when D_2s are antagonized in the tuberoinfundilbular pathway

Performance in practice: confessions of a psychopharmacologist

What could have been done better here?

- In a cross-titration, what is an ideal dosing strategy for patients switching from one antipsychotic to aripiprazole (Abilify)?
  - Although studies suggest patients do well with cross-titrations when switching from one antipsychotic to aripiprazole (Abilify), clinical experience suggests that patients can also do well if the full dose of aripiprazole (Abilify) is added to the maintenance

dose of the first antipsychotic for several days before the dose
of the first antipsychotic is slowly decreased

- Because this patient was obese and hypertensive, clinicians could
  have considered a more metabolically neutral antipsychotic than
  paliperidone palmitate IM (Invega Sustenna) initially
- Drug plasma levels should have been used to guide dosing of
  antipsychotic medications because they can confirm medication
  compliance and can determine whether the patient's plasma level is
  within a therapeutic range

What are possible action items for improvement in practice?

- Research to determine an ideal way of switching from one
  antipsychotic to aripiprazole (Abilify). Currently, there is no
  clear consensus on whether cross-titration, abrupt switching, or
  increasing aripiprazole (Abilify) to target dose before decreasing the
  dose of the first agent is superior
  - Given the high affinity of aripiprazole (Abilify) for D_2s, it is often
    noted that psychosis sometimes increases during cross-titration
    because the higher-affinity aripiprazole (Abilify) may displace
    other actively bound atypical antipsychotics which have been
    routinely lowering dopamine activity at the synapse
- Research to determine alternative methods of addressing
  antipsychotic-induced hyperprolactinemia, especially if the
  antipsychotic responsible is also very effective, in order to avoid
  antipsychotic polypharmacy
- Research available studies and case reports that have addressed
  antipsychotic-induced hyperprolactinemia by switching to other
  prolactin-sparing antipsychotics, such as quetiapine (Seroquel)
- Further investigate whether other partial D_2 agonists, such as
  cariprazine (Vraylar) and brexpiprazole (Rexulti), can also treat
  antipsychotic-induced hyperprolactinemia
- Investigate the apparent trend of prolactin-unfriendly and metabolic-
  unfriendly atypical antipsychotics continuing to be used when some
  newer agents tend to have less risk of these over the longer term

Tips and pearls

- While there is no clear consensus as to whether a pretreatment prolactin level should be measured, doing so for patients started on typical or atypical antipsychotics commonly associated with hyperprolactinemia (haloperidol [Haldol], risperidone [Risperdal], paliperidone [Invega], olanzapine [Zyprexa]) can help diagnose medication-induced hyperprolactinemia more proactively
  ○ This is achieved through establishment of a temporal relationship between prolactin level and time of initiation of antipsychotic medication
- In most cases, if a patient with high prolactin levels is asymptomatic or only mildly (less than 200 ng/mL) symptomatic, it is best not to discontinue or change the antipsychotic regimen while following prolactin levels perhaps annually. However, the risks and benefits need to be evaluated on a case-by-case basis
- It's a good practice to screen for side effects of hyperprolactinemia at regular intervals, especially when treating with agents that are more likely to elevate prolactin levels
- Some examples of symptoms associated with medication-induced hyperprolactinemia include sexual dysfunction, amenorrhea, vaginal dryness, galactorrhea, male gynecomastia, and infertility
- Treatment options for medication-induced hyperprolactinemia include changing to a prolactin-sparing antipsychotic (quetiapine [Seroquel], iloperidone [Fanapt], Aripiprazole [Abilify], brexpiprazole [Rexulti], cariprazine [Vraylar]), addition of sex steroids, and addition of D_2 agonists, and decreasing the current dose of medication can be helpful
- Work-up for a space-occupying lesion of the sellar region, such as a pituitary adenoma, should be considered if there are signs such as visual field defects or headache. This work-up typically includes MRI of the pituitary gland

Mechanism of action moment

Why do prolactin levels typically decrease when treating with aripiprazole (Abilify), when the levels increase through the use of other antipsychotics?

- The tuberoinfundibular dopamine pathway consists of dopaminergic neurons that project to the hypothalamus
  ○ This pathway, through the release of dopamine, inhibits the release of prolactin from the pituitary gland, keeping prolactin levels normal in a homeostatic manner

- Antipsychotic medications, especially strong D_2 antagonists such as risperidone (Risperdal), decrease the normal dopamine receptor agonism in the tuberoinfundibular pathway
  - This in turn decreases inhibition of prolactin release from the pituitary gland, leading to hyperprolactinemia
- Due to its unique mechanism of D_2 partial agonism, aripiprazole (Abilify) increases dopamine activity in areas with low dopamine affinity. In this manner, it may directly, pharmacodynamically, reverse the side effect
  - Brexpiprazole (Rexulti) and cariprazine (Vraylar) act similarly but are less studied
- By the same mechanism, aripiprazole (Abilify) decreases dopamine activity in areas of the brain with relatively high dopamine activity, such as the mesolimbic dopamine pathway that is implicated in causing psychotic symptoms when hyperactive
- Aripiprazole (Abilify), therefore, can theoretically increase dopamine agonism in the tuberoinfundibular pathway, causing appropriately decreased release of prolactin from the pituitary gland, decreasing prolactin levels and lowering side effects
- Also of note is that aripiprazole (Abilify) has one of the highest affinities for the D_2
  - When introduced into the plasma of a patient with another antipsychotic already on board, it will typically displace the original antipsychotic from its binding with the D_2
  - In this case, this displacement of a fully blocking antipsychotic with a partially antagonistic one will yield a net effect of less dopamine blockade which will allow prolactin to be better controlled with more normal inhibition processes
  - This same effect in the mesolimbic dopamine pathway can allow for some breakthrough psychosis as well

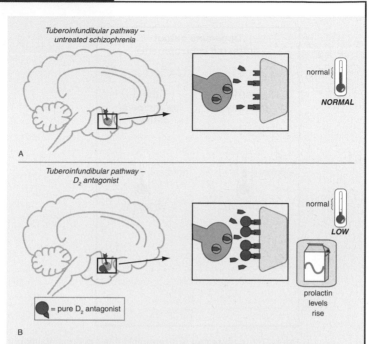

Figure 7.1 Tuberoinfundibular dopamine pathway and D₂ antagonists. (A) The tuberoinfundibular dopamine pathway, which projects from the hypothalamus to the pituitary gland, is theoretically "normal" in untreated schizophrenia. (B) D₂ antagonists reduce activity in this pathway by preventing dopamine from binding to D₂s. This causes prolactin levels to rise, which is associated with side effects such as galactorrhea (breast secretions) and amenorrhea (irregular menstrual periods).

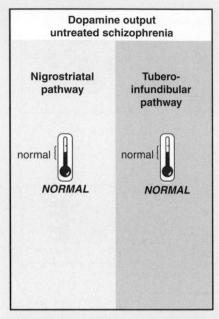

Figure 7.2 In untreated schizophrenia, the brain maintains homeostasis in the nigrostriatal and tuberoinfundibular pathways, allowing for optimal dopamine to be present to allow for normal movement and prolactin management.

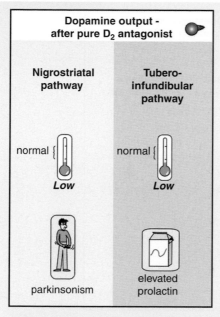

Figure 7.3 When using an antipsychotic to treat psychosis, D₂ antagonism will lower dopamine transmission in the mesolimbic pathway. Unfortunately, D₂ blockade is non-selective, and here we see that D₂ is also blocked in the nigrastriatal pathway allowing for movement disorder to occur, and in the tuberoinfundibular pathway allowing for hyperprolactinemia to occur.

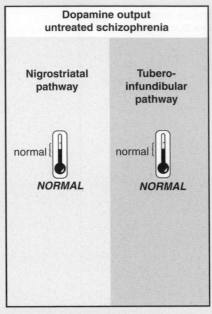

Figure 7.4 Here we will see again normal functioning of dopamine in these respective pathways.

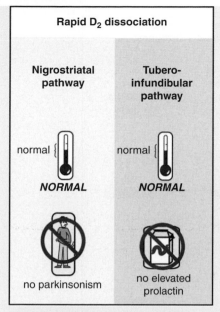

Rapid D$_2$ dissociation

| Nigrostriatal pathway | Tubero-infundibular pathway |

normal

NORMAL

normal

NORMAL

no parkinsonism

no elevated prolactin

Figure 7.5 Notice now, if an agent with low affinity for D$_2$ antagonism, such as quetiapine (Seroquel), is used, then it will bind the D$_2$ receptor briefly affording antagonism, and will tilt the nigrostriatal system toward movement disorder and the tuberoinfundibular system toward hyperprolactinemia but, with a shorter half-life and a lower affinity, the antipsychotic will lose its binding at D$_2$ and dissociate, leaving the D$_2$ to return to normal and typically reversing the trend toward creating movement disorder and prolactinemia side effects.

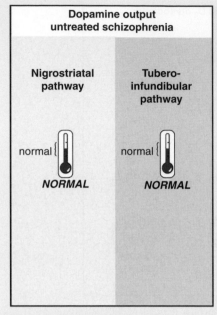

Figure 7.6 Here we will see again normal functioning of dopamine in these respective pathways.

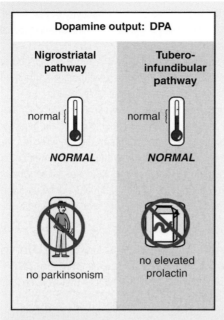

Figure 7.7 Notice now that, if an agent has partial agonism properties at the D_2 in these pathways, there should not be blockade and lowering of dopamine activity, therefore adequate dopamine neurostimulation should occur to allow for good neuromuscular movement activity and good control of blood prolactin levels.

Two-minute tutorial

Monitoring serum levels of antipsychotic medication

- Serum levels can be ordered for some antipsychotic medications, including olanzapine (Zyprexa), paliperidone (Invega), risperidone (Risperdal), and haloperidol (Haldol). Other antipsychotic levels can be ordered but it may be difficult to find a lab to perform and sometimes insurance carriers will not cover the lab order
- Plasma levels are useful if it is unclear whether the patient has been taking medication as prescribed, or when there is an insufficient response despite a therapeutic dose being issued
- If a patient is taking less medication than prescribed, this would likely result in a low serum level
- If there is an insufficient response despite a therapeutic dose, one possible explanation is that the patient has increased enzyme activity of the cytochrome p450 (CYP450) enzymes that metabolize that medication, as increased enzyme activity would cause a relatively low serum concentration

- Conversely, if a patient has decreased activity of that CYP450 enzyme, this could cause a high serum level of that medication, increasing the risk of side effects
  - Relatively high and low activity of P450 enzymes could be due to either genetics or medication interactions as some medications induce P450 enzymes and some inhibit them
- If a patient does not respond to a medication despite a therapeutic serum level, the patient may be considered a clear pharmacokinetic and pharmacodynamic non-responder to that particular medication
- In the above case, if the patient continued to experience psychotic symptoms despite an increase in the dose of paliperidone (Invega) to 9 mg/d, an FDA-approved and therapeutic dose, one option would have been to check the serum level of this medication

Improving medication compliance with LAI antipsychotics

- Some antipsychotics are available as long-acting, intramuscular formulations and have been discussed in previous cases
- The use of LAIs can increase the chances that a patient will be adherent to medication
  - Essentially, clinicians do not have to rely on patient reporting about medication adherence, as with LAIs once the patient fails to show for their injection appointment, the provider knows the patient has become non-compliant and is more at risk of a psychotic relapse
  - Their use can delay time to relapse and the need for rehospitalization
- Factors that can decrease the likelihood that a patient will be adherent to medication include:
  - Lack of social support
  - History of medication non-adherence
  - High complexity of the medication regimen
  - Poor rapport between provider and the patient
  - Lack of financial resources
  - Cognitive impairment
  - Lack of motivation
  - Low education level
  - Substance use
  - Fear of side effects
- In the above case, the patient was transitioned from oral paliperidone (Invega) to an LAI formulation of paliperidone palmitate IM (Invega Sustenna) due to her history of medication non-compliance, with good effect

Post-test questions

Which antipsychotic medications are most commonly associated with causing hyperprolactinemia?

A. Haloperidol (Haldol)
B. Olanzapine (Zyprexa)
C. Quetiapine (Seroquel)
D. Risperidone (Risperdal)
E. A and D
F. A, B, and D
G. All of the above

Answer: E

Antipsychotic medications that are associated with a relatively high risk of hyperprolactinemia include risperidone (Risperdal), paliperidone (Invega), and haloperidol (Haldol). Risperidone in particular is effectively and efficiently transported by P-glycoprotein, so appears to have easy access to the central nervous system (CNS) and tuberoinfundibular pathway compared to other antipsychotics.

What is true about antipsychotic-induced hyperprolactinemia?

A. Clinical guidelines recommend treatment of asymptomatic hyperprolactinemia
B. It can be reversed with a partial dopamine-2 receptor (D_2) agonist
C. It does not appear to be dose related
D. There appears to be equal incidence in males and females
E. A and B
F. A, B, and C
G. All of the above

Answer: B

Antipsychotic-induced hyperprolactinemia is likely dose related, can be reversed with the addition of aripiprazole, and appears to be more frequent in females. The Endocrine Society does not recommend treating asymptomatic medication-induced hyperprolactinemia.

References

1. Byerly, M, Suppes, T, Tran, QV, et al. Clinical implications of antipsychotic-induced hyperprolactinemia in patients with schizophrenia spectrum or bipolar spectrum disorders: recent developments and current perspectives. *J Clin Psychopharmacol* 2007; 27:639–61

2. Holt, RI, Peveler, RC. Antipsychotics and hyperprolactinaemia: mechanisms, consequences and management. *Clin Endocrinol (Oxf)* 2011; 74:141–7

3. Johnsen, E, Kroken, RA, Abaza, M, et al. Antipsychotic-induced hyperprolactinemia: a cross-sectional survey. *J Clin Psychopharmacol* 2008; 28:686–90

4. Keck, PE, Jr., McElroy, SL. Aripiprazole: a partial dopamine D$_2$ receptor agonist antipsychotic. *Expert Opin Investig Drugs* 2003; 12:655–62

5. Melkersson, K. Differences in prolactin elevation and related symptoms of atypical antipsychotics in schizophrenic patients. *J Clin Psychiatry* 2005; 66:761–7

6. Melmed, S, Casanueva, FF, Hoffman, AR, et al. Diagnosis and treatment of hyperprolactinemia: an Endocrine Society clinical practice guideline. *J Clin Endocrinol Metab* 2011; 96:273–88

7. Meng, M, Li, W, Zhang, S, et al. Using aripiprazole to reduce antipsychotic-induced hyperprolactinemia: meta-analysis of currently available randomized controlled trials. *Shanghai Arch Psychiatry* 2015; 27:4–17

8. Meyer, JM, Stahl, SM. *The Clinical Use of Antipsychotic Plasma Levels*. Cambridge: Cambridge University Press, 2021

9. Miyamoto, BE, Galecki, M, Francois, D. Guidelines for antipsychotic-induced hyperprolactinemia. *Psychiatr Ann* 2015; 45:266–72

10. Petty, RG. Prolactin and antipsychotic medications: mechanism of action. *Schizophr Res* 1999; 35 Suppl.:S67–73

11. Stahl, SM. *Stahl's Essential Psychopharmacology: Neuroscientific Basis and Practical Applications*, 5. Cambridge: Cambridge University Press, 2021

12. Turrone, P, Kapur, S, Seeman, MV, et al. Elevation of prolactin levels by atypical antipsychotics. *Am J Psychiatry* 2002; 159:133–5

13. Volavka, J, Czobor, P, Cooper, TB, et al. Prolactin levels in schizophrenia and schizoaffective disorder patients treated with clozapine, olanzapine, risperidone, or haloperidol. *J Clin Psychiatry* 2004; 65:57–61

14. Wang, ZM, Xiang, YT, An, FR, et al. Frequency of hyperprolactinemia and its associations with demographic and clinical characteristics and antipsychotic medications in psychiatric inpatients in China. *Perspect Psychiatr Care* 2014; 50:257–63

Case 8: To dopamine or not to dopamine, that is the question

The Question: What is the impact of using a stimulant and an antipsychotic to treat comorbid psychiatric disorders?

The Psychopharmacological Dilemma: Use of medications with potentially opposing mechanistic actions

Kathryn Myers

Pretest self-assessment question

What neurotransmitter system is routinely influenced by both antipsychotics and stimulants?

A. Norepinephrine
B. Serotonin
C. γ-aminobutyric acid (GABA)
D. Dopamine
E. Glutamate

Patient evaluation on intake

- A 13-year-old male with history of Attention-Deficit/Hyperactivity Disorder (ADHD), schizoaffective disorder, and subsyndromal autism spectrum disorder (ASD) admitted to an inpatient psychiatry unit for acute psychotic decompensation
- Presented with increased aggression, hallucinations, and paranoid delusions

Psychiatric history

- Diagnosed with ADHD 4 years ago, with several stimulant trials showing limited benefits so far
- Was hospitalized 6 months ago for similar aggression, paranoia, and mood lability but without hallucinations
- He has had difficulties socially engaging with peers since early childhood and often found to be "in his own world"

Social and personal history

- Adopted at age 3 and living with biological sister, adoptive mother, and one non-biological sibling
- Biological mother died from an accident when patient was an infant
- A prior hospitalization 6 months ago occurred as he became overly focused on a female peer at school, trying to monopolize time with

her in socially unacceptable ways, including waiting for her outside of the bathroom
- He is in regular classes with a 504 educational plan allowing extra time for testing

Medical history

- No acute or chronic conditions

Family history

- Biological mother has history of bipolar disorder (BP) or schizophrenia, and substance use disorder (SUD)
- Biological sister diagnosed with possible schizophrenia

Medication history

- Previous trials of methylphenidate (Ritalin) and dextroamphetamine (Dexedrine) stimulants discontinued due to ineffectiveness or increased irritability and aggression
- Started on lisdexamfetamine (Vyvnase) for hyperactivity and inattention 4 months ago
- Started also on an atypical antipsychotic, risperidone (Risperdal), and lithium (Eskalith) 6 months ago at prior hospitalization for aggression and mood lability, which initially appeared to be helpful before recent regression in symptoms noted at intake
- Clonidine (Catapres) added to help with sleep disturbance a month after hospital discharge

Current medications

- Lisdexamfetamine (Vyvanse) 40 mg/d, a stimulant for inattention and hyperactivity
- Risperidone (Risperdal) 4 mg/d, an atypical antipsychotic for psychosis and aggression
- Lithium (Eskalith) 600 mg/d, a mood stabilizer for his mood lability
- Clonidine (Catapres) 0.15 mg/d, an α_2 agonist antihypertensive agent used for insomnia

Patient evaluation

- Worsening aggression toward adoptive mother and siblings over the last 2 months
- Increasing paranoia including toward food being poisoned. Adoptive mother reports he has been refusing to eat with a 10-pound weight loss noted over the last month

- Reports seeing "demons" and fighting them by throwing fireballs
- He is refusing to sleep because of the demon attacks and he needs to "protect the world"
- He is seen pacing around exam room "throwing" fireballs. He becomes agitated when attempts are made to redirect him

Question

What would be your next steps in changing medication? Choose all that apply.

- Give the atypical antipsychotic olanzapine (Zyprexa) for acute agitation
- Increase dose of risperidone (Risperdal) with goal of 6 mg/d in mind
- Add another antipsychotic while continuing the risperidone (Risperdal) at current dose
- Decrease risperidone (Risperdal) and start cross-titrating to another antipsychotic
- Stop lisdexamfetamine (Vyvanse)
- Obtain a lithium level and increase lithium (Eskalith) to a therapeutic dose
- Obtain a risperidone level to check for compliance
- Increase clonidine (Catapres) to help more with sleep and agitation
- Do not change his medications. Place in a quiet room and observe to see whether his symptoms improve in the morning

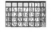

Further investigation

Is there anything else that you would like to know about the patient?

- Does patient have "subsyndromal autism" or are these behaviors actually the development of negative symptoms associated with schizophrenia?
- Was history of mood lability influenced in either direction by prior stimulant trials?
- Will discontinuation of current stimulant trial, lisdexamfetamine (Vyvanse), improve psychosis, aggression, and mood lability?

Case outcome: initial evaluation

- Olanzapine (Zyprexa) 5 mg oral dissolving tablet (ODT) was given for acute agitation to maintain safety in the emergency room (ER) as a one-time as-needed medication dose

- Lisdexamfetamine (Vyvanse) was discontinued as there was concern that some of his aggression and mood lability may have been influenced or generated by the stimulant
  - Increased aggression and irritability had been seen in other stimulant trials this patient had previously
  - This could also drive psychotic symptoms as a side effect
- Risperidone (Risperdal) was decreased to 2 mg/d to start a cross-taper ultimately to quetiapine (Seroquel) instead
  - This atypical antipsychotic agent has a potent norepinephrine reuptake inhibitor (NRI) property which might help ADHD symptoms similar to the approved NRI atomoxetine (Strattera)
- Risperidone (Risperdal) taper was started because there was felt to be only a limited benefit likely from further titration
  - For children and adolescents, usual dosing for aggression or irritability related to ASD is 0.5 – 3 mg/d in split dosing
  - For bipolar mania in children and adolescents, typical dosing is 1–2.5 mg/d in split dosing
  - For schizophrenia, the goal is 3 mg/d with usually a range of 1–6 mg/d in split dosing
- Quetiapine (Seroquel) was started at 25 mg/d
- Quetiapine (Seroquel) was chosen as the new antipsychotic due to its sedating side effects as patient has not been sleeping
  - For bipolar mania in children and adolescents, typical dosing is 400–600 mg/d in split dosing
  - For schizophrenia in children and adolescents, typical dosing is 400–800 mg/d in split dosing

Attending physician's mental notes: initial psychiatric evaluation

- Wow, that's a lot of medications and medication changes
- Sometimes polypharmacy helps and sometimes it can make the diagnosis, symptom outcome, and side-effect burden more confusing, especially when this approach fails

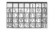

Case outcome: interim follow-ups through 3 days

- He was admitted to a child and adolescent inpatient psychiatric unit as ER stabilization failed
- Three nights after admission, he was still pacing in the hallway and reported to nursing that supernatural beings were controlling his eyes
- On examination, he was found to be in acute distress. His eyes were gazing upward and appeared to be stuck in place

Question

What is happening to the patient? What would you do?

- He is purposely doing this for attention. Do nothing and wait for the day team to decide whether his medications should be changed
- His psychosis is worsening and his gaze is like this because of his delusions or catatonia. He needs an extra dose of antipsychotic
- He is experiencing a dystonic extrapyramidal symptom (EPS) side effect from his medication, sometimes called oculogyric crisis (OC). He needs to be treated with an anticholinergic medication now

Attending physician's mental notes: interim follow-ups through 3 days

- Unfortunately, in trying to streamline medications we have created a new side-effect issue
- Likely has the extrapyramidal syndrome (EPS) called dystonia
- This is urgent and needs to be treated with an anticholinergic

Case outcome: interim follow-up day 4

- Diphenhydramine (Benedryl) 25 mg for dystonia, and quetiapine (Seroquel) 25 mg for acute agitation, are now being combined
- Within 30 minutes, acute dystonia escalated OC plus retrocollis, stridor, and laryngeal spasms, making this a medical emergency
- Diphenhydramine (Benedryl) 50 mg intramuscular (IM) started, and patient sent to the ER for observation and to protect airway

Attending physician mental notes: day 4

- When EPS symptoms progressed, there was concern that his airway could be compromised needing urgent medical management not afforded on the psychiatric unit
- Anticholinergics were needed ASAP to treat this dystonia
  - Diphenhydramine (Benedryl) is an anticholinergic that restores the balance between acetylcholine and dopamine activity in the basal ganglia
    - It is most often used in children to lower this type of EPS
- Quetiapine (Seroquel) was used for two reasons:
  - Treatment plan in place includes cross-taper to this antipsychotic
  - It is one of the antipsychotics with lowest risk of causing EPS moving forward

Question

What changes, if any, would you make after he is medically cleared and returned to the psychiatric unit?

- Lower risperidone (Risperdal) more quickly
- Maintain routine use of diphenhydramine (Benedryl)
- Start routine use of a different anticholinergic such as benztropine (Cogentin) when giving antipsychotic medications

Case outcome: day 5

- On return to the unit, diphenhydramine (Benedryl) 50 mg/d was started for EPS prevention
- The antipsychotic cross-taper from risperidone (Risperdal) to lower-EPS-risk quetiapine (Seroquel) was continued more quickly, with goal of reaching 400–600 mg/d for better symptom control

Attending physician mental notes: day 5

- Now that EPS emergency is over, we do need to move away from atypical antipsychotic polypharmacy to avoid EPS and focus on quetiapine (Seroquel) monotherapy
- Anticholinergics, like diphenhydramine (Benedryl), need to be used routinely for a period of time
- The stimulant likely needs to be fully removed to determine whether the psychosis apparent is iatrogenic or not
- May need to continue clonidine (Catapres) for insomnia and agitation for a while
- The goal should be to lower the number of psychotropics, ideally to a monotherapy, and readdress symptoms after some prolonged observation

Case outcome: through day 14

- Patient was slowly titrated to 400 mg/d of quetiapine (Seroquel)
- He experienced better sleep and mild daytime sedation so clonidine (Catapres) was gradually removed
- No other side effects were noted and no EPS returned
- Gradually, hallucinations and delusions resolved
- Agitation would occur randomly and appeared not to be driven by psychosis but rather rigidity from ASD and frustration tolerance difficulty when limits were being set
- Patient was able to be discharged back home on quetiapine (Seroquel) monotherapy

Case debrief

- Sometimes in our efforts as a pscyhopharmacologist, we *see the tree instead of the forest* in our quest for rapid symptom reduction
- This case shows where polypharmacy for several different disorders likely led to creation of a new psychotic state or the triggering of an underlying psychotic disorder
  - Trying to treat ADHD with a dopaminergic stimulant likely led to dopamine mesolimbic pathway overactivity and the generation of both hallucinations and delusions
  - The patient had a clear family history of psychotic disorder likely making him susceptible to new-onset psychosis
  - Trying to control the psychosis with multiple agents rapidly caused a dystonic reaction that was life threatening, etc.
- The inpatient psychiatrist needed to triage the problems at hand from most dangerous to least – dystonia, psychosis, ADHD, autism – and develop a treatment plan based on this order
- The case outlines using this approach instead of a DSM-5 disorder-based approach, with successful outcomes likely in all areas except for ASD

Take-home points

- Cross-titration of antipsychotics, or other classes of psychotropics, is considered polypharmacy
  - Even a true cross-titration can result in higher pharmacokinetic drug levels or higher pharmacodynamic impacts
  - In this case, even though the dose of quetiapine (Seroquel) was low and its affinity is lower than that of the longer half-life and higher-affinity risperidone (Risperdal), there was still a cumulative and additive effect of dopamine-2 receptor (D_2) blockade in the nigrostriatal dopamine pathway system that afforded the onset of a dystonia
  - When cross-titrating, the clinician must think through the affinities and half-lives of both agents in certain cases
- Using a stimulant can also change dopamine balance in the mesolimbic pathway and can create psychosis in those who are at risk for psychosis, and at higher doses during intoxication in any individual
  - Perhaps in these patients with ADHD and psychotic propensity, non-stimulant medications should more strongly be considered, such as NRIs (atomoxetine [Strattera]) or α_2 receptor agonists (clonidine ER [Kapvay] / guanfacine ER [Intuniv])

Performance in practice: confessions of a psychopharmacologist

What could have been done better here?

- On the surface everything seemed to make sense
  - ○ Use a stimulant for ADHD
  - ○ Use an atypical antipsychotic for ASD aggression
  - ○ Use more atypical antipsychotic for psychosis and escalating agitation
- When the clinical situation changes rapidly, it may make sense to jettison the DSM-5 and frankly triage based on target symptoms as was done in this case
  - ○ Pace is slower in the outpatient setting but this clinician could have taken a deep breath, thought through psychosis being more important than inattention, and lowered off the stimulant, possibly avoiding the robust psychosis that developed
  - ○ Pace is faster in the inpatient service, but, similarly, this clinician, due to an urgent situation, had to take a deep breath, step back, and analyze the situation based on the medical problems or symptoms at hand, in a descending order of urgency
- Sometimes this target symptom approach is needed more than an absolute disorder-based approach

Tips and pearls

Dystonic reactions

- OC and laryngospasm (LC) are both rare types of dystonic movement disorder caused by sustained contractions of ocular or larynx/pharynx musculature that may last minutes to hours
  - ○ This is usually seen after the initiation or dose increase of an antipsychotic agent
  - ○ Even some of the least EPS-prone atypical antipsychotics (quetiapine [Seroquel], iloperidone [Fanapt], lumaterperone [Caplyta]) can cause this
- OC is characterized by uncontrolled deviation of the eyes, most commonly upward
- Laryngospasm is characterized by throat constriction, stridor, and difficulty breathing
- Both occur due to acute changes in the production, storage, and reuptake of DA resulting in a net hypodopaminergic state, likely in the nigrostriatal dopaminergic pathway
- Both cause significant pain

- The most common causes of dystonia, specifically for OC, include:
  - Medications
    - Most commonly D_2 blocking agents such as the antipsychotics discussed above, and antiemetics such as metoclopramide (Reglan) or prochlorperazine (Compazine)
  - Neurodegenerative disorders
  - Neurometabolic disorders
    - Monoamine neurotransmitter disorders or enzyme deficiencies in the dopamine pathway
    - Usually autosomal-recessive inheritance and may be misdiagnosed as cerebral palsy

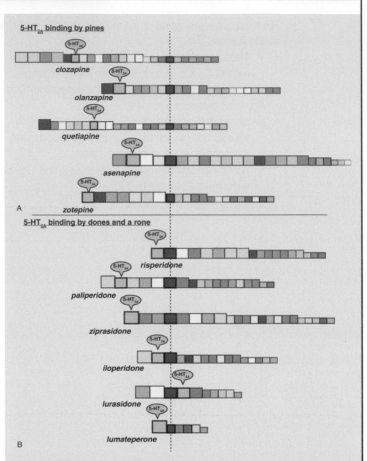

Figure 8.1 How likely is a dystonia theoretically? Shown here is a visual depiction of the binding profiles of drugs used to treat psychosis. Each colored box represents a different binding property, with the size and positioning of the box reflecting the binding potency of the property (i.e., size indicates potency relative to a standard K_i scale, while position reflects potency relative to the other binding properties of that drug). The vertical dotted line cuts through the D_2 binding box, with binding properties that are more potent than D_2 on the left and those that are less potent than D_2 on the right. Therefore, agents with higher serotonin 5-HT$_{2A}$ receptor antagonism affinity (larger boxes to the left of the red dotted line) are less likely to cause dystonia and other EPS syndromes. Note the "dones" usually will have a greater D_2 affinity and more EPS as a result. The "pines" are shifted to the left above and have lower antagonist D_2 affinity paired with greater 5-HT$_{2A}$ antagonist affinity, allowing less EPS generally to occur. The net effect of this is greater dopamine activity can occur in the nigrostriatal pathway.

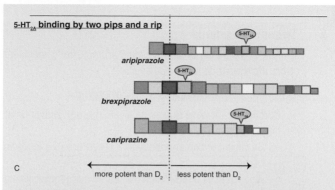

aripiprazole

brexpiprazole

cariprazine

C

more potent than D$_2$ | less potent than D$_2$

Figure 8.1 (cont.) The pips and rips are unique as they are partial D$_2$ agonists which means they are net partial antagonists when treating high dopaminergic states such as psychosis. They will lower dopaminergic neuronal firing partially, but not as aggressively as a full antagonist. In this diagram, it is a bit misleading as they have very high D$_2$ receptor affinity but they do not aggressively block D$_2$ receptors.

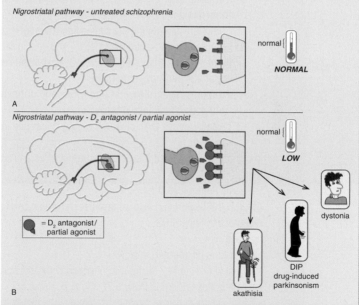

Nigrostriatal pathway - untreated schizophrenia

normal {

NORMAL

A

Nigrostriatal pathway - D$_2$ antagonist / partial agonist

normal {

LOW

= D$_2$ antagonist/ partial agonist

dystonia

DIP
drug-induced
parkinsonism

akathisia

B

Figure 8.2 How antipsychotics cause dystonia. (A) The nigrostriatal dopamine pathway is theoretically unaffected in untreated schizophrenia. (B) Blockade of D$_2$s prevents dopamine from binding there and can cause motor side effects such as drug-induced parkinsonism (tremor, muscle rigidity, slowing or loss of movement), akathisia (motor restlessness), and dystonia (involuntary twisting and contractions).

143

Two-minute tutorial

Can the combination of stimulant and antipsychotic agents lead to more movement disorder side effects?

Stimulants, antipsychotics, and dopamine

- Stimulants: increase dopamine levels through activation of the limbic system and cortex
  - Strongest action at dopamine-1 receptors (D_1) in the frontal cortex
  - Also robustly effect D_2s in the limbic and nigrostriatal areas
- In this case
  - Lisdexamfetamine (Vyvanse) (discontinued 40 mg daily in this case)
    - Prodrug of d-amphetamine
    - Becomes metabolically active after absorption by intestinal wall
    - Converted to d-amphetamine and L-lysine in the liver
    - D-amphetamine:
      - Competitively inhibits the dopamine transporter (DAT), norepinephrine transporter (NET), and vesicular monoamine transporter 2 (VMAT2) to prevent reuptake of dopamine and norepinephrine
      - Promotes rapid release of dopamine and norepinephrine from presynaptic nerve terminals
      - Likely reverses DAT, also increasing dopamine in the synapse
- Antipsychotics: antagonize D_2s, with strongest effects in the limbic system
  - Primarily antagonize D_2s
  - Atypical antipsychotics also antagonize serotonin 5-HT_{2A} receptors to lower EPS
- In this case
  - Risperidone (Risperdal) 4 mg/d
    - Typical dosing is 2–4 mg/d in children with psychosis
    - At this dose, there is likely a 70–80% D_2 occupancy
    - EPS occurs in a dose-dependent manner. The higher the dose, the greater the risk for EPS, especially if 80% or more occupancy
  - Olanzapine (Zyprexa) (prn dose of 5 mg on admission)
    - Moderate binding to D_2 resulting in possibly lower EPS risk compared to risperidone (Risperdal). Only clozapine (Clozaril), iloperidone (Fanapt), quetiapine (Seroquel), and lumateperone (Caplyta) have lower risk for EPS

- Stronger binding and antagonism to H1 (histamine), 5-HT$_{2C}$ (serotonin), and anticholinergic muscarinic receptors
- Risks of weight gain, hyperglycemia, sedation, dizziness, constipation, dry mouth, dyspepsia, etc., are elevated
  - Quetiapine (Seroquel) 400 mg/d
    - Typical dosages in children and adolescents:
      - Schizophrenia 400–800 mg/d
      - Bipolar mania 400–600 mg/d
    - Weaker antagonistic binding affinity for the D$_2$, this reduces risk for EPS
    - Strong antagonistic binding to H1 (histamine) and moderate binding to 5-HT$_{2C}$ allow for more sedation and increased appetite
    - Additive effects likely occurred with the atypical antipsychotics having overlapping half-lives and elevated plasma levels, allowing for greater D$_2$ blockade and EPS to occur

Combination may cause stimulant–antipsychotic syndrome

- Explains the interaction between stimulants and antipsychotics as related to their pharmacodynamic actions on the dopamine system
  - This interaction can actually increase risk for dystonic reactions
- Dopamine is released from the presynaptic terminal at a steady tonic or background level
- When these neurons are activated by a stimulus, they release a larger burst of dopamine into the synapse which activates postsynaptic receptors primarily directed toward motor behavior and also impacts the reward pathway
- Stimulants activate the dopamine system further by increasing tonic dopamine levels with presynaptic action
  - This can decrease the burst size needed to activate the postsynaptic receptors and eventually results in downregulation and likely supersensitivity of the postsynaptic receptors
- Antipsychotics also increase tonic dopamine activity but do this through postsynaptic action by blocking dopamine receptors. This will result in upregulation (increase) of the postsynaptic receptors
- Through these mechanisms, the combined use of stimulants and antipsychotics can create a state of further increased tonic dopamine activity and decreased burst size events
- In the case discussed above, the cause of the dystonic reaction may have been the result of discontinuing lisdexamfetamine (Vyvanse) in the setting of having scheduled lower risperidone

(Risperdal), increased quetiapine (Seroquel), and a dose of olanzapine (Zyprexa), continued after patient had been taking both lisdexamfetamine (Vyvanse) and risperidone (Risperdal) for many months

- Effectively, by discontinuing the stimulant, there was likely a decrease in the release of dopamine from the presynaptic neurons acutely, and with the continuation of the antipsychotics, the postsynaptic receptors continued to be blocked to a higher degree as available dopamine had lessened
- Several case reports show this can happen when adding, switching, or removing a stimulant or antipsychotic when used in combination, as in this case

Post-test question

What neurotransmitter system is routinely influenced by both antipsychotics and stimulants?

A. Norepinephrine
B. Serotonin
C. γ-aminobutyric acid (GABA)
D. Dopamine
E. Glutamate

Answer: D

The antipsychotic class typically will diminish dopamine firing in the nigrostriatal and mesolimbic pathways, and the stimulants will increase firing more so in the mesocortical and mesolimbic pathways. Therefore, they mostly share the dopaminergic system in common.

References

1. Gough, A, Morrison, J. Managing the comorbidity of schizophrenia and ADHD. *J Psychiatry Neurosci* 2016; 41:E79–E80
2. Guler, G, Yildirim, V, Kutuk, MO, et al. Dystonia in an adolescent on risperidone following the discontinuation of methylphenidate: a case report. *Clin Psychopharmacol Neurosci* 2015; 13:115–17
3. Masliyah, T, Ad-Dab'bagh, Y. Low-dose risperidone-induced oculogyric crises in an adolescent male with autism, Tourette's and developmental delay. *J Can Acad Child Adolesc Psychiatry* 2011; 20:214–16
4. Pliszka, SR. *Neuroscience for the Mental Health Clinician*, 2nd edn. New York: The Guilford Press, 2016

5. Slow, EJ, Lang, AE. Oculogyric crises: a review of phenomenology, etiology, pathogenesis, and treatment. *Mov Disord* 2017; 32:193–202

6. Stahl, SM. Preface. In Stahl, SM, Mignon, L. *Stahl's Illustrated Attention Deficit Hyperactivity Disorder.* Cambridge: Cambridge University Press, 2009

7. Stahl, SM. *Prescriber's Guide: Stahl's Essential Psychopharmacology*, 5. Cambridge: Cambridge University Press, 2005

8. Stahl, SM. *Prescriber's Guide: Stahl's Essential Psychopharmacology*, 5. Cambridge: Cambridge University Press, 2014

9. Stahl, SM. *Stahl's Essential Psychopharmacology: Neuroscientific Basis and Practical Applications*, 5. Cambridge: Cambridge University Press, 2021

10. Stahl, SM. *Stahl's Illustrated Violence: Neural Circuits, Genetics and Treatment.* Cambridge: Cambridge University Press, 2014

11. Yanofski, J. The dopamine dilemma: using stimulants and antipsychotics concurrently. *Psychiatry (Edgmont)* 2010; 7:18–23

Case 9: The one that came out of nowhere

The Question: How do you diagnose and treat covert dyskinesia (CD)?

The Psychopharmacological Dilemma: Permanent neuromuscular side effects are common

Hassaan Gomaa

Pretest self-assessment question

What is the most common atypical antipsychotic associated with CD?

A. Risperidone (Risperidal)
B. Olanzapine (Zyprexa)
C. Aripiprazole (Abilify)
D. Quetiapine (Seroquel)
E. Lurasidone (Latuda)

Patient evaluation on intake

- A 71-year-old female with a history of major depressive disorder (MDD) with a chief complaint of "worsening depression and anxiety" who was admitted to an inpatient unit due to severity of symptoms and being unable to care for herself
- Patient has financial stress, but unable to identify other issues of concern
- Reports frustration from her involuntary abnormal movements of her lips

Psychiatric history

- History of MDD symptoms for many decades
- Unable to remember when depressive symptoms started but endorsed a lifetime history of depressed mood, insomnia, decreased appetite, fatigue, psychomotor retardation, and passive suicidal thinking, which has been fluctuating in severity for years
- On admission, patient was taking the serotonin–norepinephrine reuptake inhibitor (SNRI), duloxetine (Cymbalta) 60 mg/d; a stimulant, methylphenidate (Ritalin) 10 mg/d; a benzodiaozepine (BZ) anxiolytic, clonazepam (Klonopin) 2 mg/d; and a benzodiazepine receptor agonist (BZRA) hypnotic, zolpidem (Ambien) 5 mg/d
- Methylphenidate (Ritalin) 10 mg/d was added to her psychotropic regimen 4 years prior to this admission due to extreme fatigue related to MDD, which improved significantly with this intervention
- Prior to this hospitalization, she had taken the atypical antipsychotic aripiprazole (Abilify) 5 mg/d for 2 years for augmentation of her

antidepressant regimen. It improved her depressive symptoms but had to be stopped 4 months before admission by the patient's neurologist due to left-sided resting tremors, which were felt to be extrapyramidal syndrome (EPS) symptoms
- Tremors resolved after discontinuation of aripiprazole (Abilify) but the patient developed repetitive involuntary movements in her tongue, lips, and jaw 2 months later
- Her tongue was protruding, lips smacking, and jaw had an involuntary chewing-like movement
- These movements hindered the patient from eating appropriately and she lost approximately 10 lb

Social and personal history

- Born and raised in Ohio
- Graduated high school and worked as a store clerk most of her life
- Married and living with husband who is her main support system
- Has four children who reside out of state but call her frequently
- She has no history of tobacco, alcohol, or illicit drug use

Medical history

- Coronary artery disease (CAD)
- Atrial fibrillation
- Hyperlipidemia
- Hypertension (HTN)
- Osteoporosis
- Diabetes mellitus type 2
- Obstructive sleep apnea (currently on continuous positive airway pressure with good compliance) (OSA)
- Peripheral neuropathy

Family history

- Denied family history of any psychiatric illness

Medication history

- Previous trial of tricyclic antidepressant (TCA) nortriptyline (Pamelor) but was unable to remember the dosage
- Trial of selective serotonin reuptake inhibitor (SSRI) antidepressant fluoxetine (Prozac) up to 80 mg/d for several months but was not helpful

Current medications

- Duloxetine (Cymbalta) 60 mg/d, an SNRI
- Methylphenidate (Ritalin) 10 mg/d, a stimulant
- Clonazepam (Klonopin) 2 mg/d, a BZ anxiolytic
- Zolpidem (Ambien) 5 mg/d, a BZRA hypnotic
- Amlodipine (Norvasc) 5 mg/d
- Atorvastatin (Lipitor) 40 mg/d
- Levothyroxin (Synthroid) 50 mcg/d
- Insulin aspart (NovoLog) 12 units three times per day
- Insulin glargine (Lantus) 50 units per night
- Aspirin 81 mg/d

Psychotherapy history

- Patient reported participating in cognitive behavioral therapy (CBT) in the past for 3–4 months but was no longer in therapy at admission
- Felt CBT did not help remarkably

Patient evaluation on initial visit

- Exacerbation of chronic MDD symptoms now
- Patient has been compliant with her psychotropic regimen
- Has good insight into her illness
- Complained of dyskinetic repetitive involuntary movements in her tongue, lips, and jaw 2 months after aripiprazole discontinuation, which really bothered her
- These are prominent during initial examination here as well

Further investigation

Is there anything else that you would like to know about the patient?

How severe are her movements? How should they be monitored?

- The Abnormal Involuntary Movement Scale (AIMS) is a 12-item clinician-rated scale used to assess dyskinesias in patients taking antipsychotic medications
- Items are scored from 0 (none) to 4 (severe)
- Patient's AIMS score before starting aripiprazole (Abilify) was 0
- Two months after stopping it, her AIMS score was 5 which suggests milder tardive dyskinesia (TD) now

How often to monitor?

- Every 12 months for atypical antipsychotics such as her aripiprazole (Abilify)
- Guidelines suggest monitoring her every 3 months now as she is high risk

Attending physician's mental notes: initial psychiatric evaluation

- Patient is depressed and using polypharmacy without much effectiveness now
- She is not imminently lethal but not functioning well
- Need to continue her inpatient stay

Question

Based upon her history so far, what would you do next?

- Maximize her SNRI duloxetine (Cymbalta)
- Augment or change her antidepressant

Case outcome: interim follow-up hospital week 1

- Mirtazapine (Remeron) 7.5 mg/d, a norepinephrine antagonist / selective serotonin antagonist antidepressant (NaSSA), was added as a combination strategy to the patient's SNRI regimen for better control of her MDD symptoms
- Aripiprazole (Abilify) was not restarted, and will need to avoid future antipsychotics given her movement disorder
- Methylphenidate (Ritalin) was also discontinued as there is worry that her nigrostriatal dopaminergic system is dysfunctional, with dyskinesia induced by aripiprazole (Abilify), and stimulants are known to cause tics and other movement disorders
- Her sedative and hypnotic are continued as her sleep and agitation from depression are controlled and sometimes these GABAergic agents help treat movement disorders or the anxiety patients have about the movements
- Patient showed moderate improvement regarding her mood, sleep, and appetite symptoms within several days
- With improved MDD, patient perceived the abnormal facial movements to be of minimal distress and refused medications (vesicular monoamine transporter 2 [VMAT2] inhibitors such as valbenazine [Ingrezza] and deutetrabenazine [Austedo]) to lower her TD symptoms
- She continued to have some minimal distress with eating
- Discharged home with partial MDD improvement and to continue her treatment as an outpatient

Attending physician mental notes: interim follow-up hospital week 1

- It seems that a successful SNRI and NaSSA antidepressant combination strategy is starting to become effective for her MDD
- Removing the atypical antipsychotic had improved her abnormal movements somewhat; perhaps time off the offending atypical antipsychotic will help further
- Will need outpatient team to follow with sequential AIMS examinations to see whether her movements resolve, especially her difficulty eating
- In clinical practice, it often seems that mood disorder patients not only acquire TD more often than schizophrenia (SP) patients, but also seem bothered more by the movements
  - Mood disorder patients seem to be bothered more by these abnormal movements and have greater loss of quality of life due to them
  - Suspect that SP patients, due to their negative symptomatology, may seem to lose interest in grooming, hygiene, and appearance or be less bothered in public by the movements
- It is likely, if her abnormal movements do not resolve, she will seek and be a good candidate for treatment with a VMAT2 inhibitor such as valbenazine (Ingrezza) or deutetrabenazine (Austedo)

Question

In your clinical experience, would you expect the patient's repetitive involuntary movements to disappear?

- Yes, they will completely disappear in 4–8 weeks
- They may disappear over several weeks to several years
- No, this kind of dyskinesia is more likely to persist much longer

Case debrief

- The inpatient team worked closely with the outpatient team and alerted them about the movements detected and suggested quarterly monitoring and assessment
- Over 3 months, many of the abnormal movements dissipated, but the patient was still bothered by milder jaw movements and chewing problems
- After consent, patient agreed to a trial of deutetrabenazine (Austedo) and saw a remission of her remaining dyskinesia symptoms
- She suffered some initial headaches which resolved with over-the-counter (OTC) pain medication acetaminophen (Tylenol)

- CD is a subtype of TD that appears typically 2 weeks after discontinuing or decreasing an antipsychotic's dose and lasts several weeks post cessation of an antipsychotic
  - It is felt that this patient fits the diagnostic entity

Take-home points

- Sometimes movement disorder is missed in the outpatient setting and the inpatient team must be astute and never assume that it has been addressed
- Any history of EPS such as akathisia or parkinsonism should alert the provider that TD is more likely over the long term
- There are now effective treatments for lowering TD so that all patients with these movements should be assessed, regardless of how acute or chronic their symptoms have been

Performance in practice: confessions of a psychopharmacologist

What could have been done better here?

- This short case illustrates that TD happens with the newer, safer atypical antipsychotics, as well as older typical ones

  - AIMS testing should occur annually or by any new provider working with the patient
  - Higher-risk cases should be assessed this way quarterly
  - The history of prior movement disorder suggests this more stringent testing was likely needed

What are possible action items for improvement in practice?

- Review movement disorders created by antipsychotic use and their respective treatments

  - Parkinsonism, dystonia, akathisia, neuroleptic malignant syndrome (NMS), tardive and other dyskinesias

Tips and pearls

What if there is not time for an AIMS examination?

- Ideally an AIMS is completed, start to finish, and a score is established and documented
- If time does not permit
  - Watch the patient as they walk to and from your office, down the hallway, looking for TD or EPS
  - During your session, scan the patient's extremities and face a few times

- During COVID, when masked, you may need to have the patient take off their mask
- During COVID, when using televideo you may need the patient to show you more than their face and shoulders to monitor for TD and EPS movements axially and with the extremities
- At a minimum, have them perform the finger tapping part of the AIMS with both hands as this seems to be sensitive in unmasking mild TD orofacially

Two-minute tutorial

Part 1 – tardive dyskinesia (TD)

Guidelines about using AIMS in patients taking antipsychotics

- It is recommended that AIMS is used to follow up regularly on patients taking antipsychotics as below:
  - Every 12 months for atypical antipsychotics
  - Every 6 months for typical antipsychotics
  - Every 3 months for high-risk patients
- Assessment and scoring are as mentioned above
- If AIMS score has increased from the previous visit, some possible interventions might be:
  - Discontinuing or reducing the antipsychotic medication dose
  - Changing to a less TD-prone antipsychotic such as quetiapine (Seroquel) or clozapine (Clozaril)
  - Requesting a neurology consult
  - Diagnosing TD and starting VMAT2 inhibitor
    - Valbenazine (Ingrezza)
    - Deutetrabenazine (Austedo)
- When do we need to conduct an AIMS?
  - Prior to starting an antipsychotic
  - Following up on patients taking antipsychotics as mentioned above
  - In a week after discontinuing antipsychotics, and once again after 3 months to avoid missing CD

Use of AIMS to aid the diagnosis of tardive dyskinesia (TD)

To diagnose TD, a patient needs to meet three criteria:

1. Being exposed for 3 months or more to an antipsychotic treatment
2. Must have moderate abnormal involuntary movements in one body part, or mild abnormal involuntary movements in two or more body parts
3. Should be an absence of conditions that can mimic TD

Abnormal Involuntary Movements Scale (AIMS)

- Is a validated and guideline-suggested examination scale that helps to identify TD and its severity
- Table 9.1 provides an example of this scale, in which a clinician asks the patient to perform several voluntary physical movements while observing for abnormal involuntary movements that might arise

Table 9.1 Abnormal Involuntary Movements Scale (AIMS)

Facial and oral movements	1. **Muscles of facial expression** e.g., movements of forehead, eyebrows, periorbital area, cheeks, including frowning, blinking, smiling, grimacing	01234
	2. **Lips and perioral area** e.g., puckering, pouting, smacking	01234
	3. **Jaw** e.g., biting, clenching, chewing, mouth opening, lateral movement	01234
	4. **Tongue** Rate-only increases in movement both in and out of mouth. NOT inability to sustain movement. Darting in and out of mouth	01234
Extremity movements	5. **Upper (arms, wrists, hands, fingers)** Include choreic movements (i.e., rapid, objectively purposeless, irregular, spontaneous) and athetoid movements (i.e., slow, irregular, complex, serpentine). DO NOT INCLUDE TREMOR (i.e., repetitive, regular, rhythmic)	01234
	6. **Lower (legs, knees, ankles, toes)** e.g., lateral knee movement, foot tapping, heel dropping, foot squirming, inversion and eversion of foot	01234
Trunk movements	7. **Neck, shoulders, hips** e.g., rocking, twisting, squirming, pelvic gyrations	01234
Global judgments	8. **Severity of abnormal movements overall**	01234
	9. **Incapacitation due to abnormal movements**	01234
	10. **Patient's awareness of abnormal movements.** Rate only patient's report	01234
	No awareness 0	
	Aware, no distress 1	
	Aware, mild distress 2	
	Aware, moderate distress 3	
	Aware, severe distress 4	
Dental status	11. **Current problems with teeth and/or dentures**	No Yes
	12. **Are dentures usually worn?**	No Yes
	13. **Edentia?**	No Yes
	14. **Do movements disappear in sleep?**	No Yes

- Items should be rated from 0 (none) to 4 (severe)
  - 1 is minimal or extreme normal, 2 is mild, and 3 is moderate
  - To assess patients accurately for abnormal movements, the following procedure has to be followed:
    - Patient should remove gum or any food in his/her mouth
    - Asking about the general condition of their teeth, dentures, or any lost teeth is important, and if problems exist this should be considered while scoring

- Patient should tell if there are any bothersome involuntary movements they notice
- Patient should be observed sitting in a firm chair with hands to the knees and feet flat on the floor while observing for movements
- Patient should next be observed with hands hanging without support
- Patient's open mouth should be observed twice, then ask patient to protrude their tongue during this exercise twice again to observe abnormal movements
- Patient's body should be observed while tapping thumb with each finger as rapidly as they can for 10–15 seconds. Here the key is not to observe the tapping but to scan the whole body for abnormal movements at the same time
- Next, flex patient's arms one at a time and observe for abnormal movements
- Next, ask the patient to stand, extend his/her arms with palms down, and finally to take a few steps back and forth and observe for abnormal movements

Risk factors for TD

Risk of developing TD increases with

- Both Caucasian and Black race
- Old age
- Female gender
- Having a mood disorder
- Longer duration of illness
- Longer duration of antipsychotic exposure
- Early EPS during exposure

Part 2 – covert dyskinesia (CD)

In the presented case above where the patient had reduced movements but not remission after 3 months, which subtype of TD do you think the patient has?

- Transient TD
- Withdrawal TD
- Covert dyskinesia (CD)
- Persistent TD

The patient should be diagnosed with covert dyskinesia (CD)

- CD is a form of TD where the abnormal movements appear approximately 2 weeks after antipsychotic withdrawal or dose reduction

- The difference between CD and a withdrawal dyskinesia is that CD persists for more than 8 weeks after antipsychotic cessation
- CD is also different from withdrawal dyskinesia as CD typically does not resolve spontaneously
- Risk factors for TD and ultimately CD are Caucasian and African descent, older age, female gender, history of mood disorders, and longer illness duration. (Most of these factors are present in this case)

Managing CD

- To date, evidence for CD treatment is obtained from case reports and a few review articles
- Off-label pharmacologic treatments for CD suggest that
  ○ Tetrabenazine (Xenazine) has been used in randomized trials and may allow dyskinesia improvement
  ○ Amantadine (Symmetrel), cyproheptadine (Periactin), and clonazepam (Klonopin) show partial improvement in case studies
- But, mainly, the scarce literature up until the last few years still suggests that reinstitution of the offending antipsychotic or starting another antipsychotic to mask the CD symptoms by creating parkinsonian stiffness and rigidity may be an option to lower CD severity
- Since there is no mention of TD-approved VMAT2 inhibitor trials in CD, and as CD is likely a precursor to TD, it is worth a trial in these patients suffering from drug-induced dyskinesia
- Newer approved agents for TD, such as valbenazine (Ingrezza) and deutetrabenazine (Austedo), have not been tested for CD patients yet, but it makes sense intuitively to use them

Valbenazine (Ingrezza) and deutetrabenazine (Austedo) for TD

- Valbenazine (Ingrezza)
  ○ Commonly causes sedation
  ○ Once-daily dosing
  ○ Higher doses can be associated with subtle QTc prolongation
  ○ Recommended starting dose is 40 mg/d which usually is increased to a maximum of 80 mg/d
  ○ It is metabolized via CYP2D6 and CYP3A4 enzymes so the recommended maximum dose in the presence of a strong CYP2D6 or CYP3A4 inhibitors is 40 mg/d

- Deutetrabenazine (Austedo)
  - Common side effects include sedation, dry mouth, diarrhea, and fatigue
  - Twice-daily dosing initially approved but an extended release once-daily dose is now available
  - QTc increases initially noted above 24 mg/d dosing but recent studies have shown less
  - Recommended starting dose is 12 mg/d in divided doses which can be up-titrated to a maximum of 48 mg/d if needed, but new once-daily preparations from 6 to 24 mg will be released
  - It is metabolized via CYP2D6 enzyme so the recommended maximum dose in patients taking a strong CYP2D6 inhibitor is 36 mg/d

Mechanism of action moment: VMAT2 inhibitors for TD

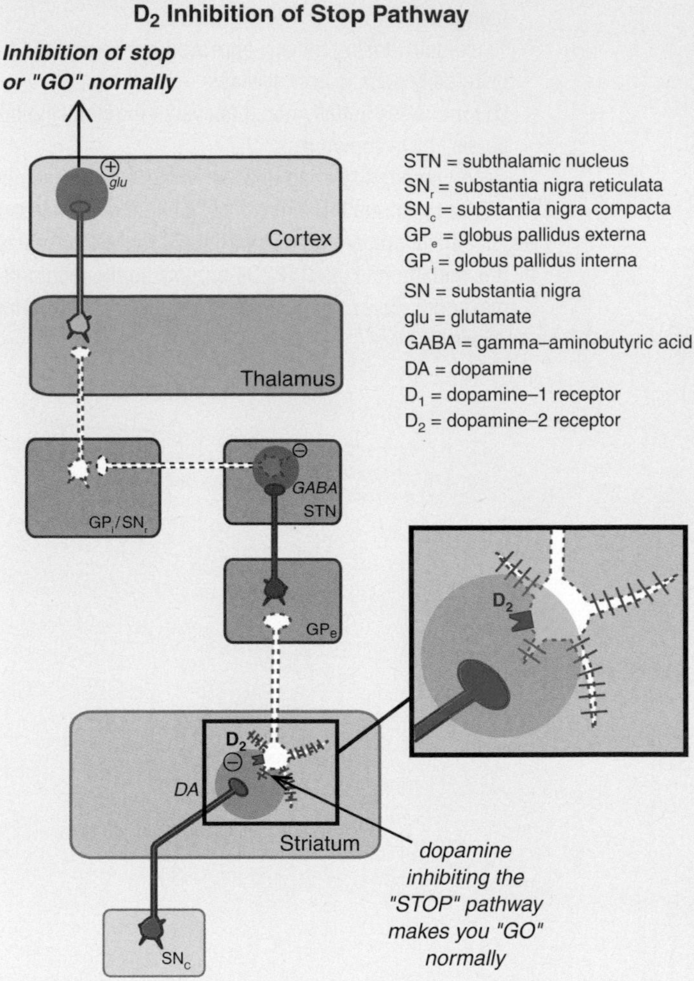

D_2 Inhibition of Stop Pathway

*Inhibition of stop
or "GO" normally*

Cortex

Thalamus

GP_i/SN_r

GABA
STN

GP_e

D_2

DA

D_2

Striatum

SN_c

STN = subthalamic nucleus
SN_r = substantia nigra reticulata
SN_c = substantia nigra compacta
GP_e = globus pallidus externa
GP_i = globus pallidus interna
SN = substantia nigra
glu = glutamate
GABA = gamma–aminobutyric acid
DA = dopamine
D_1 = dopamine–1 receptor
D_2 = dopamine–2 receptor

*dopamine
inhibiting the
"STOP" pathway
makes you "GO"
normally*

Figure 9.1 Dopamine-2 receptor (D_2) inhibition of the stop pathway. We must first understand normal functional neuroanatomy to better understand how TD, CD, and EPS side effects are generated. Dopamine released from the nigrostriatal pathway binds to postsynaptic D_2s on a γ-aminobutyric acid (GABA) neuron projecting to the globus pallidus externa. This causes inhibition of the indirect (stop) pathway, thus instead telling it to "GO." This is the normal mode and allows for smooth movements without dyskinesia, dystonia, athetosis, etc.

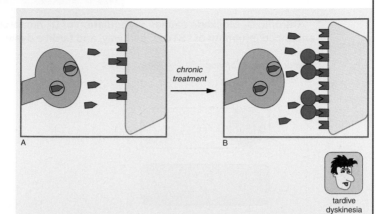

tardive
dyskinesia

Figure 9.2 Tardive dyskinesia. (A) Dopamine binds to D$_2$s in the nigrostriatal pathway. (B) Chronic blockade of D$_2$ by using antipsychotics in the nigrostriatal dopamine pathway can cause upregulation of those receptors, which can lead to CD and TD. This upregulation may alter the usual neurocircuitry noted in Figure 9.1.

Chronic D₂ blockade causes upregulation of D₂ receptors, enhanced inhibition of "STOP" pathway, and tardive dyskinesia

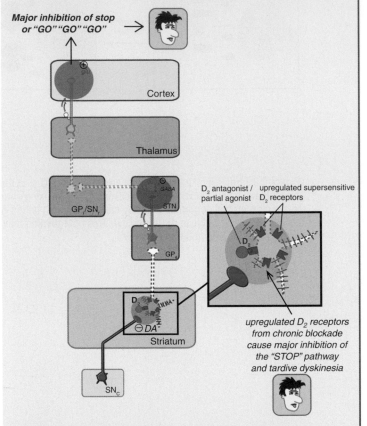

Figure 9.3 Chronic D₂ blockade and overinhibition of the stop pathway. Dopamine released from the nigrostriatal pathway is blocked from binding to postsynaptic D₂s by antipsychotics on GABA neurons projecting to the globus pallidus externa. Chronic blockade of these receptors can lead to their upregulation; the upregulated receptors may also be "supersensitive" to dopamine. Dopamine can now exert its inhibitory effects in the indirect (stop) pathway, and in fact cause so much inhibition of the "STOP" signal that the "GO" signal is now overactive, leading to the hyperkinetic involuntary movements of tardive dyskinesia. This neural circuit is now corrupted, leading to abnormal movements.

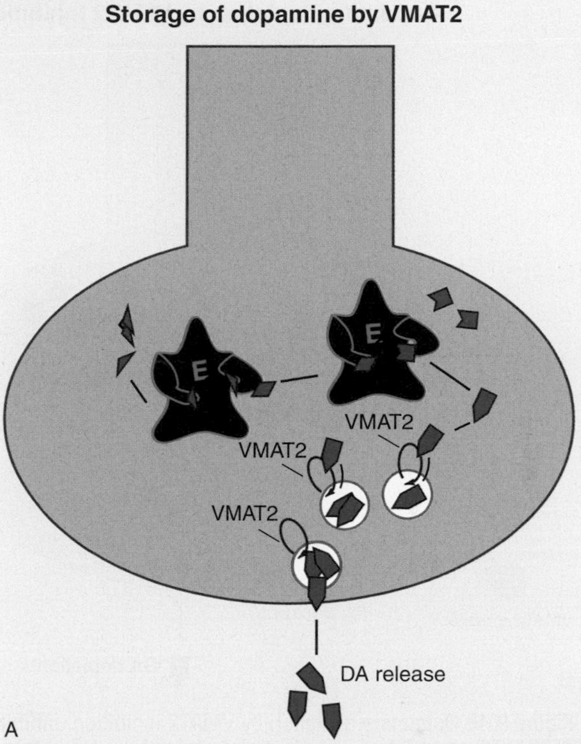

Storage of dopamine by VMAT2

A

Figure 9.4A VMAT2 and dopamine. In order to better understand how VMAT2 inhibitors help to treat TD, and likely CD, we must understand the VMAT2 system and its usual function and role. The VMAT2 is an intraneuronal transporter located on synaptic vesicles. VMAT2 takes intraneuronal monoamines, including dopamine, up into the synaptic vesicles so that they can be stored until they are needed for release during neurotransmission.

Dopamine depletion by VMAT2 inhibition

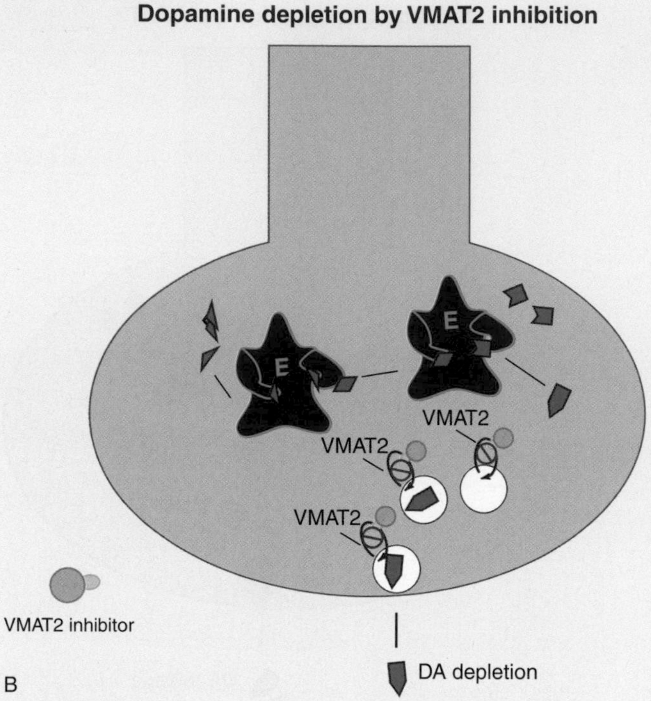

Figure 9.4B Dopamine depletion by VMAT2 inhibition. Inhibition of VMAT2 treats TD as it prevents dopamine from being taken up into synaptic vesicles. The intraneuronal dopamine is therefore catabolized, leading to depletion of dopamine stores. By removing this extra dopamine from synapsis where upregulated, supersensitive D_2 receptors exist after long-term D_2 blockade, a normal amount of dopamine/D_2 activation occurs, and abnormal TD movements dissipate as burst firing of these neurons lowers.

Post-test question

What is the most common atypical antipsychotic associated with CD?

A. Risperidone (Risperidal)

B. Olanzapine (Zyprexa)

C. Aripiprazole (Abilify)

D. Quetiapine (Seroquel)

E. Lurasidone (Latuda)

Answer: C

Interestingly, CD seems to be associated more with aripiprazole (Abilify) than with other atypical antipsychotics, and the majority of CD cases in the past 20 years are of patients taking this atypical antipsychotic. The process is still unclear but it is theorized that this atypical antipsychotic is associated with higher rates of acute akathisia compared to others and is a risk for and precursor of TD. Case reports suggest that CD is more likely to be preceded by akathisia. For an unknown reason, aripiprazole (Abilify) has the most case reports in the literature. Perhaps this is due to the high affinity of aripiprazole (Abilify) for the D_2, or due to the fact that it is one of the most commonly used atypicals and has more use and opportunity for side effects to develop and be reported in the literature.

References

1. American Psychiatric Association. *Diagnostic and Statistical Manual of Mental Disorders: DSM-5*, 5th edn. Arlington, VA: American Psychiatric Publishing, Inc., 2013

2. Braude, WM, Barnes, TR. Late-onset akathisia – an indicant of covert dyskinesia: two case reports. *Am J Psychiatry* 1983; 140:611–12

3. Burris, KD, Molski, TF, Xu, C, et al. Aripiprazole, a novel antipsychotic, is a high-affinity partial agonist at human dopamine D_2 receptors. *J Pharmacol Exp Ther* 2002; 302:381–9

4. Chang, S, Lin, Y, Pan, Y. Covert dyskinesia associated with aripiprazole: a case report. *Taiwanese Journal of Psychiatry* 2019; 33:172–3

5. Fernandez, HH, Factor, SA, Hauser, RA, et al. Randomized controlled trial of deutetrabenazine for tardive dyskinesia: the ARM-TD study. *Neurology* 2017; 88:2003–10

6. Fernandez, HH, Stamler, D, Davis, MD, et al. Long-term safety and efficacy of deutetrabenazine for the treatment of tardive dyskinesia. *J Neurol Neurosurg Psychiatry* 2019; 90:1317–23

7. Gardos, G, Cole, JO, Tarsy, D. Withdrawal syndromes associated with antipsychotic drugs. *Am J Psychiatry* 1978; 135:1321–4

8. Gomaa, H, Mahgoub, Y, Francis, A. Covert dyskinesia with aripiprazole: tip of the iceberg? A case report and literature review. *J Clin Psychopharmacol* 2021; 41:67–70

9. Guy, W. *ECDEU Assessment Manual for Psychopharmacology*, revised edn. Rockville, MD: US Dept. of Health, Education, and Welfare, Public Health Service, Alcohol, Drug Abuse, and Mental Health Administration, National Institute of Mental Health, Psychopharmacology Research Branch, Division of Extramural Research Programs, 1976

10. Moseley, CN, Simpson-Khanna, HA, Catalano, G, et al. Covert dyskinesia associated with aripiprazole: a case report and review of the literature. *Clin Neuropharmacol* 2013; 36:128–30

11. Patra, S. Tardive dyskinesia and covert dyskinesia with aripiprazole: a case series. *Curr Drug Saf* 2016; 11:102–3

12. Schooler, NR, Kane, JM. Research diagnoses for tardive dyskinesia. *Arch Gen Psychiatry* 1982; 39:486–7

13. Solmi, M, Pigato, G, Kane, JM, et al. Clinical risk factors for the development of tardive dyskinesia. *J Neurol Sci* 2018; 389:21–7

14. Stahl, SM. *Stahl's Essential Psychopharmacology: Neuroscientific Basis and Practical Applications*, 5. Cambridge: Cambridge University Press, 2021

15. Touma, KTB, Scarff, JR. Valbenazine and deutetrabenazine for tardive dyskinesia. *Innov Clin Neurosci* 2018; 15:13–16

Case 10: Darth Vaper strikes again

The Question: What are the treatment options to reduce rehospitalization for schizophrenia in the setting of treatment resistance?

The Psychopharmacological Dilemma: How to manage treatment in the setting of side effects and adverse events

Sutanaya Pal and Daniel Jackson

Pretest self-assessment question

Which is part of the criteria for treatment-resistant schizophrenia (TRS)?

A. At least two past treatments, each consisting of at least 3 weeks at a therapeutic dose

B. At least one past treatment at a therapeutic dose, with at least 80% of prescribed doses taken

C. At least two past treatments, each consisting of at least 6 weeks at a therapeutic dose

D. Gray matter decrease on imaging significantly higher compared to other schizophrenia patients

E. Ineffective response to clozapine (Clozaril)

Patient evaluation on intake

- A 34-year-old male patient with a history of schizophrenia since age 19, with ongoing psychotic symptoms for the past 6 weeks
- Refusing the atypical antipsychotic paliperidone long-acting injectable (LAI) (Invega Sustenna) 234 mg injections for the past 2 months
- Psychotic symptoms include delusions with paranoid themes, and auditory hallucinations
- The hallucinations are congruent with paranoid delusional content of being monitored by outside forces
- He has negative symptoms such as amotivation and blunted affect

Psychiatric history

- First-break psychosis and first hospitalization occurred at age 21
- No history of depressive or manic episodes
- No history of suicide attempts or suicidal ideation
- Treated with risperidone (Risperdal) at first hospitalization and was discharged on 4 mg/d
  - Discontinued it after a few weeks

- Required another hospitalization within the year, where another atypical antipsychotic, olanzapine (Zyprexa), was initiated and titrated to 20 mg/d, but it was only partially effective
- Subsequent hospitalizations resulted in adequate trials of another atypical, aripiprazole (Abilify), followed by typical antipsychotic haloperidol (Haldol)
- Hospitalizations typically yield a modest antipsychotic response, but patient often continues to be symptomatic and only able to stay out of the hospital for brief periods of time
- For the past 5 months, he had been treated with paliperidone LAI (Invega Sustenna) at 234 mg each month
  - Unfortunately, he has refused injections for the past 2 months

Social and personal history

- Lives at home with parents
- High school graduate
- Unemployed, on disability
- No history of abuse or trauma
- Smokes one pack of cigarettes daily since age 19. Cannabis use of ½ gram 2–3 times per week for the past 5 years

Medical history

- Borderline hypertension

Family history

- Mother has a history of major depressive disorder (MDD)
- Father has a history of bipolar disorder (BP), cannabis use disorder (CUD), and alcohol use disorder (AUD)
- Paternal grandfather with schizoaffective disorder, depressive type likely

Medication history

- Risperidone (Risperdal) 4 mg/d which he discontinued after a few weeks
- Olanzapine (Zyprexa) 20 mg/d, which was partially effective
- Aripiprazole (Abilify) 30 mg/d – partially effective
- Haloperidol (Haldol) 10 mg/d – partially effective
- Paliperidone LAI (Invega Sustenna) 234 mg / 4 weeks – near remission of positive symptoms before patient discontinued

Current medications

- None

Psychotherapy history

- He received some supportive psychotherapy while in hospital and attended various psychotherapy groups as well
- Attended 1–2 sessions with an outpatient therapist before discontinuing therapy

Patient evaluation on initial visit

- Patient now has concerns of "being monitored by computer and phone cameras," starting 6 weeks ago
- Increased isolation noted by family, with frequent refusal to leave his room
- Admits auditory hallucinations of "Big Brother" notifying the patient that he is being monitored
- On the day of hospitalization, the parents called 911 after the patient smashed all electronics in the house as a result of internal stimuli and delusional thinking
- Urine drug screen is negative for all substances, including cannabis

Question

Based on what you know about this patient's history and symptoms, what would you do next?

- Start electroconvulsive therapy (ECT)
- Start clozapine (Clozaril) monotherapy
- Start amisulpride (Solian) monotherapy
- Combine ECT and clozapine (Clozaril) dual therapy
- Start typical antipsychotic fluphenazine (Prolixin) LAI

Attending physician's mental notes: initial psychiatric evaluation

- While ECT has been evaluated as an intervention for treatment-resistant schizophrenia (TRS), there is insufficient evidence of whether it is any more effective than clozapine (Clozaril)
    - ECT is often more effective for people with schizophrenia with affective symptoms, which this patient does not have
- Sometimes clozapine (Clozaril) and ECT dual therapy can be effective
    - Many of these studies evaluate dual therapy in patients who are already resistant to clozapine (Clozaril) monotherapy
- Typical guidelines suggest ECT as an adjunctive treatment if an antipsychotic monotherapy fails to help resolve psychosis
- Amisulpride (Solian) is an atypical antipsychotic not available in the United States

- o It does have evidence supporting its use in overall symptom management (positive, negative, and depressive symptoms) in "multi-episode" schizophrenia
  - • It cannot be obtained for this patient unfortunately
- The patient has a long history of minimal or partial response to a variety of antipsychotics indicating clear treatment resistance despite relatively good compliance (except for this admission)
- TRS is an indication for clozapine (Clozaril) in this patient

Further investigation

Is there anything else that you would like to know about the patient?

- Does he have any significant medical problems?
  - o Medical history indicates no significant cardiac or neurological history, but rechecking for any history of arrhythmia, cardiomyopathy, or seizures is warranted, along with repeat EKG (to check his QTc). Clozapine (Clozaril) has a small effect on the QTc (<10 seconds at clinical doses)
  - o He has no cardiac conditions after evaluation
- What about his history of cannabis use?
  - o He has no recent use per patient and family, and urine screen is negative
- Is he safe to start clozapine (Clozaril) based upon baseline blood absolute neutrophil counts (ANC)?
  - o ANC is within normal limits

Attending physician's mental notes: initial psychiatric evaluation (continued)

- This patient has several admissions for ongoing psychotic symptoms
- He has never been psychosis free
- He has tried a few atypical antipsychotics and one typical antipsychotic and, despite adequate trials, continues with this difficult relapsing pattern
- He is treatment resistant and likely deserves a trial of clozapine (Clozaril) as it has been shown to be effective when other agents fail to help fully
- Outside of this admission he has been medication compliant so will hold off on using an LAI for now

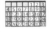

Case outcome: interim follow-up visits from 1 to 3 weeks

- Clozapine (Clozaril) was initiated per usual titration after consent
- Titrated up to 450 mg/d

- ° At this dose, there was a remission of auditory hallucinations and paranoid delusions
- ° He continued to have a blunted affect but appeared more motivated and active than before
- ° Trough plasma level was 550 ng/mL
- Weekly ANC monitoring remained normal and above 1500/microliter
- Patient was discharged to his parents' home with outpatient follow-up for continued monitoring

Case outcome: interim follow-up visit at 5 weeks

- Patient was taken to the ER by his parents
- Despite apparent medication compliance, the delusions and auditory hallucinations returned
- The patient was hospitalized again, and usual clozapine (Clozaril 450 mg/d) continued

Question

What do you think caused the relapse of symptoms?

- Drop in plasma clozapine (Clozaril) levels due to medication non-compliance
- Drop in plasma levels due to other medications and drug–drug interactions
- Drop in plasma levels due to cigarette smoking
- Exacerbation of symptoms due to cannabis use
- Psychotic symptoms secondary to organic or medical causes

Attending physician's mental notes at follow-up visit (week 5)

- The most appropriate step at this point would be to measure his plasma clozapine (Clozaril) level now
  - ° Loss of efficacy may be due to a drop in plasma levels which can be caused by several factors
    - ▪ Medication non-compliance
    - ▪ CYP1A2 enzyme-inducing medications may have been started
    - ▪ Cigarette (nicotine) smoking may have started or increased
- Both patient and family report that he had been compliant on his medications and had not been taking any other medications
- He has been abstinent from illicit substances
- While in hospital previously, he was maintained on a nicotine (NicoDerm CQ) patch
  - ° When clozapine (Clozaril) was started while he was in the hospital, he was not actively smoking

- ○ However, on discharge from the hospital, he resumed smoking
  - ▪ This likely caused his clozapine (Clozaril) plasma blood levels to drop as nicotine patches tend not to induce CYP1A2 while cigarettes do
- Given the above information, it would be appropriate to titrate his dose up by even perhaps 30% toward 600 mg/d with close clinical and plasma level monitoring

Case outcome: interim follow-up at 8 weeks

- The patient's dose was increased gradually to 600 mg/d with good compliance, tolerability, and response in the hospital. His positive symptoms remitted fully with partial improvement in his amotivation. He continued to have a blunt affect
- Plasma trough levels of clozapine (Clozaril) were approximately 570 ng/mL at steady state
- He was discharged from the hospital after a few days at these levels
- However, he was brought to the ER again by his parents, a few days after discharge, with complaints of drooling, excessive sedation (he was sleeping most of the day and stumbling in the hallways), and not oriented to time, place, or person
- Per parents, he had been compliant on his medications and had continued to smoke

Question

What do you now think resulted in his symptoms above?

- Intentional overdose on clozapine (Clozaril)
- Use of nicotine vaping
- Hepatic dysfunction
- Relapse in cannabis use
- Medication non-compliance

Attending physician's mental notes: follow-up visit (week 8)

- Suspect we are back to an issue with cigarette use changing his hepatic 1A2 metabolism through non-compliance or re-emergence of cannabis use disorder (CUD) is possible
- We seemingly had psychotic symptom remission, which is excellent, but things falling apart clinically when the patient goes home

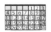

Case outcome: interim follow-up at 8 weeks (continued)

- Further history reveals that the patient had decided to quit smoking cigarettes at home and switched to vaping nicotine instead
- He took his clozapine (Clozaril) as prescribed

- History, examination, and lab findings reveal no signs of hepatic dysfunction
- Urine drug screen was negative as well

Question

How is vaping different from smoking cigarettes where clozapine (Clozaril) is concerned?

- The electronic nicotine delivery systems (or ENDSs) are a variable group of devices used for vaporizing (Vaping)
  - Of note, ENDS have a lower emission of polycyclic aromatic hydrocarbons (PAHs) than normal cigarettes
  - This is of special importance, as it is PAHs that induce CYP1A2, which controls clozapine (Clozaril) metabolism, and not nicotine itself
- Switching to ENDSs is equivalent to quitting smoking (or starting a nicotine patch) as far as clozapine (Clozaril) plasma levels are concerned
  - When his cigarette smoking stopped and vaping started, it resulted in a quick rise in clozapine (Clozaril) plasma levels and a remarkable increase in clinical side effects for the patient
  - His CYP450 1A2 enzyme activity lowered and he could not catabolize clozapine excessively anymore
  - Common dose-dependent adverse effects of clozapine (Clozaril) to watch for include sedation and hypersalivation, both of which this patient developed
- Clozapine (Clozaril) dose was decreased to 450 mg/d again
  - Steady-state trough levels then lowered to an improved 530 ng/mL
  - Adverse effects resolved
  - He was counseled to remain off cigarettes or get in touch with his outpatient doctor if his nicotine frequency of use changes or his type of nicotine used changes
  - Vaping cessation will likely need to be addressed later with this patient

Case debrief

- While the exact definition of TRS is variable, there is a general consensus among available guidelines
  - Studies which followed patients with first-episode psychosis estimate the prevalence of treatment resistance at 23–33%
  - Most studies show that a majority of those who are treatment resistant appear to be so from the beginning of their illness, advocating for earlier use of clozapine (Clozaril)

- To have TRS, there must be a failure of two adequate trials (of 6–8 weeks, therapeutically dosed) of antipsychotics
  - Treatment with clozapine (Clozaril) has been shown to decrease psychotic symptoms significantly when other agents have failed, and, additionally, lower the risk of suicidal behavior and suicide attempts (independent from antipsychotic activity)
  - Guidelines may differ on the type of antipsychotic utilized but most agree that at least one of them should be an atypical antipsychotic
- The patient was a good candidate for clozapine (Clozaril) as he had failed multiple adequate trials of other antipsychotics
- Clozapine (Clozaril) dosage, adverse effects, investigations, and monitoring were pivotal in determining why he would relapse after remission of psychotic symptoms despite clear compliance and adherence with this treatment
- One factor while prescribing clozapine (Clozaril) is the patient's smoking status, where clozapine (Clozaril) levels are over one-third lower in smokers compared to non-smokers
- Olanzapine (Zyprexa) is the other antipsychotic that is metabolized by the CYP1A2 enzyme. A meta-analysis indicated that plasma levels of olanzapine are different for smokers and non-smokers to the extent that non-smokers require a 30% dose reduction
- Some of the antipsychotics not affected by smoking include aripiprazole (Abilify) and risperidone (Risperdal) (metabolized by CYP2D6 and CYP3A4, respectively), quetiapine (Seroquel) (CYP3A4), ziprasidone (Geodon) (aldehyde oxidase and CYP3A4), and paliperidone (Invega) (glucoronidization)
- Other treatments to consider if clozapine (Clozaril) is not effective include:
  - ECT monotherapy
  - ECT/clozapine (Clozaril) combination
  - Aripiprazole (Abilify) / clozapine (Clozaril) dual therapy
  - Use of an LAI plus olanzapine (Zyprexa)

Take-home points

- The PAHs found in cigarettes decrease plasma levels of clozapine (Clozaril) due to induction of the CYP1A2 isoenzyme that is primarily responsible for its metabolism
- Nicotine replacement products such as patches and gums do not affect antipsychotic levels
- ENDSs such as e-cigarettes or vaping devices are also considered to not significantly affect levels

- Plasma levels, urine drug screens, and family corroborative history about compliance are essential in determining why psychotic relapses occur

Performance in practice: confessions of a psychopharmacologist

What could have been done better here?

- Doses of clozapine (Clozaril) greater than 500 mg/d may often require a split dose to mitigate side effects and keep peak plasma drug levels lower
  - While this would not have necessarily prevented the side effects the patient experienced, it may have lessened them
- A careful interview and informed consent regarding nicotine use habits (cigarettes, patches, vaping devices) may have helped to predict and avoid the clinical problems encountered prior to discharge
- Table 10.1 reviews common drug–drug interactions clinicians should watch for

Table 10.1 Overview of cytochrome P450 enzymes

Note that patients have inherited their ability to process medications based on their liver's ability to metabolize drugs to inactive metabolites and be excreted. Approximately 10–15% of all patients will have difficulty processing medications that pass through the 1A2 system, such as clozapine (Clozaril) in this case. Cigarette smoking will increase the activity and efficiency of 1A2, making patients process certain drugs faster, thus lowering plasma levels and effectiveness

Cytochrome P450 enzyme, and extent of activity in the human GI tract	Basic facts	Moderate/strong inducers	Ultrarapid phenotypes
CYP3A4: 30% of all hepatic cytochrome activity, 70% of all gut cytochrome activity	Chromosome 7 Relatively few functional polymorphisms Low affinity / high capacity enzyme	Carbamazepine Efavirenz Nevirapine Oxcarbazepine Phenobarbital Phenytoin Rifampin	Yes, rare
CYP2D6: 20% of all hepatic cytochrome activity, but only 1–2% by weight	Chromosome 15 Multiple polymorphisms High affinity / low capacity enzyme	Not inducible	Ethiopian 29% Saudi 19% Spanish 10% Italian 8.3% US White 3.5%
CYP2C9: 20% of liver cytochrome activity (in combination with 2C19)	Chromosome 10 Multiple polymorphisms	Carbamazepine Efavirenz Lopinavir Nelfinavir Nevirapine Phenobarbital Phenytoin Rifampin Ritonavir	Unclear whether this phenotype exists

Table 10.1 (Cont.)

Cytochrome P450 enzyme, and extent of activity in the human GI tract	Basic facts	Moderate/strong inducers	Ultrarapid phenotypes
CYP1A2: 10–15% of all CYP450 activity	Chromosome 15 Multiple polymorphisms Low affinity / high capacity enzyme Located only in the liver	Cigarette smoke (but not vaping) Omeprazole	No However, a variant (CYP1A2*1F) exists that increases the inducing effects of smoking

Tips and pearls

- Cigarettes are among a bevy of other factors that can alter clozapine (Clozaril) levels
- Had this patient been a woman, potentially taking an oral contraceptive pill (OCP), use would need to be considered, as ethinylestradiol-containing OCPs may increase clozapine (Clozaril) levels. The ethinylestradiol component of OCPs primarily affects clozapine (Clozaril) levels through inhibition of CYP1A2
- CYP1A2, CYP3A3/4, and CYP2D6 inhibitors or inducers must be considered when dosing clozapine (Clozaril). Among psychotropics, some SSRIs (fluoxetine, paroxetine, and to some extent citalopram) and the NDRI (bupropion) inhibit these enzymes
- Carbamazepine (Tegretol) induces CYP3A4 which rapidly clears other medications

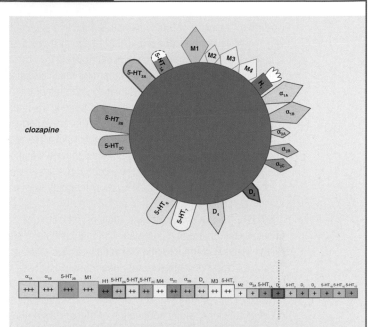

Figure 10.1 Clozapine's unique pharmacological icon and binding profile may explain its effectiveness. This figure portrays a qualitative consensus of current thinking about the binding properties of clozapine. In addition to 5-HT$_{2A/D_2}$ antagonism, numerous other binding properties have been identified for clozapine, most of which are more potent than its binding at the D$_2$. It is unknown which of these ultimately contribute to clozapine's special efficacy in TRS or to its unique side effects. Some postulate that it is weaker at D$_2$ agonism and greater for D$_4$ receptors, or that the pairing of D$_1$/ D$_2$ weak antagonism may allow for some alleviation of negative symptoms (or at least not triggering iatrogenic ones). There seems to be a greater amount of noradrenergic activity with clozapine use which may be a combination of α$_{2a}$ receptor antagonism as well. Of course, using the serotonin hypothesis of schizophrenia suggests that clozapine can lower psychotic symptoms by way of fairly aggressive 5-HT$_{2A}$ receptor antagonism as well.

Two-minute tutorial

- While there is burgeoning research on the augmentation of clozapine (Clozaril) with ECT, clozapine (Clozaril) monotherapy remains the gold standard for TRS, and it is the only antipsychotic associated with decreased suicide in schizophrenia patients and has specific FDA labeling as such

- The threshold for response to clozapine (Clozaril) is often 350 ng/mL, with levels up to 1000 ng/mL sometimes necessary for those who do not respond to lower levels and have not developed intolerability. A level of 1000 ng/mL is the point of futility for clozapine. The point of futility can be defined as the point beyond which only an insignificant proportion of patients would benefit from raising the dose for those who can tolerate it

- While neutropenia (low ANC levels) garners much attention, other severe adverse effects must be screened and monitored for: myocarditis, paralytic ileus, seizures, and pulmonary embolism
- A Cochrane review comparing clozapine (Clozaril) to other atypical antipsychotics showed that while clozapine (Clozaril) had a higher efficacy, patients being treated with it also showed a higher quit rate due to adverse effects. Nonetheless, *continuous* use of clozapine (Clozaril) is associated with a 44% lower mortality from natural and unnatural causes
- The CATIE (Clinical Antipsychotic Trials of Intervention Effectiveness) trial was a landmark National Institute of Mental Health trial that compared atypical antipsychotics (olanzapine [Zyprexa], ziprasidone [Geodon], risperidone [Risperdal], and quetiapine [Seroquel]) with the typical antipsychotic perphenazine (Trilafon). Olanzapine (Zyprexa) showed the greatest efficacy as measured by time to discontinuation of therapy, even though it had a higher incidence of metabolic side effects. Interestingly, perphenazine (Trilafon) had comparable efficacy and was the most cost-effective drug
  - However, since the trial was only for 18 months, it did not investigate longer-term motor symptoms such as tardive dyskinesia, which is among the main concerns with typical antipsychotics and certainly occurs with atypicals as well
  - At least six other atypical antipsychotics have been released since this study and it is unknown how they would compare
  - In phase 2, clozapine (Clozaril) was used for those who discontinued the first drug due to efficacy reasons, and it was found to be more effective than the other agents
- When studies have varying, relaxed classifications of treatment resistance, the benefits of clozapine (Clozaril) for TRS are obscured. However, if rigorous criteria for treatment resistance are used, clozapine demonstrates superiority over other antipsychotics
- The usual stringent criteria were developed by Kane et al., who state that in addition to a minimum treatment time frame and doses of multiple antipsychotics, a prospective trial of haloperidol (Haldol) should be conducted before treatment resistance is determined
  - If the "modified Kane criteria" are used, the benefits of clozapine (Clozaril) over other antipsychotics are clearly seen, with response rates greater than or equal to 40%, compared to less than 5% for other antipsychotics

- Marder and Yang state that the "exact mechanism of clozapine's antipsychotic action remains unknown." Despite the structures of loxapine (Loxitane), olanzapine (Zyprexa), and quetiapine (Seroquel) being similar to clozapine (Clozaril) (olanzapine [Zyprexa] and quetiapine [Seroquel] are actually derived from clozapine [Clozaril]), none has matched the efficacy of clozapine (Clozaril). Theories are discussed in the caption to Figure 10.1 above
- Up to one-third of those with schizophrenia will go on to have treatment resistance similar to the case presented here
- TRS entails ongoing psychosis despite trials and failures with at least two adequate trials of antipsychotics
- Clozapine (Clozaril) monotherapy is the gold standard for TRS; however, a subset of these patients will be resistant to clozapine (Clozaril) monotherapy
- Augmentation with ECT is increasingly studied. The latest iteration of guidelines recommends ECT as an adjunctive treatment but warns against an increased frequency of headaches and memory impairments with the combination
- Despite the efficacy of clozapine (Clozaril), it is underutilized due to concern for significant, life-threatening adverse effects as well as the need for periodic blood monitoring, a challenge for patients with poor compliance
- In addition to monitoring for adverse effects, care must be taken with concurrent use of medications or substances that can significantly affect plasma levels of clozapine

Post-test question

Which is part of the criteria for treatment-resistant schizophrenia?

A. At least two past treatments, each consisting of at least 3 weeks at a therapeutic dose
B. At least one past treatment at a therapeutic dose, with at least 80% of prescribed doses taken
C. At least two past treatments, each consisting of at least 6 weeks at a therapeutic dose
D. Gray matter decrease on imaging significantly higher compared to other schizophrenia patients
E. Ineffective response to clozapine (Clozaril)

Answer. C

At least two past treatments of at least 6 weeks at a therapeutic dose are part of the consensus criteria for TRS. Adherence of at least 80% is required for at least two of the past treatments. There is emerging neuroimaging evidence that TRS patients have decreased gray matter volume compared to those who are treatment-responsive, but this has not yet become an established criterion to define treatment resistance. Ineffective response to clozapine (Clozaril) characterizes those who are "ultra-treatment resistant." These are patients who met criteria for treatment resistance and then failed an adequate trial of clozapine (Clozaril).

References

1. Asenjo Lobos, C, Komossa, K, Rummel-Kluge, C, et al. Clozapine versus other atypical antipsychotics for schizophrenia. *Cochrane Database Syst Rev* 2010; CD006633
2. Bozzatello, P, Bellino, S, Rocca, P. Predictive factors of treatment resistance in first episode of psychosis: a systematic review. *Front Psychiatry* 2019; 10:67
3. Demjaha, A, Lappin, JM, Stahl, D, et al. Antipsychotic treatment resistance in first-episode psychosis: prevalence, subtypes and predictors. *Psychol Med* 2017; 47:1981–9
4. Gillespie, AL, Samanaite, R, Mill, J, et al. Is treatment-resistant schizophrenia categorically distinct from treatment-responsive schizophrenia? A systematic review. *BMC Psychiatry* 2017; 17:12
5. Glasser, AM, Collins, L, Pearson, JL, et al. Overview of Electronic Nicotine Delivery Systems: a systematic review. *Am J Prev Med* 2017; 52:e33–e66
6. Granfors, MT, Backman, JT, Laitila, J, et al. Oral contraceptives containing ethinylestradiol and gestodene markedly increase plasma concentrations and effects of tizanidine by inhibiting cytochrome P450 1A2. *Clin Pharmacol Ther* 2005; 78:400–11
7. Grover, S, Sahoo, S, Rabha, A, et al. ECT in schizophrenia: a review of the evidence. *Acta Neuropsychiatr* 2019; 31:115–27
8. Howes, OD, McCutcheon, R, Agid, O, et al. Treatment-resistant schizophrenia: Treatment Response and Resistance in Psychosis (TRRIP) Working Group consensus guidelines on diagnosis and terminology. *Am J Psychiatry* 2017; 174:216–29
9. Huhn, M, Nikolakopoulou, A, Schneider-Thoma, J, et al. Comparative efficacy and tolerability of 32 oral antipsychotics for the acute treatment of adults with multi-episode schizophrenia: a systematic review and network meta-analysis. *Focus (Am Psychiatr Publ)* 2020; 18:443–55
10. Kane, J, Honigfeld, G, Singer, J, et al. Clozapine for the treatment-resistant schizophrenic: a double-blind comparison with chlorpromazine. *Arch Gen Psychiatry* 1988; 45:789–96

11. Keepers, GA, Fochtmann, LJ, Anzia, JM, et al. The American Psychiatric Association practice guideline for the treatment of patients with schizophrenia. *Am J Psychiatry* 2020; 177:868–72

12. Lally, J, Ajnakina, O, Di Forti, M, et al. Two distinct patterns of treatment resistance: clinical predictors of treatment resistance in first-episode schizophrenia spectrum psychoses. *Psychol Med* 2016; 46:3231–40

13. Marder, SR, Yang, YS. Clozapine. In Schatzberg, AF, Nemeroff, CB, eds. *The American Psychiatric Association Publishing Textbook of Psychopharmacology*. Arlington, VA: American Psychiatric Publishing, Inc. 2017.

14. McEvoy, JP, Lieberman, JA, Stroup, TS, et al. Effectiveness of clozapine versus olanzapine, quetiapine, and risperidone in patients with chronic schizophrenia who did not respond to prior atypical antipsychotic treatment. *Am J Psychiatry* 2006; 163:600–10

15. Meyer, JM, Stahl, SM. *The Therapeutic Threshold and the Point of Futility*. Cambridge: Cambridge University Press, 2021, 34–59

16. Meltzer, HY, Alphs, L, Green, AI, et al. Clozapine treatment for suicidality in schizophrenia: International Suicide Prevention Trial (InterSePT). *Arch Gen Psychiatry* 2003; 60:82–91

17. Meyer, JM, Stahl, SM. *The Clozapine Handbook: Stahl's Handbooks*. Cambridge: Cambridge University Press, 2019

18. Prior, TI, Baker, GB. Interactions between the cytochrome P450 system and the second-generation antipsychotics. *J Psychiatry Neurosci* 2003; 28:99–112

19. Saffari, AA, Daher, N, Ruprecht, AA, et al. Particulate metals and organic compounds from electronic and tobacco-containing cigarettes: comparison of emission rates and secondhand exposure. *Environ Sci Process Impacts* 2014; 16(10):2259–67

20. Schatzberg, A, Nemeroff, C. *The American Psychiatric Association Publishing Textbook of Psychopharmacology*, 5. Arlington, VA: American Psychiatric Publishing, Inc., 2017

21. Sinclair, DJM, Zhao, S, Qi, F, et al. Electroconvulsive therapy for treatment-resistant schizophrenia. *Schizophr Bull* 2019; 45:730–2

22. Singh, H, Dubin, WR, Kaur, S. Drug interactions affecting clozapine levels. *J Psychiatr Intensive Care* 2015; 11:52–65

23. Smith, T, Mican, L. What to do when your patient who takes clozapine enters a smoke-free facility. *Curr Psychiatry* 2014; 13:47–8, 57

24. Stahl, SM. *Stahl's Essential Psychopharmacology: Neuroscientific Basis and Practical Applications*, 5. Cambridge: Cambridge University Press, 2021

25. Swainston Harrison, T, Perry, CM. Aripiprazole: a review of its use in schizophrenia and schizoaffective disorder. *Drugs* 2004; 64:1715–36

26. Taylor, D, Paton, C, Kapur, S. *The Maudsley Prescribing Guidelines in Psychiatry*, 11th edn. Chichester: Wiley-Blackwell, 2012

27. Tiihonen, J, Taipale, H, Mehtälä, J, et al. Association of antipsychotic polypharmacy vs monotherapy with psychiatric rehospitalization among adults with schizophrenia. *JAMA Psychiatry* 2019; 76:499–507

28. Tiihonen, J, Vartiainen, H, Hakola, P. Carbamazepine-induced changes in plasma levels of neuroleptics. *Pharmacopsychiatry* 1995; 28:26–8

29. Tsuda, Y, Saruwatari, J, Yasui-Furukori, N. Meta-analysis: the effects of smoking on the disposition of two commonly used antipsychotic agents, olanzapine and clozapine. *BMJ Open* 2014; 4:e004216

30. Vermeulen, JM, van Rooijen, G, van de Kerkhof, MPJ, et al. Clozapine and long-term mortality risk in patients with schizophrenia: a systematic review and meta-analysis of studies lasting 1.1–12.5 years. *Schizophr Bull* 2019; 45:315–29

31. Wagner, E, Löhrs, L, Siskind, D, et al. Clozapine augmentation strategies – a systematic meta-review of available evidence. Treatment options for clozapine resistance. *J Psychopharmacol* 2019; 33:423–35

32. Wagner, E, McMahon, L, Falkai, P, et al. Impact of smoking behavior on clozapine blood levels – a systematic review and meta-analysis. *Acta Psychiatr Scand* 2020; 142:456–66

33. Wang, G, Zheng, W, Li, XB, et al. ECT augmentation of clozapine for clozapine-resistant schizophrenia: a meta-analysis of randomized controlled trials. *J Psychiatr Res* 2018; 105:23–32

34. Youn, T, Jeong, SH, Kim, YS, et al. Long-term clinical efficacy of maintenance electroconvulsive therapy in patients with treatment-resistant schizophrenia on clozapine. *Psychiatry Res* 2019; 273:759–66

Case 11: First-time Mom's struggle with postpartum post-traumatic stress disorder (PTSD)

The Question: What do you do when postpartum PTSD is resistant to treatment?

The Psychopharmacological Dilemma: Finding an effective regimen for postpartum PTSD with comorbid depression

Sabahath Shaikh

Pretest self-assessment question

Which of the following treatments for PTSD has the most compelling outcomes for lowering core PTSD symptoms?
A. Clonidine (Catapres)
B. Prazosin (Minipress)
C. Quetiapine (Seroquel)
D. Sertraline (Zoloft)

Patient evaluation on intake

- A 24-year-old female with a chief complaint of "I have these nightmares"
- Was doing fine until the birth of her baby 8 months ago
- Nervous, traumatized due to birth experience, and scared for future pregnancies

Psychiatric history

- Suffered no major psychiatric symptoms until the birth of her infant
- Was scheduled for vaginal delivery under epidural anesthesia but ended up going into C-section under general anesthesia as epidural did not work and she had failure to progress
  - She suffered from anesthesia awareness and was able to feel pain, hear, and remember events that happened during the C-section
- Anxiety symptoms developed after this event
  - Has not been able to sleep due to nightmares, flashbacks related to delivery. Is hypervigilant and tries to avoid triggers related to trauma
  - Has anxiety and fear about future pregnancies
- Admits to full depressive symptoms
  - Guilt about not being able to care for her family, hopeless about future pregnancies, fatigued, amotivated, decreased appetite and sleep

- Now finds herself worrying about "everything, all the time," feels irritable, restless, cannot focus, and is tense. She was not a "worrier" prior
- Additionally, she can barely leave her house
  - Has panic attacks just thinking about running errands by herself
  - Finds it difficult to attend family gatherings and rushes back home
  - Feels being negatively judged in public by others but is not delusional
- Stays at home more and feels her husband has been very supportive throughout

Social and personal history

- Graduated with bachelor's degree in accounting
- Currently a stay-at-home Mom but was working part-time in retail
- Spouse is employed and they have no financial difficulties currently
- Does not use drugs or alcohol

Medical history

- 10 lb of weight gain during pregnancy
- C-section 8 month ago
- No acute or chronic medical issues

Family history

- Denies any known mental illness in any family member

Medication history

- Was trialed on the selective serotonin reuptake inhibitor (SSRI) sertraline 25 mg/d and had possible seizure activity
- Her primary care provider recommended genetic testing and she was found to have CYP2D6 "poor metabolizer" status
- Later her primary care provider prescribed her a benzodiazepine (BZ) sedative anxiolytic clonazepam (klonopin) 0.5 mg/d as needed for anxiety. Patient stopped taking after few days considering the negative side-effect profile of medication
- Currently on desvenlafaxine (Pristiq) 25 mg/d, a serotonin–norepinephrine reuptake inhibitor (SNRI)
  - Perhaps seeing a 10% improvement in symptoms of anxiety and depression despite the subtherapeutic dosing
    - Feels less irritable and panicky
    - Continues to experience nightmares, flashbacks
    - She still gets anxious thinking about stepping out of the house

Current medications

- Desvenlafaxine (Pristiq) 25 mg/d
- Melatonin 3 mg/d

Psychotherapy history

- Recently, started a few sessions of outpatient trauma-focused therapy with an adept clinician
- Has noticed mild improvement with this intervention, and is hopeful

Patient evaluation on initial visit

- Acute onset of PTSD symptoms with associated symptoms of major depressive disorder (MDD) with postpartum onset and generalized anxiety disorder (GAD) roughly 8 months ago
  - It is possible that the MDD and GAD are solely driven by and manifestations of her PTSD as she had no clear premorbid dysfunction in these areas
- Now has elevated anxiety while interacting with friends and being in public as she feels judged
  - This seems more guilt-based ideation, possibly from depression rather than social anxiety fearing embarrassment
- Has been non-compliant with medication management for various reasons, mostly due to the possibility and worry about developing side effects
- Reports no current side effects from desvenlafaxine (Pristiq)
- Has started eye movement desensitization and reprocessing (EMDR) therapy
- Good insight regarding illness and wants to get better

Question

Do you expect a patient with these symptoms to recover?

- Yes, she had no mental health disorder prior to delivery, and she has been suffering for only a short term – several months now
- No, sometimes a traumatic event can cause chronic PTSD with chronic, unremitting depression

Attending physician's mental notes: initial psychiatric evaluation

- This patient recently experienced traumatic labor and is experiencing likely postpartum PTSD as a result
- She seems to suffer from major MDD with postpartum onset too, which seems greater than the cognitive–emotional change usually afforded to PTSD-driven symptoms

- It seems her anxiety and depression stem clearly from her trauma as she was highly functional before delivery without any symptoms
- Genetic testing revealed she is a CYP2D6 poor metabolizer so she may tolerate some medications poorly unless dosing is kept low
- She has recently been started on a sub-therapeutic SNRI and continues with EMDR therapy, fostering a good prognosis hopefully
- Responsibility of caring for her infant given her current symptoms is concerning. However, her spouse is supportive and helps with childcare

Question

Which of the following would be your next step?

- Increase the desvenlafaxine (Pristiq) to the therapeutic US Food and Drug Administration (FDA) dose of 50 mg/d for MDD despite treating her for PTSD, and encourage her to be compliant
- Increase the melatonin to a higher, more effective dose for insomnia
- Augment the current medications with a third agent to accelerate response
- Do nothing additionally outside of waiting for the low-dose SNRI and EMDR therapy effectiveness to occur

Attending physician's mental notes: initial psychiatric evaluation (continued)

- Patient currently seems to be on a standard approach to treating comorbid PTSD with its resultant depression and anxiety
- She failed initial trial on SSRI due to side effects but was never on therapeutic dose
- Currently started on low dose of an SNRI with plan to titrate
  - The SNRI is approved for treating MDD, and theoretically has the same serotonergic potential as the approved SSRI products for alleviating PTSD symptoms
  - Also, this SNRI will have no issue with her 2D6 enzyme system as it is not metabolized further by this pathway
- Patient receiving EMDR therapy
- This looks like a good prognosis as she is less irritable and denies any current side effects
- However, she needs to continue to be compliant with her medications
- Her insomnia is also a concern, as that can exacerbate her anxiety and depression
- Does meet criteria for PTSD with comorbid MDD and think her GAD symptoms may be better ascribed to agitation components driven by both her MDD and PTSD

PATIENT FILE

Further investigation

Is there anything else that you would like to know about the patient?

What about details concerning past medication treatment and current EMDR therapy?

- Had taken sertraline (Zoloft) 25 mg/d and clonazepam (Klonopin) 0.5 mg/d for 15 days – both subtherapeutic in nature
  - Did not tolerate sertraline (Zoloft) well and had seizures after taking for 10 days
  - Tolerated clonazepam (Klonopin) well but discontinued given its possible addictive properties, which she was worried about
- Started EMDR 2 months ago
  - Follows up weekly and has had eight sessions so far
  - She has a good rapport with her therapist and notices mild improvement
  - The therapist has a good reputation

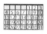

Case outcome: first interim follow-up visit at 4 weeks

- She is not compliant with her medications and forgets to take them daily
- Encouraged to set up phone reminders and educated on importance of medication compliance
- She has noticed mild improvement in her symptoms of MDD and no change in PTSD symptoms
- She has no side effects and is hopeful to notice improvement with improved compliance
- She now has attended more EMDR therapy sessions

Question

Would you consider continuing her current medications or change strategies?

- Yes, continue both desvenlafaxine (Pristiq) and melatonin at same doses
- Continue desvenlafaxine (Pristiq) at a higher dose but keep melatonin as is
- Continue melatonin at higher dose as only change
- Continue desvenlafaxine (Pristiq) at current dose given her non-compliance, and add prazosin (Minipress), a norepinephrine α_1 receptor antagonist for her nightmares
- No, discontinue both agents as they have now failed to allow for a clinical response and start a new regimen

Case outcome: second interim follow-up visit at 8 weeks

- She is more compliant with her medications and reports no current side effects
- Desvenlafaxine (Pristiq) is increased to 50 mg/d and she tolerates well
- MDD symptoms remit except for insomnia and psychomotor agitation, but these may be attributable more to PTSD rather than to residual MDD symptoms
- She continues with nightmares and flashbacks regarding her delivery, unfortunately
- She now has attended more EMDR therapy sessions

Attending physician's mental notes: second interim follow-up visit (week 8)

- Patient seems to be doing very well and is no longer depressed
- PTSD continues
  - She may need a higher dose of her SNRI
  - She may need better insomnia and agitation control
- Continuing with comorbid PTSD is a risk factor for an MDD relapse if not addressed
- EMDR seems helpful regarding the emotional and cognitive aspects of her PTSD but not the reliving and hyperarousal symptoms

Question

Would you consider continuing her current medications or change strategies?

- Yes, continue both desvenlafaxine (Pristiq) and melatonin at same doses
- Continue desvenlafaxine (Pristiq) at a higher dose but keep melatonin as is
- Continue melatonin at higher dose as only change
- Add prazosin (Minipress) for nightmares
- Add an atypical antipsychotic for agitation
- Add a BZ for insomnia/agitation

Case outcome: third interim follow-up visit at 12 weeks

- Desvenlafaxine (Pristiq) is increased to 100 mg/d and reliving events have improved remarkably but insomnia is increased now
- MDD symptoms continue in remission except for insomnia, which is likely side effect-based
- Outside of side effect-based insomnia, she has slight increase in blood pressure now at 140/90 mmHg on several measures during the week

Attending physician's mental notes: third interim follow-up visit (week 12)

- Patient seems to be doing very well and is no longer depressed and most of her PTSD has improved
- Remarkable and worsening insomnia continues and she still reports nightmares
- Continuing with comorbid PTSD is a risk factor for an MDD relapse if not addressed
- Patient given options of increasing melatonin at bed, adding a hypnotic, adding prazosin (Minipress) for nightmares, or adding an atypical antipsychotic for insomnia/agitation

Case outcome: fourth interim follow-up visit at 16 weeks

- Desvenlafaxine (Pristiq) is continued at 100 mg/d as her key monotherapy given her near remission of symptoms
- Melatonin increased to 10 mg/d without improvement and is discontinued
- Zolpidem (Ambien), a benzodiazepine receptor agonist (BZRA) hypnotic is used 5–10 mg/d for insomnia with good effect now, but the patient begins sleepwalking
  - Insomnia and nightmares now are alleviated
- MDD symptoms continue in remission
- Blood pressure remains borderline elevated

Attending physician's mental notes: fourth interim follow-up visit (week 16)

- MDD and PTSD seem remitted, which is excellent
- Has side effects of somnambulism and borderline hypertension
- Often, blood pressure will normalize over a few months on SNRI medications
- The sleepwalking is concerning and distressing to the patient
- Patient given options of adding another BZRA hypnotic, adding a sedating antidepressant, or adding an atypical antipsychotic for insomnia/agitation
  - Might consider doxepin (Silenor), an antihistamine hypnotic, or a dual orexin antagonist hypnotic such as suvorexant (Belsomra), lemborexant (Dayvigo), or daridorexant (Quuiviq)

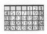

PATIENT FILE

Case outcome: fifth interim follow-up visit at 20 weeks

- Desvenlafaxine (Pristiq) is continued at 100 mg/d
- Doxepin (Silenor) 6 mg/d, a low-dose tricyclic antidepressant (TCA) which is approved for insomnia and is antihistaminergic at low doses, is used for insomnia but she awakens with a hangover effect and discontinues
- Suvorexant (Belsomra), a DORA, 10 mg/d is started but she develops headaches
- Lemborexant (Dayvigo), a DORA, is started and she reports restorative sleep, minimal nightmares and has no side effects while taking 5 mg/d
  ○ PTSD felt to be in remission
- MDD symptoms continue in remission
- Blood pressure seems to be lowering without treatment

Case debrief

- This patient had comorbid PTSD and MDD that, despite side-effect burden, seems to have reached remission of both disorders
- Interestingly, it was later determined that the patient is a CYP2D6 poor metabolizer which may explain some of her side-effect sensitivity, and starting desvenlafaxine (Pristiq) was a good choice as it avoids the P450 enzymatic system.
  ○ It undergoes oxidative N-demethylation via cytochrome P4503A4 to a minor extent. CYP2D6 is not involved in the metabolism of desvenlafaxine (Pristiq)
- Patient was non-compliant with her medications due to fear of side effects, which improved
- She developed greater insomnia as a side effect, which was mitigated by attempting to use different hypnotic agents until one with minimal, to no, side effects was utilized, and her nightmares greatly diminished as well

Take-home points

- Depressive and anxiety disorders are often comorbid
- Remission is generally felt to occur when both disorders are fully remitted, as residual symptoms of either likely create relapse and recurrence in the other disorder
- It is often more important to assess and mitigate adverse effects as a key intervention to keep a patient on their medication, so that a good therapeutically dosed trial can be continued for an adequate duration of time

Performance in practice: confessions of a psychopharmacologist

What could have been done better here?

- Sometimes it is difficult to tell which patients are side-effect sensitive due to their worry and expectations about getting side effects vs. their possible real pharmacokinetic inability to process medications via hepatic degradative metabolism
- Pharmacogenetic testing is not warranted in every patient (exc. CYP450 2D6 testing) but perhaps can be used earlier in those with medication sensitivities

What are possible action items for improvement in practice?

- Review which antidepressants require active CYP2D6 activity to be metabolized
- Use lower drug dosing in those who may be sensitive

Tips and pearls

- Regardless of whether a patient is psychologically or biologically sensitive to a prescribed medication, two skill sets may be used both to improve their expectations and to lower suffering by way of systemic side effects
- First, consider starting the dose below what the FDA says
  - For example, the use of the SSRI sertraline (Zoloft) is approved to start at 50 mg/d
  - Clinically, it may make sense to explain this to the patient: that you, as a clinician, *prefer a safer*, more conservative approach where you usually start your patients on a *tiny* dose, *way below* what the FDA suggests, so that the patient and his/her body can *get used to it more gradually* and that you find many day-to-day side effects tend to happen much, *much* less often
  - This sets the clinician to be seen as benevolent and truly looking out for the patient which aids in rapport building, and patients will be more forgiving if side effects do occur
  - This likely changes the patient's expectations from thinking they *will definitely* get side effects over to *maybe thinking they won't*
  - By starting doses lower for a few days like this, you build trust and can reduce side effects if the patient is worried and getting psychological nocebo side effects, and if they truly are CYP2D6 or other enzyme deficient the much lower dose is likely the correct dose and may be pushing towards therapeutic as the patient cannot process and metabolize the drug
  - Remember that lower than usual doses are usually not therapeutic and likely delay time to onset and symptom relief

- ○ Finally, even tiny doses can have a robust placebo effect and up to 40% of our patients may actually respond to lower doses and have fewer side effects
- Second, consider micro-titrating the most sensitive patients
  - ○ Take the example above to a further extreme, where you can often use a liquid drug preparation and start at an even lower dose
  - ○ Using sertraline (Zoloft) as above, it comes in a 25 mg tablet as the lowest strength and perhaps, if it is scored, it can be snapped in half to 12.5 mg/d, or quartered down to 6.25 mg/d
  - ○ The liquid solution of this medication comes in a 20 mg/mL version
  - ○ A patient can be issued a 1 mL (1 cc) syringe without a needle and can draw up one-tenth of a mL (cc) which is about 2 mg of drug, where they can increase by one-tenth of a cc every few days
  - ○ Not only can you use a lower than normal dose, you can microtitrate or use an eye dropper essentially to deliver a much, much, much smaller dose
  - ○ Psychologically, this is very powerful in convincing the patient you are kind and caring and gives them very fine control over dose escalation in a very graded fashion

Mechanism of action moment

Promoting sleep

To promote sleep

Enhance
▼ GABA

Inhibit
◯ hypocretin/orexin
◇ acetylcholine
◣ dopamine
▶ norepinephrine
⬚ serotonin
⊚ histamine

insomnia

asleep

deficient arousal   excessive arousal

Figure 11.1 Promoting sleep. To treat insomnia, one can administer medications that enhance the sleep drive, such as the GABAergic BZs or Z drugs. The primary action of these drugs is to increase the effectiveness and activity of the sleep center of the brain called the ventrolateral preoptic area (VLPO). Alternatively, one can administer medications that reduce arousal by inhibiting neurotransmission involved in wakefulness. If we remove wakefulness drive, the net effect is to become fatigued and then somnolent. Antagonists at orexin OX1 R/OX2 R (suvorexant and lemborexant) and histamine (doxepin) H1 receptors have this particular effect.

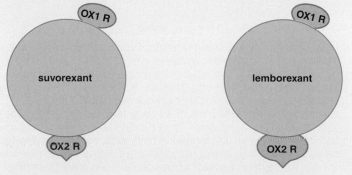

Figure 11.2 Orexin receptor antagonists.The dual orexin receptor antagonists suvorexant (Belsomra) and lemborexant (Dayvigo) are shown here. Suvorexant has comparable affinity for orexin 1 (OX1 R) and orexin 2 (OX2 R) receptors, while lemborexant has higher affinity for OX2 R than for OX1 R.

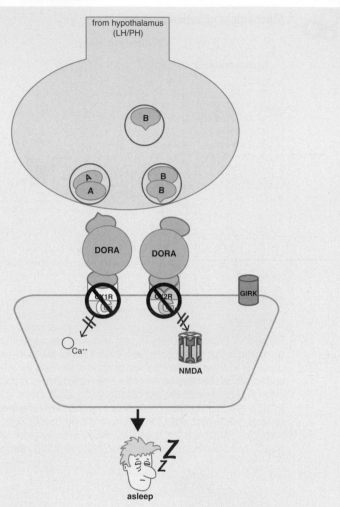

Figure 11.3 Blockade of orexin receptors. Orexin neurotransmission is mediated by two types of postsynaptic receptors, orexin 1 (OX1 R) and orexin 2 (OX2 R). OX1 R are particularly expressed in the noradrenergic locus coeruleus, which suggests that activity here may potentiate increased noradrenergic activity to promote wakefulness. OX2 R are highly expressed in the histaminergic tubero-mammillary nucleus (TMN) where, similarly, histamine activity may be stimulated to promote further wakefulness. Theoretically, the orexin system may serve as a backup in case the noradrenergic or histaminergic wakefulness systems falter; orexin can boost their activity to avoid falling asleep at inopportune times during the day. Furthermore, blockade of the wakefulness/arousal-promoting orexin receptors by dual orexin receptor antagonists (DORAs) prevents the excitatory effects and fatigue and somnolence may occur. Finally, blockade of OX2 R leads to decreased expression of NMDA (N-methyl-D-aspartate) glutamate receptors which may further lower arousal to help promote sleep.

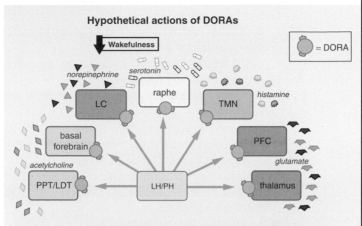

Hypothetical actions of DORAs

Figure 11.4 Hypothetical actions of dual orexin receptor antagonists (DORAs). By blocking orexin receptors, and particularly orexin 2 receptors, DORAs prevent orexin from promoting the release of other wake-promoting neurotransmitters. Above, we discussed the actions of orexin lowering or noradrenergic and histaminergic activity, but orexin blockade may also lower activity in other arousal centers of the brain where acetylcholine, serotonin, and other neurotransmitter activity may also be dampened to lower wakefulness and arousal.

Two-minute tutorial

PTSD pharmacotherapy

- Although some treatments, such as certain SSRIs, are approved for PTSD, psychopharmacological treatments for PTSD are not as effective as these same treatments when used in other disorders
- Often, patients with traumatic histories will require more psychotherapy-driven treatment protocols, given the relative ineffectiveness of medication-based PTSD treatments
- The selective serotonin reuptake inhibitors (SSRIs) paroxetine (Paxil) and sertraline (Zoloft) are the only well-studied FDA approvals, and when they fail to provide PTSD remission, then many off-label, less studied approaches may be needed
- Also, PTSD is so highly comorbid that many of the psychopharmacological treatments are more effectively aimed at comorbidities such as depression, insomnia, substance abuse, and pain, than at the core symptoms of PTSD, often leaving the patient with residual symptoms and on polypharmacy
- BZs are to be used with caution for treating PTSD agitation, hyperarousal, and insomnia
  - There is limited evidence from clinical trials for efficacy in PTSD
  - Many PTSD patients abuse alcohol and other substances

- Antihistamines may be repurposed
  - Hydroxyzine (Vistaril) is approved for anxiety neurosis and is often used as a pre-anesthetic
    - It is sedating, removes arousal, and can improve sleep and hyperarousal and vigilance
  - Quetiapine (Seroquel), an atypical antipsychotic, is also sedating in this manner
    - It further antagonizes serotonin 2a receptors ($5\text{-}HT_{2A}$) to promote deeper sleep, and antagonizes dopamine-2 receptors (D_2s) to provide a calming effect
  - Likely has the most compelling data of any atypical antipsychotic for use in PTSD but brexpiprazole (Rexulti) is under active investigation as well
- Antihypertensives may be repurposed
  - α_1 antagonists (prazosin [Minipress]) may be used at night to prevent nightmares specifically
  - α_2 agonists (clonidine [Catapres]) may be used for agitation
- Experimental use of techniques to block reconsolidation of emotional memories with the combination of psychotherapy and drugs (especially MDMA/ecstasy) are in testing now

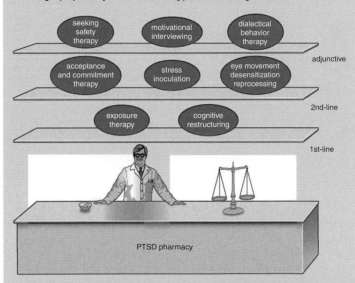

Figure 11.5 This image shows the range of psychotherapy approaches that should be considered for treating patients with PTSD. As noted, medication outcomes for PTSD tend to be lower than for other disorders in general, and patients should be informed that combining psychotherapy and medications is likely warranted in most cases. Those therapies outlined on the lowest shelf have the most supportive evidence regarding positive outcomes in PTSD.

Post-test question

Which of the following treatments for PTSD has the most compelling outcomes for lowering core PTSD symptoms?

A. Clonidine (Catapres)

B. Prazosin (Minipress)

C. Quetiapine (Seroquel)

D. Sertraline (Zoloft)

Answer: D

Sertraline is one of the only approved medications for PTSD and is the most correct answer. Paroxetine is the other approval. Prazosin has very focused data for treating nightmares only in PTSD, but the overall data seems to be equivocal. Clonidine is often used for its sedating/calming effects and in lieu of riskier BZ sedatives, but it has very little supporting evidence. Quetiapine is an atypical antipsychotic with smaller controlled studies that shows some effectiveness, but it is not officially approved for use.

References

1. Abdallah, CG, Averill, LA, Akiki, TJ, et al. The neurobiology and pharmacotherapy of posttraumatic stress disorder. *Annu Rev Pharmacol Toxicol* 2019; 59:171–89

2. Canfield, D, Silver, RM. Detection and prevention of postpartum posttraumatic stress disorder: a call to action. *Obstet Gynecol* 2020; 136:1030–5

3. Dekel, S, Ein-Dor, T, Dishy, GA, et al. Beyond postpartum depression: posttraumatic stress–depressive response following childbirth. *Arch Womens Ment Health* 2020; 23:557–64

4. Hamblen, JL, Norman, SB, Sonis, JH, et al. A guide to guidelines for the treatment of posttraumatic stress disorder in adults: an update. *Psychotherapy (Chic)* 2019; 56:359–73

5. Stahl, SM. *Stahl's Essential Psychopharmacology: Neuroscientific Basis and Practical Applications*, 5. Cambridge: Cambridge University Press, 2021

6. Watkins, LE, Sprang, KR, Rothbaum, BO. Treating PTSD: a review of evidence-based psychotherapy interventions. *Front Behav Neurosci* 2010; 12:258

Case 12: Why so down?

The Question: What is the cause of the sexual problems?

The Psychopharmacological Dilemma: How to diagnose and manage sexual side effects of antidepressants

Sutanaya Pal

Pretest self-assessment question

Which of the following are a common cause of sexual problems in patients with depression?
A. Decreased libido due to depression
B. Relationship problems
C. Sexual side effects of antidepressants
D. Comorbid medical or neurological problems
E. All of the above

Patient evaluation on intake

- A 38-year-old man with a recurrent major depressive disorder (MDD) and sexual problems (decreased libido, and delayed ejaculation)
- Admitted for depression in the context of a recent abrupt increase in social isolation
- Was recently tapered from previous antidepressant due to absence of depressive symptoms (remission of several months) and reported sexual side effects he could not tolerate
- His previous depressive symptoms had included depressed mood, anhedonia leading to social withdrawal, and loss of interest in outdoor activities which he had enjoyed before. Early morning awakening and poor appetite were also noted. Also suffered from fatigue, trouble focusing on tasks, and feeling worthless, leading to recurrent thoughts of suicide

Psychiatric history

- Has carried diagnoses of generalized anxiety disorder (GAD), MDD, opioid use disorder (OUD)
- Multiple hospitalizations for suicidal ideation in past but nothing recent
- One past suicide attempt

Social and personal history

- Grew up with parents
- While his childhood on the surface was described as "good," his presentation was significant for difficulties surrounding appropriate development regarding separation–individuation
- Completed high school
- Substance use
  - Smokes cigarettes
  - Occasional alcohol use
  - OUD on maintenance buprenorphine (Subutex)
    - Abstinent for 2 years
- Currently on social security disability but works random odd jobs when able
- Is currently in a stable relationship with his girlfriend

Medical history

- History of hypertension, hypercholesterolemia
- Lower back pain, with neurological symptoms such as urinary retention that now requires him to self-catheterize

Family history

- No significant family psychiatric history

Medication history

- Had been on multiple medications in the past including lurasidone (Latuda), risperidone (Risperidal), trazodone (Desyrel)
- No history of psychosis, despite being on multiple antipsychotics
- Takes buprenorphine (Subutex) for opioid maintenance
- Had adverse reaction to the naloxone in Suboxone which included vomiting and headaches

Current medications

- Fluoxetine (Prozac) 40 mg/d, a selective serotonin reuptake inhibitor (SSRI)
- Buprenorphine (Subutex) 12 mg/d, a mu (μ)-opioid partial receptor agonist
- Gabapentin (Neurontin) 2700 mg/d for chronic back pain, a calcium channel blocking agent for neuropathic pain management

Psychotherapy history

- Tried supportive harm reduction psychotherapy and now is in Narcotics Anonymous, which seems to work better for him regarding maintaining abstinence
  - He has been abstinent as such for 2 years

Patient evaluation on initial visit

- MDD is in full remission. Good mood. Engaged with work and family
- His GAD is at baseline mild to moderate in severity and fluctuates, mostly with social stressors
  - He endorses worries about multiple matters, including work, finances, and relationships
  - Feels irritable, tired, with muscle tension
  - Has struggled with GAD since childhood, and says that his anxiety "is always there"
- Sexual symptoms reported of decreased libido and delayed ejaculation
  - Notes that his libido worsens during exacerbations of his back pain
  - Reports that the delayed ejaculation predated the back injury and was unrelated to the exacerbation
  - It also predated the buprenorphine (Subutex)

Further investigation

Is there anything else that you would like to know about the patient?
Assess for causes of sexual dysfunction
- Is decreased libido secondary to MDD or to relationship problems?
- Are there comorbid medical, neurological conditions present?
- Is there ongoing substance use?
- Are there side effects of medications?

Attending physician's mental notes: initial psychiatric evaluation

- It was decided to stop fluoxetine (Prozac) and switch from this SSRI to a norepinephrine–dopamine reuptake inhibitor (NDRI), bupropion XL (Wellbutrin XL), as it has a lower risk of sexual side effects as it is devoid of serotonin enhancing activity
  - It is indicated for MDD, but not for GAD, though
  - Typically without serotonergic activity, this NDRI is felt to be less effective than other antidepressants such as selective serotonin–norepinephrine reuptake inhibitors (SNRIs) and SSRIs for GAD

- History and physical exam showed that the patient's MDD was in remission and he has no current relationship problems
- Investigations showed no diabetes, which is a common cause of sexual dysfunction, and there is no spinal cord radiculopathy that can explain his problem
- No ongoing OUD, urine screens are negative
- Expressed wish to stop smoking which is also an indication for bupropion (Wellbutrin)
- His history of delayed ejaculation is most consistent with known sexual side effects of SSRIs

Case outcome: at 4 weeks

- He was started on bupropion XL (Wellbutrin XL) 150 mg/d, which was increased to 300 mg/d after 2 weeks
- He tolerated the drug well but complained of worsening depression within 4 weeks of stopping fluoxetine (Prozac)
  - Presented as sad, anhedonic, with decreased sleep, trouble concentrating
- Unfortunately, was admitted to the hospital for suicidal ideation and a self-aborted suicide attempt
- Continued to complain of decreased libido, but reported that it worsened with exacerbations of his back pain
  - Delayed ejaculation had improved after stopping the fluoxetine (Prozac)
- Continued to remain abstinent from substances other than nicotine

Question

What are your options for evaluating and treating the patient at this point?

- Continue safety assessment and hospitalization
- Increase dose of bupropion XL (Wellbutrin XL)
- Start another antidepressant
- Restart fluoxetine (Prozac)

Attending physician's mental notes: follow-up (week 4)

- He was hospitalized for safety and stabilization, which is a priority
- He had been on a therapeutic dose of bupropion XL (Wellbutrin XL) for only 2 weeks
  - Perhaps that was not a sufficiently long duration
  - Perhaps it could be increased to the 450 mg/d dose
  - It should be continued given its relative lack of sexual dysfunction, but he may need an augmentation or combination strategy

- ◦ Might consider adding his fluoxetine (Prozac) back as it clearly had made his MDD better, and hope the continued bupropion XL (Wellbutrin XL) will alleviate his sexual problems
- ◦ Could also switch to an SNRI or a norepinephrine antagonist / selective serotonin antagonist (NaSSA) antidepressant

Case outcome: at 8 weeks

- At the hospital, he was started on the NaSSA antidepressant mirtazapine (Remeron) 15 mg/d
  - ◦ It generally has a low risk for sexual side effects as it has no serotonin reuptake inhibitor properties
  - ◦ It was started to help with sleep, and for its additional antidepressant effects as a combination strategy
  - ◦ May be a good drug to augment bupropion XL (Wellbutrin XL) as they have different mechanisms of action which result in elevations of serotonin, norepinephrine, and dopamine activity
- After a 5-day stay, he was discharged on these two medications
- At his next outpatient visit, he reported that he felt tired during the day despite getting better sleep, and has increased coffee drinking to no avail
- He also reports he had gained several pounds in weight

Question

What would you do about his new side effects?

- Increase dose of bupropion XL (Wellbutrin XL)
- Stop mirtazapine (Remeron)
- Add a stimulant such as methylphenidate (Ritalin)
- Add a wakefulness agent such as modafinil (Provigil)
- Suggest diet and exercise routines

Attending physician's mental notes: follow-up visit (week 8)

- It is great that his MDD is in remission
- His sexual problems have resolved as well
- It makes sense to continue his combination of NDRI and NaSSA antidepressants
- Suspect his new fatigue is a side effect of mirtazapine (Remeron)
- Suspect his new weight gain is a side effect
- Will need to see if he can tolerate these side effects, will likely need to treat and ameliorate the side effects because changing antidepressants yet again risks a relapse and a possible return to hospital after only a short remission period

Case outcome at 12 weeks

- Bupropion XL (Wellbutrin XL) was increased to 450 mg/day and fatigue resolved gradually
- Weight gain halted but he was 8 lb heavier and unhappy with this
- He declined prescription weight loss agents as they were too expensive, after his insurance refused to pay for cosmetic agents
- Despite this, the patient seemed committed to a portion-controlled diet and agreed to start walking daily for a new exercise regimen

Case debrief

- This MDD patient had some typical side effects that seemed to interfere with his treatment plan
- This intolerability forced a medication change that unfortunately led to a worsening of MDD symptoms
- He had multiple treatment options available to better balance out the good effects vs. negative effects of depression medication management
- Sometimes combining two agents can have a win-win effect where effectiveness is improved while counteracting the side effects associated with one or both agents

Take-home points

- Consider the different causes of sexual dysfunction in patients with MDD
- It is important to keep in mind that antidepressants are a major cause of sexual dysfunction, but not the only cause
- Sexual dysfunction is commonly associated with MDD and can have multiple causes
  - Decreased libido and erectile dysfunction are common
  - These signs and symptoms may also be secondary to comorbid substance use disorders, in this case opioid maintenance with buprenorphine (Subutex)
  - Buprenorphine (Subutex) has been known to be associated with decreased libido, for example
- Clinicians must take a history that juxtaposes the onset of sexual dysfunction to a time frame after an antidepressant initiation or dose increase, otherwise the patient may have had premorbid sexual difficulties
- Regarding antidepressants, the SSRIs and SNRIs have the highest rate of sexual dysfunction

- Antidepressants with a lower incidence of sexual side effects include: bupropion XL (Wellbutrin XL), mirtazapine (Remeron), trazodone (Desyrel), vilazodone (Viibryd), and vortioxetine (Trintellix)

Performance in practice: confessions of a psychopharmacologist

What are possible action items for improvement in practice?

What could have been done better here?

- Investigate which antidepressant combinations may create a win-win situation in which MDD may be better treated, perhaps with less overall side-effect burden
- Use bupropion XL (Wellbutrin XL)
  - As an NDRI, it has an absence of serotonergic activity which is often associated with weight gain, sexual dysfunction, and sometimes fatigue
  - Its side-effect profile is more activating, meaning patients will have more energy and sometimes develop anxiety and insomnia
  - It has a side-effect profile of creating nausea and/or curbing appetite
  - Therefore, it can be given in combination with almost any other antidepressant that is producing side effects of fatigue or increased appetite
- Use mirtazapine (Remeron)
  - As a NaSSA antidepressant, it does antagonize serotonin 2A (5-HT_{2A}) and 3 (5-HT_3) receptors
    - 5-HT_{2A} receptor antagonism generally reduces headaches, insomnia, and activating side effects created by other pro-serotonergic drugs
    - 5-HT_3 receptor antagonism generally reduces gastrointestinal side effects created by other pro-serotonergic drugs
  - Mirtazapine (Remeron) also antagonizes histamine (H1) receptors, causing fatigue and somnolence
  - Therefore, it can be combined with most other antidepressants to reduce side effects of insomnia, agitation, or stomach upset

Tips and pearls

- Literature suggests several methods to deal with antidepressant-induced sexual dysfunction. Some obvious ones include waiting for spontaneous reduction over time, or reducing the antidepressant dose at risk of MDD relapse

- Switching to another antidepressant with a lower incidence of sexual dysfunction is possible but it is often unknown whether the MDD will get better, get worse, or remain the same symptomatically, compared with the originally used antidepressant
- There are also multiple options for supplemental therapy to alleviate sexual dysfunction but the only clearly evidence-based options are: to add another antidepressant such as bupropion XL (Wellbutrin XL), mirtazapine (Remeron), or nefazodone (Serzone); and to add approved phosphodiesterase inhibitors (sildenafil, tadalafil, vardenafil)

Two-minute tutorial

Side effects and switching antidepressants

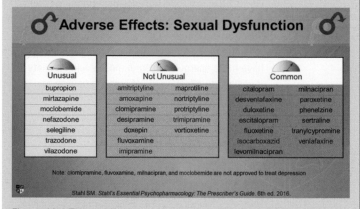

Figure 12.1 The antidepressants on the left have very little serotonin reuptake inhibition and therefore produce much less sexual dysfunction as a result. In patients with pre-existing sexual problems (except for premature ejaculation), choosing from this list makes sense. In those patients who are treated with agents in the other columns and develop sexual side effects, sometimes a switch to an agent on the left is also warranted. Interestingly, vilazodone (Viibryd) is a very weak SSRI and its 5-HT$_{1A}$ pre/postsynaptic partial agonism lend to its lower sexual dysfunction risk compared to other SSRIs. Figures 12.2–12.6 will discuss how this antidepressant works mechanistically and how it may avoid sexual side effects in a majority of patients who take it.

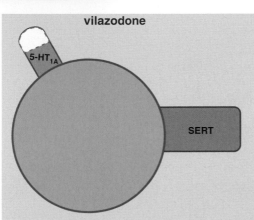

vilazodone

Figure 12.2 Vilazodone is a partial agonist at the serotonin 1A receptor and also inhibits serotonin reuptake; thus, it is referred to as a serotonin weakly partial agonist / reuptake inhibitor (SPARI).

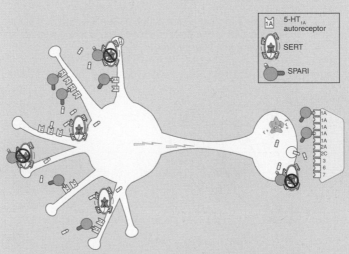

SPARI action: first, about half of SERTs and half of 5-HT$_{1A}$ receptors are occupied immediately

Figure 12.3 Mechanism of action of serotonin partial agonist / reuptake inhibitors (SPARIs), part 1. When a SPARI is administered, about half of serotonin transporters (SERTs) and half of serotonin 1A (5 HT$_{1A}$) receptors are occupied immediately.

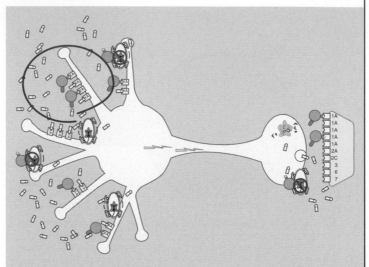

SPARI action: second, 5-HT increases at 5-HT₁A somatodendritic receptors on the left

Figure 12.4 Mechanism of action of SPARIs, part 2. Blockade of the SERT causes serotonin to increase initially in the somatodendritic area of the serotonin neuron (left).

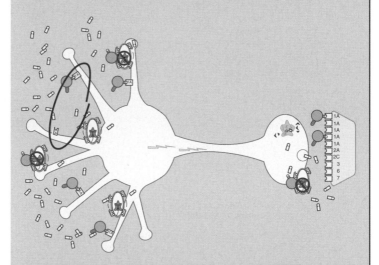

SPARI action: third, 5-HT actions on the left cause 5-HT₁A autoreceptors to desensitize/downregulate

Figure 12.5 Mechanism of action of SPARIs, part 3. The consequence of serotonin increasing in the somatodendritic area of the serotonin (5-HT) neuron is that the somatodendritic 5-HT₁A autoreceptors desensitize or downregulate (red circle).

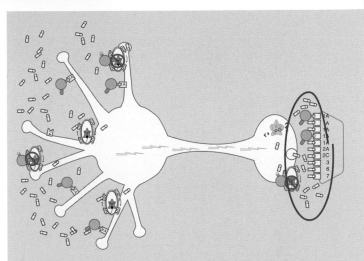

SPARI action: fourth, neuronal firing and serotonin release are disinhibited at the synapse on the right

Figure 12.6 Mechanism of action of SPARIs, part 4. Once the somatodendritic receptors downregulate, there is no longer inhibition of impulse flow in the 5-HT neuron. Thus, neuronal impulse flow is turned on. The consequence of this is release of 5-HT in the axon terminal (red circle).

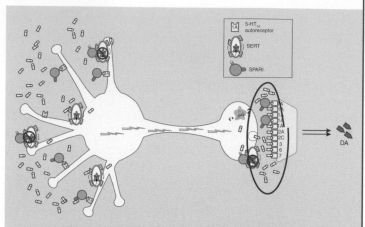

SPARI action: finally, antidepressant actions begin, and downstream enhancement of DA release may mitigate sexual dysfunction

Figure 12.7 Mechanism of action of SPARIs, part 5. Finally, once the SPARIs have blocked the SERT, increased somatodendritic 5-HT, desensitized somatodendritic 5-HT$_{1A}$ autoreceptors, turned on neuronal impulse flow, and increased release of 5HT from axon terminals, the final step (shown here, red circle) may be the desensitization of post-synaptic 5-HT receptors. This timeframe correlates with antidepressant action. In addition, the addition of 5-HT$_{1A}$ partial agonism may lead to downstream enhancement of dopamine (DA) release. There is an ascending serotonin neuronal pathway that leads from the raphe nuclei in the midbrain with projections to the limbic system, cortex, and other central nervous system structures that is felt to lower MDD symptoms.

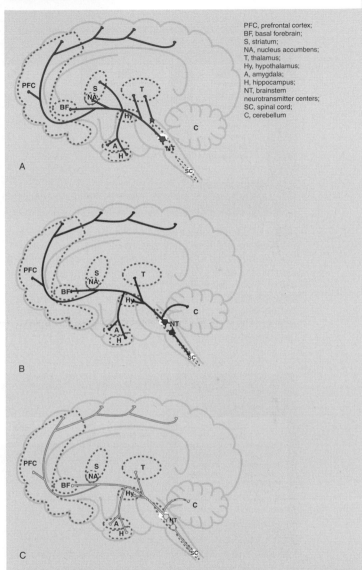

PFC, prefrontal cortex;
BF, basal forebrain;
S, striatum;
NA, nucleus accumbens;
T, thalamus;
Hy, hypothalamus;
A, amygdala;
H, hippocampus;
NT, brainstem
neurotransmitter centers;
SC, spinal cord;
C, cerebellum

Figure 12.8 Major monoamine projections. A – dopaminergic pathways in blue; B – noradrenergic pathways in red; C – serotonergic in yellow. Notice that all monoamine pathways can ascend into brain structures or descend into the spinal cord. Serotonin (C) has both ascending and descending projections. The descending pathway leads to the spinal cord. These serotonergic projections extend down from the brainstem and through the spinal cord, and 5-HT$_{1A}$ partial agonism afforded by vilazodone use here is felt to allow greater dopaminergic neurotransmission at the level of spinal segments, possibly lowering the incidence of sexual dysfunction side effects.

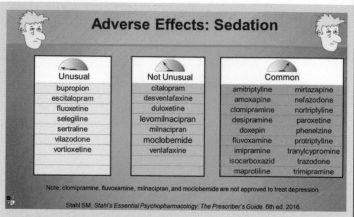

Figure 12.9 In this image, again on the left, are antidepressants with the least amount of sedating side effects. In patients who are already fatigued from their MDD or those who have medical conditions lending to increased burden of fatigue, one of these antidepressants may be a good initial choice. Patients who develop sedation on their initial antidepressant may need to be switched to one of the agents again on the left. Note that sometimes sedating side effects are actually welcome positive effects. These side effects may improve insomnia or agitation, for example, in certain patients.

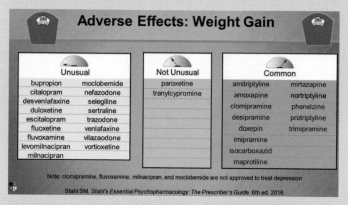

Figure 12.10 Here on the left are agents associated with less antidepressant-induced weight gain. These may be started in those patients already overweight or showing signs of metabolic disorder. Similar to the side effects mentioned above, if the first antidepressant utilized promotes weight gain in a patient, a switch to one of the antidepressants on the left may be warranted.

Factors to Consider in Choosing Between Switching or Augmenting

Consider switching to another antidepressant when:	Consider an adjunctive medication when:
• It is the first antidepressant trial • There are poorly tolerated side effects to the initial antidepressant • There is no response (< 25% improvement) to the initial antidepressant • There is more time to wait for a response (less severe, less functional impairment) • Patient prefers to switch to another antidepressant	• There have been 2 or more antidepressant trials • The initial antidepressant is well tolerated • There is partial response (> 25% improvement) to the initial antidepressant • There are specific residual symptoms or side effects to the initial antidepressant that can be targeted • There is less time to wait for a response (more severe, more functional impairment) • Patient prefers to add on another medication.

Kennedy SH et al. Can J Psychiatry 2016;61(9):540-60.

Figure 12.11 Clinically there has been no clearly proven benefit in large studies to help us determine when to switch monotherapy antidepressants vs. combining and augmenting with a polypharmacy approach. Outside of changing antidepressants due to side-effect intolerability, other reasons are noted on the left above. On the right, as treatment resistance in MDD increases, there generally is more latitude to use polypharmacy in clinical practice.

Post-test question

Which of the following are a common cause of sexual problems in patients with depression?

A. Decreased libido due to depression
B. Relationship problems
C. Sexual side effects of antidepressants
D. Comorbid medical or neurological problems
E. All of the above

Answer: E

Sexual dysfunction in MDD may be pre-existing in nature due to medical causes or relational causes. MDD itself may cause decreased libido. Certainly, antidepressants with serotonin reuptake inhibition as a key mechanism of action are associated with sexual dysfunction. Some studies reveal that decreased libido and sexual arousal problems were more commonly associated with depression, but impaired orgasm was less common prior to taking antidepressants. Most commonly associated with SSRI use (60–70% – delayed orgasm and decreased libido being the most common), SNRIs (70% – delayed orgasm and decreased libido being the most common), tricyclic antidepressants (TCAs: 30% – decreased libido, erectile dysfunction, delayed orgasm, and impaired ejaculation), and monoamine oxidase inhibitors (40% –

similar to TCAs). A meta-analysis showed the various rates of sexual dysfunction with different drugs: citalopram (Celexa), venlafaxine (Effexor), and sertraline (Zoloft) had the highest incidence at around 80%.

References

1. Carvalho, AF, Sharma, MS, Brunoni, AR, et al. The safety, tolerability and risks associated with the use of newer generation antidepressant drugs: a critical review of the literature. *Psychother Psychosom* 2016; 85:270–88

2. Kumsar, NA, Kumsar, Ş, Dilbaz, N. Sexual dysfunction in men diagnosed as substance use disorder. *Andrologia* 2016; 48:1229–35

3. La Torre, A, Giupponi, G, Duffy, D, et al. Sexual dysfunction related to psychotropic drugs: a critical review – part I: antidepressants. *Pharmacopsychiatry* 2013; 46:191–9

4. Laumann, EO, Paik, A, Rosen, RC. Sexual dysfunction in the United States: prevalence and predictors. *JAMA* 1999; 281:537–44

5. Mago, R, Mahajan, R, Thase, ME. Medically serious adverse effects of newer antidepressants. *Curr Psychiatry Rep* 2008; 10:249–57

6. Ramdurg, S, Ambekar, A, Lal, R. Sexual dysfunction among male patients receiving buprenorphine and naltrexone maintenance therapy for opioid dependence. *J Sex Med* 2012; 9:3198–204

7. Sadock, B, Sadock, V, Ruiz, P. *Synopsis of Psychiatry: Behavioral Sciences / Clinical Psychiatry*. Philadelphia: Lippincott Williams & Wilkins, 2015

8. Stahl, SM. *Stahl's Essential Psychopharmacology: Neuroscientific Basis and Practical Applications*, 4. Cambridge: Cambridge University Press, 2013

9. Stahl, SM. *Stahl's Essential Psychopharmacology: Prescriber's Guide*, 7. Cambridge: Cambridge University Press, 2020

10. Taylor, D, Paton, C, Kapur, S. *The Maudsley Prescribing Guidelines in Psychiatry*, 11th edn. Oxford: Wiley-Blackwell, 2012

Case 13: It's confusing, isn't it?

The Question: What caused the acute change in mental status?

The Psychopharmacological Dilemma: Lithium side effect or not?

Sutanaya Pal

Pretest self-assessment question

What are the common adverse effects of lithium (Lithobid, Eskalith) that can lead to an acute change in mental status?

A. Lithium toxicity
B. Hypothyroidism
C. Changes in sodium levels
D. Drug interactions
E. A,C,D
F. All of the above

Patient evaluation on intake

- A 40-year-old lady with a 15-year history of schizoaffective disorder who presented with worsening symptoms of psychosis on the first anniversary of her husband's death
- Admits delusions of reference and psychotic denial of the death of her husband
- Has auditory hallucinations in which she would hear her dead relative's voice calling to her in a negative, accusatory manner
- Prior mood episodes were consistent with full depressive episodes
  - She has no prior manic episodes
- As a result, she was prescribed the selective serotonin reuptake inhibitor (SSRI) fluoxetine (Prozac) 20 mg/d and the atypical antipsychotic olanzapine (Zyprexa) up to 15 mg/d, which resulted now in a switch to mania after a week of being on this combined regimen
- She abruptly began to exhibit irritability, psychomotor agitation, excess talkativeness, increased involvement in sexual activities, decreased need for sleep, and increased distractibility
- Her psychotic symptoms persisted: auditory hallucinations and a psychotic denial of her husband's death
- She presented to the emergency room as her symptoms were sufficiently severe for her to be unable to care for herself and maintain safety at home

Psychiatric history

- Patient has well-diagnosed history of schizoaffective disorder, depressive type
- Symptoms typically well controlled on medications
  - Olanzapine (Zyprexa) 10 mg/d for psychosis until her current presentation
- She had an exacerbation of her symptoms and presented with depression and psychotic symptoms
  - She insists her husband is alive (psychotic denial)
  - Endorses depressed mood; anhedonia; severe psychomotor retardation; decreased sleep, appetite, and energy; and had suicidal ideations without a plan or intent
  - Neglectful now in caring for her 11-year-old son
- As a result, she was prescribed fluoxetine (Prozac) 20 mg/d and olanzapine (Zyprexa) 15 mg/d which has resulted now in a switch to mania after a week of being on this regimen
- No prior suicide attempts, or psychiatric hospitalization

Social and personal history

- Childhood described as "normal"
- Grew up with both biological parents and siblings
- No history of childhood abuse or neglect
- Completed high school
- Married twice, divorced and widowed, respectively
- Currently lives with her father and her 11-year-old son
- No alcohol, nicotine, or drug use

Medical history

- Arthritis and back pain

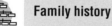

Family history

- Schizophrenia in mother and grandmother

Medication history

- No medication trials prior to preadmission use of olanzapine (Zyprexa) and fluoxetine (Prozac)

Current medications

- Olanzapine (Zyprexa) 15 mg/d taken for years
- Fluoxetine (Prozac) 20 mg/d taken for 1 week

Psychotherapy history

- No history of psychotherapy

Patient evaluation on initial visit

- Symptoms of psychosis have been gradually worsening since the death of her husband but were always depressive in nature
- Now is manic
- She was unable to care for herself and was extremely disinhibited and disorganized, frequently wandering out in the street late at night and almost walking into traffic a few times
- She was brought to the emergency room by the police who prevented her from wandering onto a busy intersection

Question

Based on what you know about this patient's symptoms what would you do next?

- Admit to an inpatient psychiatric unit for observation
- Stop fluoxetine (Prozac) antidepressant
- Increase olanzapine (Zyprexa) atypical antipsychotic
- Start another mood stabilizer
- All of the above

Attending physician's mental notes: initial visit

- She likely needs an admission to an inpatient psychiatry unit for safety and stabilization
- She is floridly manic and psychotic, unfortunately
- The addition of the SSRI antidepressant seemed to create this manic event, so stopping fluoxetine (Prozac) is an option
- Given historical response to olanzapine (Zyprexa), and its ability to treat mania and psychosis, best course of action might be to increase it for now
- Given her distinct change now from schizoaffective disorder depressive type to bipolar type, it may make sense to use an atypical antipsychotic known to treat bipolar depression as a monotherapy, or perhaps use a mood stabilizer such as lithium (Eskalith) which has some evidence for the treatment of depression as well, because the olanzapine/fluoxetine combination strategy has been problematic so far

Case outcome: interim follow-up at 10 days

- Olanzapine (Zyprexa) increased to 20 mg/d to treat psychosis
- Fluoxetine (Prozac) was maintained as it seemed to help depression until mania occurred
  - Felt the increased atypical antipsychotic could stabilize into euthymia alone
- Lithium (Eskalith, Lithobid) 600 mg/d started given its ability to treat mania and possibly maintain euthymia by acting as an antidepressant, with a goal of monotherapy use later
- Haloperidol (Haldol) was needed for agitation (receiving 10–20 mg daily)
- No change in her symptoms noted
- Patient developed tremors that were initially fine resting tremors, which became coarse tremors over the course of a few days
- Dysarthria and ataxia developed
- Became confused and was disoriented to time, place and person

Further investigation

Is there anything else that you would like to know about the patient?

Does she have any underlying or predisposing medical conditions or medications that may lend toward developing delirium?

- No. Though olanzapine (Zyprexa) does have some anticholinergic potential compared to other atypical antipsychotics, it typically is not enough to cause delirium

Does lithium cause delirium?

- Yes, if toxic, patient can present with confusion, ataxia, and tremors

Can mania present as delirium?

- Yes, manic delirium is well documented and is often co-occurring with catatonia

Question

What would you do next?

- Check lithium levels to see whether she has lithium toxicity, and lower dosage as needed
- Check electrolytes to determine sodium levels and clinical signs of dehydration
- Check thyroid functions
- Rule out new medical causes of delirium
- Remove fluoxetine (Prozac), given that its long half-life may now be creating delirious mania as it still may be building up in her system

Attending physician's mental notes: follow-up (day 10)

- Lithium level was 0.9 mmol/L which is therapeutic and usually not toxic
- Lithium (Lithobid, Eskalith) has a very narrow therapeutic index. Lithium levels above 1.5 mmol/L are considered toxic
  - Neurotoxicity can, however, be seen when normal lithium levels are recorded
- Common symptoms of lithium toxicity are nausea, vomiting, diarrhea, cerebellar signs (tremors, ataxia, dysarthria, nystagmus)
  - Extrapyramidal signs such as myoclonus, fasciculation, and fibrillation may be seen as well
- Need to check a basic metabolic panel as she could be either sodium depleted as an SSRI side effect or dehydrated causing lithium levels to increase via concentration
- Thyroid was normal at admission, doubt any acute change here even with lithium use
- The patient has received haloperidol (Haldol) as needed for dangerous agitation, and there are well-defined reports of its use with lithium causing toxicity even at normal lithium levels and this must be considered now
- Her neurological findings suggest an organic toxicity cause to be more likely than a psychotic delirious mania

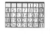

Case outcome: interim follow-up through 21 days

- Early toxicity due to lithium (Lithobid) and haloperidol (Haldol) was diagnosed given the confusion and neurological symptoms noted in the presence of normal lithium levels
- Both agents discontinued
  - The patient's delirium and motor symptoms resolved within a few days
- She was started on divalproex (Depakote) which helped to control her elevated mood symptoms
- Her irritability, increased talkativeness, distractibility, sexual indiscretion, and sleep improved gradually
- She continued to believe that her husband was alive, and continued to hear his voice, which might be her new baseline, where her affective state is controlled while the schizophrenia part of her schizoaffective disorder is not
- She denied current depressive symptoms other than mild depressed mood

- She was discharged from the inpatient unit on the following regimen:
  - Divalproex (Depakote) ER 1000 mg/d (with a blood level of 63 mcg/mL)
  - Olanzapine (Zyprexa) 20 mg/day

Case debrief

- This patient has a relatively stable schizoaffective disorder, depressive type. Patient stable for many years on olanzapine (Zyprexa) but the stress of her spouse dying and his anniversary date pushed her into a depressed state
- In response, fluoxetine (Prozac) was added and mania ensued
- This required an inpatient stay and medication adjustment
- It was felt that lithium (Lithobid) could be introduced and ultimately could become her monotherapy
- She developed toxicity when haloperidol (Haldol) was used as needed for her agitation
- Ultimately, both were discontinued and divalproex (Depakote) was used instead with good clinical antimanic effect but with subtle psychosis continuing, which will require future treatment as outpatient.

Take-home points

- Although very effective for controlling affective symptoms, lithium (Lithobid) has a narrow therapeutic index and needs close monitoring of lithium levels
- Often, clinicians worry about drug–drug interactions with lithium and non-steroidal anti-inflammatory drugs (NSAIDs) and diuretics, but haloperidol has a well-defined potential to create lithium toxicity in certain patients when combined
- Quickly reversible neurotoxicity is precipitated mostly at normal lithium levels by pre-existing neurological disease or combination with antipsychotics in the acute setting
- It is important to be cognizant of probable interactions with lithium which can lead to acute worsening of agitation and mental status
- Lithium may react more often with haloperidol (Haldol), clozapine (Clozaril), risperidone (Risperdal)

Performance in practice: confessions of a psychopharmacologist

What could have been done better here?

- Investigate the risk of switching to mania with antidepressant use with and without a mood stabilizer or antipsychotic being present

  ○ This patient was on olanzapine (Zyprexa) 10 mg/d which is likely the minimum therapeutic dose to halt mania or psychosis, but it can be used up to 20 mg/d for this purpose. Perhaps the recognition of hypomania and a dose escalation could have been instituted earlier?

  ○ When a bipolar patient begins to switch into mania, the clinician may either remove the mania driver (the antidepressant fluoxetine in this case) or increase the mood stabilizer (in this case, olanzapine) or both

  ○ It may have made sense here to have discontinued fluoxetine (Prozac) while gently increasing the olanzapine (Zyprexa) in this case because, in hindsight, the institution of two new variables (lithium and haloperidol) led to major complications

  ○ Sometimes keeping it simple is a best practice

What are possible action items for improvement in practice?

- Investigate and learn the minimum therapeutic dose for mania treatment and prevention across the atypical antipsychotic class of medication
- Investigate which atypicals can treat depression and psychosis, ideally as a monotherapy

Tips and pearls

- Serum and tissue levels of lithium may not always correlate so it is important to consider the whole clinical picture while assessing for signs of lithium toxicity
- For example, patients on safe levels of lithium can develop mild to serious side effects, while those with excessive levels may show few to none
- Serial lithium trough blood levels should be obtained while titrating, as well as electrocardiograms (EKGs) and performing pertinent focused physical examinations

Two-minute tutorial

Lithium toxicity versus delirious mania

- It is helpful to conceptualize lithium toxicity in terms of the circumstances, as acute, acute-on-chronic, and chronic toxicity
  - Acute toxicity involves acute ingestion which may be intentional or accidental, which is relatively rare
  - Clinical manifestations here include:
    - gastrointestinal (GI) symptoms (nausea, vomiting, diarrhea)
    - central nervous system (CNS) symptoms (altered mental status and cerebellar signs)
    - cerebrovascular system (CVS) symptoms (arrhythmias and low blood pressure) and renal symptoms (polyuria and polydipsia)
- Most cases of acute ingestion lead to acute-on-chronic toxicity
  - These cases have more severe symptoms at comparatively lower serum concentrations as brain levels of lithium have already reached an equilibrium
- Chronic toxicity can occur at any time during long-term treatment with lithium
  - Increasing the lithium (Lithobid) dose, change in the patient's hydration status or sodium levels, renal disease, infection or surgery, and drug interactions are some of the precipitating factors
- Neurotoxicity can be reversible or irreversible
  - Reversible neurotoxicity has been discussed in detail above
  - Irreversible toxicity is also known as SILENT (Syndrome of Irreversible Lithium Effectuated Neurotoxicity)
  - In some cases, even after lithium is removed from the body after acute toxicity, neurological symptoms persist
  - Demyelination of multiple sites in the brain might be the mechanism of this condition
  - Patients have cerebellar symptoms, extrapyramidal symptoms, and even dementia

Delirious mania

- Briefly, the DSM-5 criteria for catatonia use primarily motor symptoms for its diagnosis
- However, autonomic symptoms are common in the condition – such as fever, tachycardia, hypertension, and motor rigidity
  - When autonomic symptoms co-occur with catatonia, it is known as malignant catatonia

- ○ Other syndromes which have symptoms that overlap with catatonia and respond to similar treatments include neuroleptic malignant syndrome (NMS), toxic serotonin syndrome, delirious mania, and periodic catatonia
- Catatonia has two clinical subtypes – stuporous/akinetic (more common) and excited catatonia
- Previously, catatonia was considered to be a part of schizophrenia, but it has since been seen to be a much broader syndrome associated more with mood disorders, as well as the other conditions mentioned
- Delirious mania is a heterogeneous condition which meets the criteria for both delirium and mania
- Patients with delirious mania develop confusion, day/night reversal, stereotypic movements, and fluctuations in consciousness that may mimic a medical delirium
- A significant percentage of these patients have motor disturbances typical of catatonia
- As with other forms of delirium, clinicians should rule out medical causes first, with the usual array of tests including blood tests, brain imaging, and EEG
- Even after medical causes have been ruled out, it is important to monitor for complications by checking for vitals, dehydration, aspiration, infection, and rhabdomyolysis
- It is best to avoid antipsychotics, particularly first-generation typical agents
- Treatment is dictated by whether they have autonomic symptoms or not
  - ○ Those with autonomic symptoms require monitoring on the medical floor or in the ICU
- Benzodiazepines (BZs) and/or electroconvulsive therapy (ECT) are the first lines of treatment
  - ○ ECT is preferred if BZs do not improve symptoms or are contraindicated, or there is an emergent need to control symptoms
- For non-malignant delirious mania (or those without autonomic symptoms), mood stabilizers with or without antipsychotics are most effective
- Most experts recommend delaying the use of antipsychotics as much as possible, and only using atypical antipsychotic agents with careful monitoring for development of NMS as these patients are at a higher risk here
  - ○ There is evidence that ECT and BZs are beneficial in this sub-group as well

- Manic delirium patients typically would not have CNS findings such as ataxia, dysarthria, or tremor. They might have other motor symptoms like those typical of catatonia
  - This is an important clue to differentiate it from delirious mania

Table 13.1 Bradford Hill Criteria for judging cause and effect

Criteria	Relevance
Strength of apparent association	Bigger associations = bigger effects
Consistency (reproducibility)	Consistent findings across settings = more likely a true association
Specificity	Specific population with specific disease, unlikely other explanations
Temporality	Exposure precedes outcome
Dose effect	Greater exposure imparts greater risk (but there could also be a necessary threshold level of exposure)
Plausibility	Is there a plausible pharmacological mechanism?
Coherence	An explanation for likely association makes sense given existing knowledge
Experiment	Experimental interventions can alter the conditions
Alternate explanations	Do other likely explanations exist for the observed association?

This table shows the Bradford Hill Criteria, which can be used to better determine whether a new set of symptoms is a side effect of a drug that was initiated or increased. In this case, haloperidol was added to lithium and neurological symptoms / side effects developed. There was an abrupt onset of significant mental status and physical examination findings where the exposure preceded the outcome. The dosing of the haloperidol was high across a short amount of time. Given the literature on this drug interaction, the pattern of symptom development seems consistent, and clinically the toxicity symptoms were not as consistent with catatonia or delirium, suggesting this in fact was most likely to be a case of lithium/haloperidol toxicity. Initial studies suggested that haloperidol may increase lithium levels acutely, but this has largely not been shown through later studies. Haloperidol may blunt the neuroprotective effect of lithium whereby it lowers oxidative stress upon neurons in the CNS.

Conclusion

- Lithium (Lithobid) is the one of the first-line treatments for an acute manic episode, either as monotherapy or in combination with antipsychotics for severe cases
- There is mixed evidence for the efficacy of lithium (Lithobid) in the acute phase of bipolar depression
  - It is not FDA-approved for use in the acute phase of bipolar depression
  - Most of the evidence supporting its use in bipolar depression comes from level 2 evidence from controlled trials
  - Clinical practice guidelines from across the world give varying recommendations as to whether lithium (Lithobid) should be used *first line* for the acute phase of bipolar depression (especially since there are other options with more evidence)

- However, there is unequivocal evidence that lithium (Lithobid) is effective in reducing suicidality in patients with bipolar disorder (BP)
- It can be an excellent monotherapy in bipolar patients and an adjunct to antipsychotics in those with schizoaffective disorder, bipolar type conditions
- Like BP patients, schizoaffective disorder patients can develop mixed features, rapid cycling, or, as in this case, mania with or without psychosis

Post-test question

What are the common adverse effects of lithium (Lithobid, Eskalith) that can lead to an acute change in mental status?

A. Lithium toxicity
B. Hypothyroidism
C. Changes in sodium levels
D. Drug interactions
E. A,C,D
F. All of the above

Answer: E

The efficacy of lithium (Lithobid, Eskalith) is dose-dependent, and corresponds to the serum concentration. Most maintain it between 0.6 and 1.2 mmol/L. Blood levels > 1.5 mEq/L are considered to be toxic. Signs of toxicity include primarily GI symptoms (nausea, vomiting, diarrhea) and neurological symptoms (ataxia, tremors and other signs of neuronal hyperactivity, confusion, or altered mental status). Its use has been associated with hypothyroidism, with an incidence of 4% of the patients who are prescribed lithium. However, this is a slow process clinically and rarely creates acute mental-state changes. While the most common effect of lithium (Lithobid, Eskalith) on the kidney is reduced urinary concentrating capacity, it also causes nephrogenic diabetes insipidus resulting in loss of free water and hypernatremia. Finally, common interactions with lithium (Lithobid, Eskalith) that result in a change in lithium levels include those with thiazide diuretics, ACE inhibitors, and NSAIDs. Caffeine reduces lithium levels by as much as 24% in some individuals, resulting in a possible worsening of symptoms. Caffeine withdrawal will cause a rise in lithium levels. Lithium-induced neurotoxicity has been associated with pre-existing neurological disease and combination therapy with antipsychotics.

References

1. Fink, M. Delirious mania. *Bipolar Disord* 1999; 1:54–60
2. Fink, M, Taylor, M. The many varieties of catatonia. *Eur Arch Psychiatry Clin Neurosci* 2001; 251 Suppl. 1:I8–13
3. Foulser, P, Abbasi, Y, Mathilakath, A, et al. Do not treat the numbers: lithium toxicity. *BMJ Case Rep* 2017; 2017:bcr–2017
4. Frigerio, S, Strawbridge, R, Young, AH. The impact of caffeine consumption on clinical symptoms in patients with bipolar disorder: a systematic review. *Bipolar Disord* 2021; 23:241–51
5. Grandjean, EM, Aubry, JM. Lithium: updated human knowledge using an evidence-based approach. Part II: clinical pharmacology and therapeutic monitoring. *CNS Drugs* 2009; 23:331–49
6. Grandjean, EM, Aubry, JM. Lithium: updated human knowledge using an evidence-based approach. Part III: clinical safety. *CNS Drugs* 2009; 23:397–418
7. Karmacharya, R, England, ML, Ongür, D. Delirious mania: clinical features and treatment response. *J Affect Disord* 2008; 109:312–16
8. Kelly, T. Lithium and the Woozle effect. *Bipolar Disord* 2019; 21: 302–8
9. Malhi, GS, Gessler, D, Outhred, T. The use of lithium for the treatment of bipolar disorder: Recommendations from clinical practice guidelines. *J Affect Disord* 2017; 217: 266–80
10. McIntyre, JS, Charles, SC, Anzia, DJ, et al. *American Psychiatric Association Steering Committee on Practice Guidelines.* Washington, DC: APA, 2010
11. McKnight, RF, Adida, M, Budge, K, et al. Lithium toxicity profile: a systematic review and meta-analysis. *Lancet* 2012; 379:721–8
12. Netto, I, Phutane, VH. Reversible lithium neurotoxicity: review of the literature. *Prim Care Companion CNS Disord* 2012; 14(1):PCC.11r01197
13. Sadock, B, Sadock, V, Ruiz, P. *Synopsis of Psychiatry: Behavioral Sciences / Clinical Psychiatry.* Philadelphia: Lippincott Williams & Wilkins, 2015
14. Schou, M. Long-lasting neurological sequelae after lithium intoxication. *Acta Psychiatr Scand* 1984; 70:594–602
15. Shah, VC, Kayathi, P, Singh, G, et al. Enhance your understanding of lithium neurotoxicity. *Prim Care Companion CNS Disord* 2015; 17(17):10.4088/PCC.14l01767
16. Taylor, D, Paton, C, Kapur, S. *The Maudsley Prescribing Guidelines in Psychiatry*, 11th edn. Oxford: Wiley-Blackwell, 2012
17. Timmer, RT, Sands, JM. Lithium intoxication. *J Am Soc Nephrol* 1999; 10:666–74

Case 14: The adolescent who just can't stay awake

The Question: What psychopharmacological options exist for hypersomnia and residual depressive vegetative symptoms?

The Psychopharmacological Dilemma: Finding effective regimen to boost motivation and energy in a psychomotor-retarded, vegetative depressed adolescent

Fairouz Ali

Pretest self-assessment question

What is the impact of the selective serotonin–norepinephrine reuptake inhibitor (SNRI) venlafaxine (Effexor XR) on weight?

A. Unlike other antidepressants with serotonergic effects, venlafaxine (Effexor XR) can cause weight loss
B. Venlafaxine (Effexor XR) causes dose-dependent weight loss up to 5% of the body weight
C. Weight loss caused by venlafaxine (Effexor XR) in pediatric patients is related to decreased appetite, i.e., treatment-emergent anorexia
D. All of the above are true

Patient evaluation on intake

- A girl in 12th grade presents with her mother, seeking help for worsening major depressive disorder (MDD) with notable psychomotor retardation and hypersomnolence, resulting in moderate impairment in academic and social functioning

Psychiatric history

- At age 12, 6th grade, started feeling anxious about going to school following a transfer from a small-sized classroom in a school with fewer expectations/requirements and less students/friends to a larger-size classroom in a private college preparatory school with high expectations and different social settings
- At that time, she would still go to school and perform well academically, yet would not engage in social relationships and tended to isolate herself, and when in a social setting she would be shy and withdrawn, limiting her friendships. This was a change from her norm
- At age 15, 9th grade, she lost a close relative through a long process, to immunodeficiency. This loss seems to have triggered

her first episode of MDD, for which she was evaluated for the first time by psychiatry. Her symptoms then included:

- ○ Feeling sad, decreased motivation, decreased concentration, decreased energy, anhedonia, feelings of guilt and worthlessness, decreased appetite, increased sleep, self-deprecating thoughts, and fleeting passive suicidal ideation
- 7 months ago, on presentation to the outpatient clinic, she continued to endorse depressive symptoms that have worsened – per her and her mother's report –following COVID pandemic stress
- She presented with a 2-year history of chronic depression with low mood and anxiety
- Decline in school participation and her grades is noted
- Impairment in her social life and her ability to socialize with friends due to her increased isolation and lack of motivation

Social and personal history

- Patient is now a 12th grader
- Parents are married and she has two younger siblings
- She enjoys reading and dancing as well as playing soccer
- Normal delivery, initially diagnosed with failure to thrive due to low breast milk supply, yet met developmental milestones without delay

Medical history

- No acute medical problems
- Congenital bicuspid cardiac valve
- Febrile seizures
- Incidentally found to have idiopathic thrombocytopenia with no manifestations or complications
- Surgical procedures: wisdom teeth extraction
- Recently developed low BMI of 18.9 secondary to poor appetite from Venlafaxine (Effexor XR), currently tapered off also as it was only partially effective
- Currently receiving treatment for acne, isotretinoin (Accutane)

Family history

- Father has history of MDD with a brief trial of medications in his 20s. Recovered with psychotherapy

Medication history

- On her first contact with psychiatry at age 15, she was tried on multiple selective serotonin reuptake inhibitors (SSRIs), including sertraline (Zoloft), fluoxetine (Prozac), and escitalopram (Lexpro), which resulted in fatigue and development of paradoxical severe suicidal ideation leading to emergency room visits. These SSRIs were discontinued
- Started next on the SNRI duloxetine (Cymbalta) 20 mg/d, with the atypical antipsychotic MDD augmentation aripiprazole (Abilify) 2 mg/d, with some improvement in overall mood yet residual depressive symptoms in the context of low motivation, low energy, increased sleep, decreased appetite, and poor self-image persist
- 1 month prior to her clinic presentation, her prescriber added the norepinephrine–dopamine reuptake inhibitor (NDRI) bupropion (Wellbutrin) 75 mg/d, and increased the duloxetine (Cymbalta) to 40 mg/d, in addition to aripiprazole (Abilify) 2 mg/d
- Per the patient and her mother, no benefits were observed with this regimen and patient continued to endorse the same depressive symptoms with worsening vegetative component

Current medications

- Bupropion (Wellbutrin) 75 mg/d (NDRI)
- Duloxetine (Cymbalta) 40 mg/d (SNRI)
- Aripiprazole (Abilify) 2 mg/d (atypical antipsychotic)

Psychotherapy history

- At age 15, she first sought psychiatric help and was engaged in supportive psychotherapy on a bi-weekly basis while following up with medication management on a monthly basis
- At age 17, prior to her evaluation at the clinic, she was following a "life coach" for social support
- Currently attending weekly psychodynamic psychotherapy (PDP) sessions for the past 7 months

Patient evaluation on initial visit

- The patient presents with a 2-year history of MDD and social anxiety disorder vs. low self-esteem from MDD, with current symptoms as follows
  - Decreased motivation
  - Decreased concentration
  - Decreased interest

- ○ Increased sleep to the degree of limiting her participation in schoolwork
- ○ Feelings of worthlessness and guilt
- ○ Self-deprecating thoughts with fleeting sporadic passive thoughts of giving up on life
- ○ Psychomotor retardation
- ○ Fear and anxiety about social situations accompanied by fear of scrutiny by others
- ○ Anxiety attacks in social settings only, lasting less than 5 minutes, with symptoms of gagging, shortness of breath, and tachycardia
- ○ Avoiding social settings and missing weeks from school due to marked anxiety, which led to impairment in academic and social functioning
- ○ Denies having homicidal thoughts
- ○ Does not endorse hallucinations or delusions
- ○ Denies eating disorder
- ○ Denies physical, sexual, emotional abuse
- ○ No evidence of psychosis, bipolar disorder, and no history of prior mania/hypomania episodes
- ○ Moderate degree of impairment of functioning in both academic and social settings
- These symptoms failed to respond to SSRI use, and minimally responded to a combination of subtherapeutic SNRI plus NDRI along with a subtherapeutic dose of atypical antipsychotic, in addition to supportive psychotherapy

Question

How would you proceed?

- Remove the SNRI duloxetine (Cymbalta) as it has not shown benefit
- Remove the atypical antipsychotic aripiprazole (Abilify) for lack of benefit and given its risk of extrapyramidal symptoms (EPS) and tardive dyskinesia (TD)
- Switch to a novel antidepressant to target residual depressive symptoms
- Maximize dose of NDRI bupropion (Wellbutrin) and assess
- Make sure the SNRI and NDRI are dosed therapeutically

Attending physician's mental notes: initial psychiatric evaluation

- The patient's constellation of symptoms of social isolation, multiple worries with trouble relaxing, worrying about being liked by people, oversleeping episodes, low mood, low energy, low motivation, and difficulty with concentration met criteria for MDD, generalized anxiety disorder (GAD), and social anxiety disorder
- Must consider MDD with anxious distress vs. MDD with atypical features, diagnostically
- This was further confirmed by thorough evaluation, as well as data gathered via rating scales
- Patient Health Questionnaire-9 (PHQ-9) score at intake was 15 indicating moderate depression severity, and Generalized Anxiety Disorder-7 (GAD-7) score at intake was 14 indicating clinically significant moderate anxiety. Screen for Child Anxiety-Related Disorders (SCARED) confirmed diagnosis of social anxiety disorder with a score of 8 in that section, and confirmed diagnosis of GAD with a score of 9 in that section
- Despite her low doses, patient had given up hope on her current medications and wished to stop some
  - It may not make sense to push for full dosing, as such
- Plan was to first discontinue aripiprazole (Abilify) 2 mg/d
- Then to taper her off duloxetine (Cymbalta) 40 mg/d
- At the same time, aim to increase bupropion (Wellbutrin) to 150 mg/d and change to the XL slower-release preparation
- Aim to target low motivation, low energy, and poor concentration that resulted in her academic decline
- Will need to see whether other atypical and anxious MDD symptoms respond

Case outcome: initial visit

- Parents are fully informed and educated about the risks and benefits of proceeding with tapering of two medications, SNRI and atypical antipsychotic, while maximizing NDRI medication
- Patient and parents are hopeful about NDRI helping in boosting energy and motivation, with hope in decreasing hypersomnolence and improving academic performance
- Patient is motivated to streamline medications and engage in weekly PDP sessions
- Aripiprazole (Abilify) discontinued with no reported side effects or changes

- This was followed by a taper off of duloxetine (Cymbalta) successfully, without withdrawal symptoms or major mood changes
- Bupropion (Wellbutrin) was then switched to extended release (XL) and dosed at 150 mg/d

Further investigation

Is there anything else that you would like to know about the patient?

- Is there a likelihood of her history of febrile seizures predisposing this patient for future seizures on bupropion XL (Wellbutrin XL), given the lowering of the seizure threshold with bupropion XL (Wellbutrin XL)?
  - A history of febrile seizure is independent and typically not related to epilepsy or primary seizure disorder
  - A one-time febrile seizure episode does not indicate higher risk of seizure development through the course of this patient's life
  - There is no indication that this patient would be at higher risk of developing seizure on bupropion XL (Wellbutrin XL) as she does not qualify for a seizure disorder
  - It is thus safe to postulate the patient is not at risk of developing a seizure more than the normal population. Proceeding with maximizing the dose is warranted

Case outcome: first interim follow-up 2 weeks later

- Patient and parents reported observing benefits from bupropion XL (Wellbutrin XL) 150 mg/d, with mild improvement in motivation, energy, and concentration as anticipated
- Patient's academic performance improved with ability to participate in school and being more able to meet deadlines for assignments
- In terms of school setting, patient opted for attending school 100% virtually, in the midst of COVID pandemic
  - Although school generally adopted 50% in-school and 50% virtual setting, the patient preferred full virtual setting as she continued to endorse social anxiety
- Additionally, the patient and parents reported episodes of oversleeping in early mornings, and afternoon napping, still occurring. Per report, patient failed to wake up in the morning for school, thus preferred virtual school setting given flexibility of time to accommodate her oversleeping episodes
- Parents reported concern about the patient's oversleeping episodes and ongoing social isolation leading to difficulty in her engaging with friends and family even for a simple dinner meal

Question

For the patient's residual MDD symptoms, social anxiety disorder, and oversleeping episodes, what might you do next?

- Increase bupropion XL (Wellbutrin XL) dose until maximized (300–450 mg/d), if needed, while monitoring effects and side effects
- Provide psychoeducation for the family regarding proper sleep and wakefulness hygiene
- Encourage social engagements, such as dance recitals and other activities and/or friends' outings, to expose the patient to more social encounters, and work with her emotions in weekly psychotherapy sessions
- Add modafinil (Provigil) or armodafinil (Nuvigil) as a wakefulness agent
- Add a true stimulant such as methylphenidate (Ritalin) or mixed amphetamine salts (Adderall XR)
- Add thyroid hormone such as triiodothyronine (Cytomel)

Case outcome: interim follow-up visit 1 month later

- Bupropion XL (Wellbutrin XL) dose is increased to 300 mg/d to further target depressive symptoms of low motivation, hypersomnolence, poor concentration, and decreased energy and interest in socialization
- After this, patient reported some improvement in energy and motivation with further improvement academically
- However, no effect on oversleeping episodes; patient would still sleep 12 hours or more and nap in the afternoon
- The parents and the patient were educated about proper sleep and wakefulness hygiene and then implementing a sleep schedule with limitation of screen time (i.e., smart phones, laptops, TV, etc.) at least 1 hour prior to sleep, with some witnessed benefit in awakening the patient in the mornings
- Patient was able to participate in dance recitals weekly and worked through exploring her emotions in weekly psychotherapy sessions

Attending physician's mental notes: follow-up visit (month 2)

- Increased bupropion XL (Wellbutrin XL) dose to 300 mg/d has shown improvement in MDD symptoms (70%), improving school performance, energy level, and motivation, thus decreasing frustration and guilt / feelings of worthlessness
- Residual depressive vegetative symptoms, oversleeping episodes, and social isolation warrant a further increase in bupropion XL (Wellbutrin XL) dosage to 450 mg/d

- SSRI class is not recommended given the patient's prior side effect of developing suicidal ideation with three consecutive trials from this class of medicine
- Suspect any antidepressant with remarkable serotonin reuptake inhibition may cause similar side effects. If used, would dose gingerly and monitor closely

Case outcome: interim follow-up visit 2–4 months later

- Increase in bupropion XL (Wellbutrin XL) to 450 mg/d has shown further improvements in motivation, energy, and concentration
- Ongoing residual depressive symptoms still included hypersomnolence, and difficulty with sustaining motivation and energy, resulting in problems with meeting academic assignments' deadlines and missing a test
- At this time, venlafaxine (Effexor XR) 37.5 mg/d (SNRI) was discussed with the family and was added to increase serotonergic tone slightly to help residual MDD symptoms
- With this intervention, her energy level improved along with her motivation. She was able to keep up with her school assignments
- Social anxiety has decreased as now contemplating going back to in-person school after 6 months of virtual school
- While on venlafaxine (Effexor XR) 37.5 mg/d, she suffered from poor appetite and nausea, resulting in over 10 lb weight loss over the course of 1 month, with concerns about a low BMI of 18.9
  ○ Likely both antidepressants increase noradrenergic activity via reuptake inhibition, curbing her appetite
- However, no paradoxical suicidal ideation occurred at this low dose

Attending physician's mental notes: follow-up visit (month 4)

- Venlafaxine (Effexor XR) risks outweigh benefits. Weight loss with low BMI and falling off the growth curve resulted in fatigue and the patient's energy level dropping. Tapering off was initiated
- Discontinuation resulted in improved appetite and fatigue, but worsened depressive symptoms and anxiety attacks, within a few days
- Patient was started on a slower taper with daily 25 mg venlafaxine (Effexor) immediate-release trial as a lower dose, with improvement of symptoms. This dose was continued for 2 weeks, followed by 12.5 mg/d immediate release for 1 week. This was followed by complete discontinuation with no reported side effects afterwards
- Patient likely suffered from serotonin discontinuation syndrome, which was alleviated with the slow taper approach

Question

Which of the following would be your next step?

- Add mirtazapine (Remeron), a norepinephrine antagonist / selective serotonin antagonist (NaSSA) antidepressant
- Add modafinil (Provigil), a wakefulness agent
- Add a low-dose stimulant

Attending physician's mental notes: follow-up visit (month 4) (continued)

- Continue bupropion XL (Wellbutrin XL) 450 mg/d as it has resulted in moderate durable improvement of depressive symptoms and improved academic performance
- Venlafaxine (Effexor XR) discontinued due to side effects of nausea and low BMI of 18.9
- Patient is encouraged to eat healthy meals and was provided vitamins and supplements through her pediatrician as she was found to have vitamin D deficiency
- Discussed adjunct medication options noted above
- Mirtazapine (Remeron) was suggested, at a starting dose of 7.5 mg nightly to help with modifying the sleep schedule at night, rather than a stimulant during daytime, to help with improving appetite and normalizing her weight. Patient and family provided informed consent and they opted for medication trial
  - This felt ideal as it increased serotonin and norepinephrine activity via the novel non-SNRI mechanism
    - Antagonizing α_2 noradrenergic autoreceptors
    - Antagonizing serotonergic 2a, 2c, 3 receptors
- Will need to monitor for sedating daytime side effects, but hope improved sleep will alleviate hypersomnolence

Case outcome: interim follow-up visits 6 to 8 months later

- With the addition of mirtazapine (Remeron) 7.5 mg/d at night, the patient's appetite improved, with restoration of normal weight and body mass index (BMI) ensuing
- Vitamin D level was corrected as well via supplementation
- Energy level improved
- Patient continued to attend weekly for PDP with remarkable progress toward goals, targeting affect phobia with some cognitive behavioral therapy (CBT) exposure and desensitization of feared affects, including grief of losing her grandmother. Explored themes of loss of control in sessions, as well as transitioning into adult role and the conflict of autonomy vs. dependency

- Patient's motivation and overall anxiety improved as a result of combination between psychopharmacology and weekly PDP
- Toward the end of this interval:
  - The patient was engaging in full in-person school attendance, weekly dance recitals, weekend gatherings with friends, and was able to excel academically and receive scholarships for college
  - The patient ultimately discontinued mirtazapine (Remeron) as she recognized it was not needed as she was sleeping well and needed no daytime naps
  - The patient took on a new sport, golfing. She was accepted to a reputable college of her preference. She is still engaged in weekly psychodynamic psychotherapy sessions

Case debrief

- This patient suffered from MDD, GAD, and social anxiety disorder, all of which went into remission owing to a combined treatment of psychopharmacology, via NDRI antidepressant bupropion XL (Wellbutrin XL), along with PDP and with CBT techniques targeting social phobia through affect exposure and desensitization (affect phobia guidelines include a combination of cognitive behavioral techniques and psychodynamic techniques)
- Mirtazapine (Remeron) was also used as a bona fide antidepressant combination, but essentially acted as a hypnotic and restored her sleep cycle, thus putting her into MDD full remission
- She was suffering no current acute side effects and was functioning well at home and at school, and was engaged in multiple social activities
- She appeared to be maintaining normal weight for her height now
- She was less anxious in social settings, with fewer ruminations and a less negative view of herself
- She was less isolated and more engaged with family and friends
- She was no longer complaining of oversleeping episodes

Take-home points

- Augmentation of psychopharmacology with psychotherapy techniques may sometimes work better than combining medications, with the benefit of eliminating side effects such as weight loss, decreased appetite, and nausea, as depicted in this case
- Sometimes improving sleep and circadian function can be a remarkable short-term intervention

- It is crucial to monitor for side effects such as accelerated weight loss, and its impact on overall functioning and wellbeing. This is particularly important for child and adolescent cases
- Collaboration with a pediatrician is key. Vitamin D replacement has added benefit to this patient's overall functioning by improving her energy level
- Family inclusion is also of great value as they complement the picture through their input from their observations. Additionally, they have a key role in progress of treatment. Psychoeducation and informed consent are to be provided throughout the process

Tips and pearls

- Sleep hygiene was first formulated by Peter Hauri in an attempt to promote proper sleep conditions to improve insomnia
- Inappropriate sleep environment showed the highest correlations with problems going to bed
- At the onset of puberty, a daily endogenous rhythm of hormones leads to late onset of sleep (labeled as eveningness). Morningness–eveningness has a biological underpinning
- Adolescents' eveningness orientation is associated with many sleep-related problems, including extreme difficulties in returning to wakefulness
- Adequate sleep hygiene behavior in the hour before going to bed and an adequate sleep environment are the most important steps to promote early bedtimes and to cushion adolescents' drift to eveningness
- Parents' discipline by removing electronic devices from the adolescents' bedroom could promote a better sleep environment. On the downside, this may impede adolescents' development, with the impingement on autonomy
- Delay in school start time to synchronize adolescents' circadian rhythms to their daily educational and social demands could be beneficial for adolescent health and might lead to better academic performance
- This was achieved in this patient due to the flexibility applied by virtual school setting during COVID pandemic
- The following is a list of of possible sleep hygiene recommendations as per Peter Hauri
  1. Curtail time in bed
  2. Never try to force self to sleep
  3. Eliminate the bedroom clock

4. Exercise in the late afternoon or early evening
5. Avoid coffee, alcohol, and nicotine
6. Regularize the bedtime routine and wake-up time
7. Eat a light bedtime snack
8. Explore the use of short strategic napping
9. Monitor use of PRN hypnotics

Performance in practice: confessions of a psychopharmacologist

What could have been done better here?

- Finish what you start when you prescribe

  ○ When starting a psychotropic, if it is dosed too low, at a level that has been shown not to provide an outcome over placebo, your patient will not get better

  ○ The minimum therapeutic dose is the one that must be reached, where the drug has been statistically shown to beat a placebo in multiple regulatory trials

    ▪ This dose ideally must be reached in every patient

  ○ Many drugs have a dose response curve where higher doses can be more effective statistically for all, or based on case-by-case examples

  ○ Side-effect burden also tends to increase with higher doses

What are possible action items for improvement in practice?

- Investigate minimum therapeutic doses for agents used most in practice
- Investigate full dose ranges, and whether there is a dose-response curve for agents used most in practice

Two-minute tutorial

The history and effect of the FDA black box warning for prescribing antidepressants in young adults

- Multiple reports and studies showed increased rates of suicidality in young patients with MDD while prescribed SSRIs
- Suicidality or suicidal behavior is defined as serious thoughts about taking one's own life, or planning or attempting suicide
- The US Food and Drug Administration (FDA) conducted meta-analyses of 372 randomized controlled trials of antidepressants involving nearly 100,000 participants
- The rate of suicidality was higher among patients assigned to antidepressants, when compared with placebo

- In age-stratified analyses, the increased risk was shown to be significant mostly among children and adolescents under the age of 18 years
- In October 2003, the FDA issued a series of health advisories and warnings regarding prescribing SSRIs for children, adolescents, and yong adults up to age 24
- In 2004, the FDA announced a requirement of a black box warning on all antidepressants regarding the increased risk of suicidal behavior, particularly in children
- In January 2005, the warning was implemented
- In 2006, the FDA extended the warning to include young adults up to 25 years of age
- Consequently, healthcare providers' prescription of antidepressant drugs declined, resulting in an increase in the rate of suicidal incidents among patients with severe MDD
- To date, despite the FDA acting with good intentions, there is controversy regarding the validity of the industry-sponsored randomized controlled placebo trials conducted by the FDA
- Methodologically, there has been an argument regarding outcome results, given that suicidal behavior was not a primary outcome of these trials
- Additionally, the FDA did not determine any conclusive causal relationship
- The FDA did not seem to comment on or show that untreated MDD risk of suicide is likely higher than that with taking an SSRI
- Researchers have been evaluating the impact of the FDA's antidepressant black box warning over the past decade, with a resulting documented increase in rates of suicidal events in multiple studies, as shown in Figure 14.1, raising suspicion of a correlation between increased suicide rates and a decline in antidepressant prescription following the implementation of the black box warning
- In 2018, the Centers for Disease Control and Prevention announced that suicide attempts among teenagers have doubled in the last decade
- Further revision may be warranted to weigh up the data compiled over the last decade, especially as some longer-term naturalistic studies show a protective effect of up to 15% or greater in relation to completed suicide over the lifetime of SSRI takers vs. others

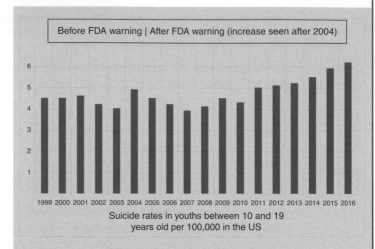

Figure 14.1 Suicide rates in youths from 1999 to 2016

The black box warning and precautions – original text used as an example of FDA boxed warning of sertraline (Zoloft)

Warning: Suicidal Thoughts and Behaviors

– Antidepressants increased the risk of suicidal thoughts and behavior in pediatric and young adult patients in short-term studies
– Closely monitor all antidepressant-treated patients for clinical worsening, and for emergence of suicidal thoughts and behaviors

Suicidal Thoughts and Behaviors in Pediatric and Young Adult Patients

– In pooled analysis of placebo-controlled trials of antidepressant drugs (SSRI and other antidepressant classes) that included approximately 77,000 adult patients and over 4,400 pediatric patients, the incidence of suicidal thoughts and behaviors in pediatric and young adult patients was greater in antidepressant-treated patients than in placebo-treated patients
– It is unknown whether the risk of suicidal thoughts and behaviors in pediatric and young adult patients extends to longer-term use, i.e., beyond 4 months. However, there is substantial evidence from placebo-controlled maintenance

trials in adults with MDD that antidepressants delay the recurrence of depression

- Monitor all antidepressant-treated patients for clinical worsening and emergence of suicidal thoughts and behaviors, especially during the initial few months of drug therapy and at times of dosage changes
- Counsel family members or caregivers of patients to monitor for changes in behavior and to alert the health care provider. Consider changing the therapeutic regimen, including possibly discontinuing SSRI, in patients with depression whose symptoms get persistently worse, or who are experiencing emergent suicidal thoughts or behaviors

Mechanism of action moment

How does mirtazapine (Remeron) work to promote better sleep?

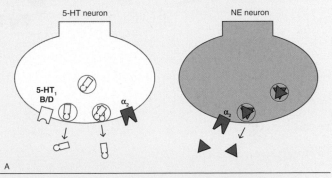

Figure 14.2 Mirtazapine's main antidepressant therapeutic action is designed to promote greater noradrenergic activity in the CNS to improve depressive symptoms. Alpha-2 antagonism increases serotonin and norepinephrine release in raphe and cortex. (A) On the left, a serotonergic neuron is shown with 5-HT$_{1B/D}$ autoreceptors and α_2-adrenergic heteroreceptors. On the right, a noradrenergic neuron is shown with presynaptic α_2 autoreceptors. (B) 5-HT$_{1B/D}$ autoreceptors and α_2-adrenergic heteroreceptors on serotonergic neurons both function as "brakes" to shut off serotonin release when bound by their respective neurotransmitters (left). Likewise, when norepinephrine binds to α_2 autoreceptors on the norepinephrine neuron, this shuts off further norepinephrine release (right). (C) Alpha-2 antagonists "cut the serotonin brake cable" when they block presynaptic α_2 heteroreceptors, thus leading to enhanced serotonin release (left). Alpha-2 antagonists also "cut the norepinephrine brake cable" by blocking presynaptic α_2 autoreceptors, leading to enhanced norepinephrine release (right).

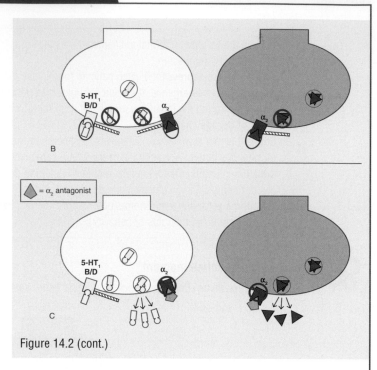

Figure 14.2 (cont.)

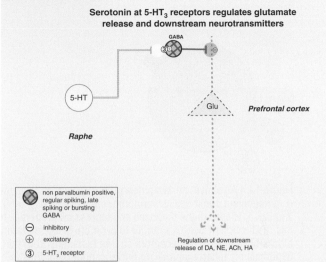

Serotonin at 5-HT$_3$ receptors regulates glutamate release and downstream neurotransmitters

5-HT$_3$ antagonists disinhibit glutamate release and enhance the release of downstream neurotransmitters to improve depression

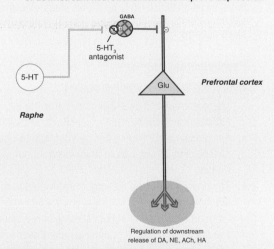

Figure 14.3 Additionally, mirtazapine antagonizes 5-HT$_3$ receptors. 5-HT$_3$ receptors regulate glutamate and downstream neurotransmitters. Serotonin (5-HT) binding at 5-HT$_3$ receptors on GABA interneurons is stimulatory; thus, it increases GABA release. GABA, in turn, inhibits glutamate pyramidal neurons, reducing glutamate output. Decreased release of excitatory glutamate means that there may be a resultant decrease in downstream release of neurotransmitters, since pyramidal neurons synapse with the neurons of most other neurotransmitters. Antagonism at the 5-HT$_3$ receptor removes GABA inhibition and thus disinhibits pyramidal neurons. The increase in glutamate neurotransmission may in turn increase the downstream release of neurotransmitters. Antagonism of 5-HT$_{2C}$ allows for increases in norepinephrine and dopamine in the frontal cortex as well.

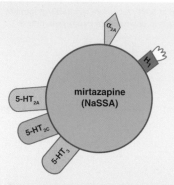

Figure 14.4 As above, mirtazapine's primary therapeutic action is α_2 antagonism and it blocks serotonin receptors 5-HT$_{2A}$, 5-HT$_{2C}$ and 5-HT$_3$. These are the theorized antidepressant properties for this medication. However, in order to promote sleep, mirtazapine blocks histamine 1 (H$_1$) receptors so that histamine from the hypothalamic tuberomammillary nuclei cannot bind, thus removing CNS arousal. A loss of arousal results in fatigue and then likely somnolence. It also blocks 5-HT$_{2A}$ serotonin receptors causing initial sedation which likely promotes sleep efficiency so that, once asleep, patients may spend more time in deeper stage 3 and 4 sleep patterns.

Psychotherapy moment

How and why does psychotherapy help?

- There is interest in identifying, and growing evidence of, the biochemical and neurobiological effects of psychotherapy
- Functional neuroimaging has been of help in visualizing the neurobiological changes in brain–behavior circuits that occur during therapy
- The prefrontal–limbic network is implicated in the process of emotion regulation
- Emotion regulation is of critical value in reversing psychopathology and is a main target of multiple psychotherapeutic approaches, whether cognitive or psychodynamic psychotherapies
- Psychotherapy is found to cause a more active prefrontal cortex, promoting effectiveness of control processes of an executive nature, which leads to an increase in cognitive control over emotional stimuli
- Studies show evidence of correlation between psychotherapy and increased activation of neural circuitry in prefrontal areas which are associated with executive functioning, such as the dorsolateral prefrontal cortex (DLPFC), dorsal anterior cingulate cortex (dACC), and ventrolateral prefrontal cortex

- Activation of such prefrontal areas represents successful recruitment of top-down cognitive control processes in the context of emotion regulation
- As a result of psychotherapy, in the prefrontal–limbic network, activated prefrontal areas act by inhibiting subcortical areas associated with emotional reactivity, such as the amygdala. This leads to successful implementation of emotion regulation strategies
- Meta-analyses of neuroimaging studies of the impact of psychotherapy show major changes in the temporal cortex, a key node of the semantic system as well
- Medial prefrontal areas and the inferior parietal lobe have also been associated with emotional semantic representations in tasks involving stimuli of expressed emotion
- Semantic representations are templates of past experiences, current interpersonal relationships, of self and others whereby patients organize and interpret the emotional significance of their daily experience. Semantic representations are viewed as a crucial aspect of psychotherapeutic interventions

Cognitive therapy, psychodynamic therapy, and associated neurobiological changes

- In CBT, distorted thoughts, feelings, and behaviors are explained as cognitively constructed maladaptive schemas (implicit or explicit). Schemas may lead to automatic thinking and behaviors
- CBT aims at increasing the patient's awareness of such schemas in therapy, and to enhance emotion regulation by implementing cognitive control processes. On neuroimaging, this is seen as activation of DLPFC, dACC, and VLPFC
- In psychodynamic approaches, in attempts to alleviate anxiety created by intrapsychic conflicts, patients implement unconscious defense mechanisms. Defenses can be viewed as an implicit form of emotion regulation in the face of evoked difficult emotions concerned with semantic representations of past traumatic experiences
- Psychodynamic therapy thus focuses on increasing the patient's awareness of such defenses to be able to identify the underlying emotions and contain them, rather than avoid them. Similar neuroimaging findings of activation in prefrontal areas are observed here as well. This indicates that the implemented reflective capacity allows for activation of executive functioning areas leading to enhanced emotion regulation
- PDP also highlights the importance of targeting semantic representations with corrective emotional experiences

- Other neuroimaging changes observed during psychotherapy are related to areas linked to emotional semantic representations, such as the inferior parietal lobe, the temporo-parietal junction (TPJ), the anterior/middle temporal lobes, and the medial prefrontal areas

Post-test question

What is the impact of the selective serotonin–norepinephrine reuptake inhibitor (SNRI) venlafaxine (Effexor XR) on weight?

A. Unlike other antidepressants with serotonergic effects, venlafaxine (Effexor XR) can cause weight loss
B. Venlafaxine (Effexor XR) causes dose-dependent weight loss up to 5% of the body weight
C. Weight loss caused by venlafaxine (Effexor XR) in pediatric patients is related to decreased appetite, i.e., treatment-emergent anorexia
D. All of the above are true

Answer: D

Venlafaxine is an SNRI. It can lead to robust norepinephrine increases in the CNS and the periphery. This can lead to nausea with subsequent appetite loss, and also can suppress appetite of its own accord. Appetite loss can lead to weight loss, which is generally a well-tolerated adverse effect until too much weight is lost and it becomes an ongoing side effect and a clinical problem to manage. However, in certain patients, the SRI property can cause an increase in weight gain similar to that caused by SSRIs

References

1. Fornaro, M, Anastasia, A, Valchera, A, et al. The FDA "Black Box" warning on antidepressant suicide risk in young adults: more harm than benefits? *Front Psychiatry* 2019; 10:294
2. Hauri, P. *Sleep Hygiene, Relaxation Therapy, and Cognitive Interventions*. New York: Plenum, 1992.
3. Katz, LY, Kozyrskyj, AL, Prior, HJ, et al. Effect of regulatory warnings on antidepressant prescription rates, use of health services and outcomes among children, adolescents and young adults. *CMAJ* 2008; 178:1005–11
4. Lu, CY, Penfold, RB, Wallace, J, et al. Increases in suicide deaths among adolescents and young adults following US Food and Drug Administration antidepressant boxed warnings and declines in depression care. *Psychiatric Res Clin Pract* 2020; 2:43–52

5. Messina, I, Sambin, M, Beschoner, P, et al. Changing views of emotion regulation and neurobiological models of the mechanism of action of psychotherapy. *Cogn Affect Behav Neurosci* 2016; 16:571–87

6. Stahl, SM. Treatments for mood disorders: so-called "antidepressants" and "mood stabilizers. In *Stahl's Essential Psychopharmacology: Neuroscientific Basis and Practical Applications*, 5. Cambridge: Cambridge University Press, 2021, 283–358

7. Stahl, SM. *Venlafaxine*, 7. Cambridge: Cambridge University Press, 2020, 841–6

8. Stepanski, EJ, Wyatt, JK. Use of sleep hygiene in the treatment of insomnia. *Sleep Med Rev* 2003; 7:215–25.

9. Vollmer, C, Jankowski, KS, Díaz-Morales, JF, et al. Morningness–eveningness correlates with sleep time, quality, and hygiene in secondary school students: a multilevel analysis. *Sleep Med* 2017; 30:151–9.

Case 15: The lady with bipolar disorder (BP), borderline personality disorder (BPD), and myasthenia gravis (MG)

The Question: Should you use mood stabilizers in patients with myasthenia gravis?

The Psychopharmacological Dilemma: Medication management of patients with Axis I, II, and III disorders and diseases

Nevena Radonjić and Elena Cappello

Pretest self-assessment question

Which medication is least likely to precipitate a myasthenic crisis in a patient with MG?

A. Lithium (Eskalith)

B. Lamotrigine (Lamictal)

C. Carbamazepine (Equetro)

D. Quetiapine (Seroquel)

Patient evaluation on intake

- A 27-year-old female with depression and suicidal ideation
- She states, "No one understands me"

Psychiatric history

- In mental health treatment since age 10 due to behavioral difficulties in school
- History of suicidal ideation since age 17
- History of four suicide attempts at age 19 via overdose, cutting, and lastly via hanging
  - The latter resulted in her first hospital admission
- Previous medication trials: fluoxetine (Prozac), sertraline (Zoloft), lamotrigine (Lamictal), bupropion XL (Wellbutrin XL), and risperidone (Risperdal)

Social and personal history

- Broke up with significant other a while back, amicably
- Graduated high school, struggled at college, on social security disability
- History of alcohol use in the early 20s, occasional alcohol intake in past 5 years
- Medical marijuana card, daily use, usually 2–3 times per day via inhalation, which she finds beneficial for chronic pain

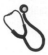

Medical history

- MG
- Migraines
- Irritable bowel syndrome (IBS)

Family history

- Father has a clear history of BP type I (BP1) and alcohol use disorder (AUD), in remission 20 years

Current medications

- Lamotrigine (Lamictal) 100 mg/d, an antiepileptic mood stabilizer
- Bupropion XL (Wellbutrin XL) 300 mg/d, a norepinephrine–dopamine reuptake inhibitor (NDRI)
- Pyridostigmine (Mestinon) 60 mg/d
- Meloxicam (Mobic) 15 mg/d

Psychotherapy history

- In weekly supportive psychotherapy for many years

Attending physician's mental notes: initial psychiatric evaluation

- The patient reports anhedonia, depressed mood, impaired sleep, fatigue, low energy, difficulty focusing, and acute suicidal ideation without a plan or intent to act on it
- She disclosed struggling with fear of abandonment, poor sense of self, chronic sense of emptiness, and affective lability
- On further interview, reports history of hypomanic episodes characterized by decreased need for sleep, increase in goal-oriented activity, engaging in risky behaviors, and having racing thoughts lasting up to 4 days, which appear independently of her BPD mood lability
- Appears that she is currently presenting with a depressive episode of bipolar II disorder (BP2) and BPD
- Patient also has a positive family history of BP
- During an initial evaluation, it is challenging to determine if this patient has BP2 with comorbid BPD, or has been misdiagnosed with BP due to symptom overlap between two disorders

Question

Is there a way to differentiate BP from BPD symptoms to make a more accurate diagnosis?

- Differentiating between BPD and BP is a frequent clinical diagnostic dilemma
- Both disorders can present with affective lability, impulsivity, suicidality, and risky behaviors
- Approximately 20% of patients with BPD have comorbid BP
- Likewise, approximately 20% of patients with BP2 have been diagnosed with BPD, while only 10% of patients with BP1 have been diagnosed with BPD
- Patients with BP2 are more likely to have a first-degree relative with BP2, the onset of symptoms in late teenage years, episodic presentation of symptoms that do not remit with age and that respond well to mood stabilizers and atypical antipsychotic drugs
- Patients with BPD are more likely to have relatives with impulse control disorders and borderline features, presence of emotional difficulties since early childhood, interpersonal sensitivity, chronic presence of symptoms that tend to improve over time, and not a clear-cut response to mood stabilizers
- Obtaining detailed psychiatric history is key in order to differentiate BPD from BP and vice versa
- The initial assessment aims to establish whether the patient is safe to be at home and to understand how she has tolerated previous medication trials, but further diagnostic clarity is needed
- Patient is currently on a mood stabilizer and NDRI, and doses of both medications could be adjusted for greater effectiveness as a first step

Further investigation

Is there anything else you would like to know about the patient?

- Does she have suicidal thinking or behaviors?
  - ○ The patient reports that she has a long history of suicidal ideation
    - Describes these as chronic in nature
    - Often exacerbated by interpersonal stressors
    - Reports that she used to cut to self-soothe in youth but stopped 10 years ago
- Does she have good social support now?
    - Reports that she has a stable income from social security payments and supportive friends

- Have any medications helped her as yet?
  - Previous antidepressant trials with fluoxetine (Prozac) and sertraline (Zoloft) were activating, resulting in an increase in energy, irritability, and impaired sleep
  - A recent trial of risperidone (Risperdal), an atypical antipsychotic, provoked an acute MG crisis
  - Her MG flare-up presented with acute muscle weakness and difficulty breathing, requiring evaluation in the emergency room
  - The patient is wary and reluctant to have *any* medication change due to this experience

Which psychiatric medications can precipitate a myasthenic crisis in patients with MG?

- Myasthenia gravis is an autoimmune disease in which antibodies against postsynaptic nicotinic acetylcholine (ACh) receptors at the neuromuscular junction (NMJ) cause fatigue and muscle weakness
- Typical symptoms of MG include ptosis, diplopia, proximal muscle weakness, respiratory muscle weakness (dyspnea), and bulbar muscle weakness (dysphagia, difficulty chewing)
- Due to increased ACh consumption, these symptoms progressively worsen during the day with muscle use
- Certain symptoms, such as fatigue, decreased energy, memory disturbance, sleep disorders, and shortness of breath, overlap with symptoms of psychiatric disorder
- These may confound MG diagnosis, present secondary to MG diagnosis, or occur in response to medical management of MG (e.g., corticosteroids)
- Approximately 20% of patients with MG are initially diagnosed with a psychiatric disorder and many patients with MG are initially placed on psychiatric medications to address their symptoms
- These medications include but are not limited to antidepressants, benzodiazepines (BZs), mood stabilizers, and antipsychotics, which can unmask or exacerbate MG symptoms
- Mood stabilizers may pose a pharmacological challenge to management of patients with MG
  - Lithium (Eskalith) may precipitate new myasthenic symptoms and exacerbate myasthenic crisis (MC)
  - Although the mechanism is not completely clear, it is hypothesized that lithium presynaptically reduces synthesis and release of ACh and postsynaptically decreases the number of ACh receptors

- Carbamazepine (Equetro) can interfere with the bioavailability of immunosuppressive treatments in MG by increasing cytochrome P450 and subsequent liver oxidation and metabolism
- There are currently no known effects of divalproex (Depakote), lamotrigine (Lamictal), and topiramate (Topamax) on MG and MG therapy
- Certain antipsychotics have been associated with worsening of MG symptoms
  - Chlorpromazine (Thorazine) was the first reported typical antipsychotic associated with MG exacerbation, and it was shown that it impairs neuromuscular transmission at both the presynaptic and postsynaptic membranes
  - Dose-dependent effects on neuromuscular transmission were also demonstrated for atypical antipsychotics clozapine (Clozaril), olanzapine (Zyprexa), sulpiride (Dolmatil), and risperidone (Risperdal)
  - Pimozide (Orap), thioridazine (Mellaril), haloperidol (Haldol), quetiapine (Seroquel), and long-acting risperidone (Consta) were also reported to cause deterioration of symptoms in patients with myasthenia gravis
  - Although antipsychotics can cause worsening of MG symptoms, MG exacerbation is not frequently reported with antipsychotic use
- BZs have the potential to induce respiratory depression and are considered contraindicated in patients with MG as they already have an increased risk for respiratory distress

Attending physician's mental notes: initial psychiatric evaluation (continued)

- Given her self-injurious behavior (SIB), a safety plan should be developed in the case of a crisis
- Education on BPD and its treatment has been provided to the patient
- Given a history of interpersonal sensitivity and affective lability, evidence-based psychotherapy for BPD should be recommended
  - If possible, we should consider psychodynamic psychotherapy (PDP) or dialectical behavioral therapy (DBT), if available
- Patient provided consent for her neurologist to be included in treatment planning given the history of MG and sensitivity to psychiatric medications

- She is on a subtherapeutic NDRI antidepressant, bupropion XL (Wellbutrin XL) and subtherapeutic mood stabilizer, lamotrigine (Lamictal)
  - She is happy with both of these because they have not worsened her MG
  - Antidepressants are not often greatly effective for BPD and may worsen BP
  - Mood stabilizers and antipsychotics may be more globally effective for BPD
  - It is typically good practice to escalate medications through their full dosing range before deciding whether they are a failed approach

Case outcome: interim follow-ups through 1 month

- The patient has agreed to increase the dose of lamotrigine (Lamictal) gingerly to 125 mg/d for 2 weeks, then 150 mg/d
  - Titrating slowly makes sense to improve both her rapport with the prescriber and her compliance with medications
- Psychoeducation on lamotrigine (Lamictal) was provided, and the possibility of developing severe rash has been discussed
- Discussed with the patient that full dosing of lamotrigine (Lamictal) is typically 200 mg/d for BP maintenance treatment, but sometimes is used higher for both epilepsy and BPD
- Patient has responded well initially to increased dosing
- Denies any appreciable side effects
- Reports that her mood improved and that suicidal ideation markedly decreased in frequency and intensity over a few weeks
- The patient shared that the relationship with her parents is very challenging
  - Historically, she found parents hypercritical, which she has described as "traumatic"
  - She seems able to appreciate how, although she cares about them, she needs to set boundaries
- The patient reports that she has reached out to a DBT psychotherapy program and plans to start therapy soon

Case debrief

- Many patients with BPD have been diagnosed with BP and vice versa
- A detailed longitudinal or corroborative history is often needed to discern between symptoms of affective lability and impulsivity in BPD vs. BP

- This patient has both, and a medication that is approved for BP was also used for BPD with some initial success, and a good referral for an evidence-based psychotherapy approach occurred
  ○ This likely is in accordance with most guidelines to use psychotropics to treat both target BPD symptoms and comorbid disorders while attempting to provide weekly psychotherapy in an outcomes-based model

Take-home points

- The pharmacological treatment of BPD remains controversial as some guidelines, such as the UK National Institute for Health and Care Excellence, recommend no drug use in BPD treatment. At the same time, American Psychiatric Association guidelines state that antidepressants, mood stabilizers, and antipsychotics could be considered in BPD treatment
- Long-term psychotherapy is considered critical in the treatment of BPD
- BPD is the most common personality disorder treated in clinical settings
- Patients with BPD commonly experience suicidal ideation, and 8–10% of BPD patients die by suicide
- Almost 90% of BPD patients engage in non-suicidal SIB
- A comprehensive approach combining psychotherapy and psychopharmacology is often needed
- The primary treatment for BPD is psychotherapy, complemented by symptom-targeted pharmacotherapy
- Psychiatric management for patients with BPD includes responding to crises often without acute medication adjustments, monitoring patients' safety, establishing and maintaining a therapeutic framework and alliance, providing education on the disorder and its treatment, monitoring progress, and re-assessing effectiveness of the treatment so as not to accumulate ineffective psychotropics and irrational polypharmacy

Performance in practice: confessions of a psychopharmacologist

What could have been done better here?

- Avoiding the use of agents known to exacerbate MG is critical
  ○ This avoids worsening of MG and more functional impairment
  ○ Builds rapport with the psychopharmacologist and improves future adherence during medication management

What are possible action items for improvement in practice?

- Use a review article to increase knowledge about psychotropic use in MG to become aware that:
  - Mood disorders are the most common comorbidity in MG
  - Starting or switching psychotropic medications can worsen symptoms of MG
  - Sometimes presenting symptoms of MG such as difficulty breathing can be misdiagnosed as anxiety
  - After initiation of antipsychotics, prescribers may erroneously diagnose MG symptoms as an extrapyramidal syndrome (EPS) and initiate anticholinergic medication that can further symptomatically worsen MG
  - Symptoms of MG are precipitated by psychotropic medications targeting nicotinic AChR and not muscarinic AChR
  - Autonomic dysfunction is reported in MG, hence sympatholytics such as prazosin and doxazosin used in the treatment of anxiety and post-traumatic stress disorder (PTSD) can cause adverse effects such as lightheadedness or orthostatic hypotension

Tips and pearls

- Avoiding anticholinergic effects (blurred vision, dry mouth, constipation, etc.) in any patient will improve compliance with taking medications
- In the treatment of MG, it is important to differentiate between medications affecting nicotinic vs. muscarinic ACh receptors
- Older psychotropics such as tricyclic antidepressants (TCAs) have selectivity for muscarinic ACh receptor antagonism and in low doses generally do not pose a risk of producing muscle weakness in patients with MG

Psychotherapy moment

- Four major therapies have been established as evidence-based treatments for BPD
  - DBT
  - Mentalization-based therapy
  - Transference-focused psychotherapy
  - Systems training for emotional predictability and problem-solving
- DBT is the most common and mainstay therapy for BPD, developed by Marsha Linehan to treat highly suicidal patients who have not responded to conventional eclectic treatment
  - DBT utilizes mindfulness, interpersonal effectiveness, emotional regulation, and stress tolerance techniques to assist patients

- Research has shown that patients with BPD who practice DBT form new neural connections from the amygdala to the dorsolateral prefrontal cortex (DLPFC) and ventromedial prefrontal cortex (VMPFC) allowing patients to respond to stressful stimuli and reflect on their emotional experiences more rapidly and efficiently
- Mentalization-based therapy has been developed by Anthony Bateman and Peter Fonagy and is focused on the reciprocal relationship between attachment security and mentalizing capacity
  - Mentalization is a term used to describe the complex ability that one develops to understand the mental activity underlying social interactions
  - Mentalization-based therapy exercises enable patients to visualize their mental state in order to construct and interpret their own perceptions and responses during stressful times
- Transference-focused psychotherapy (TFP) was developed by Frank Yeomans, John Clarkin, and Otto Kernberg
  - In this type of therapy, focus is on the reduction of suicidal ideation and self-harm via internalized object transference and introspection
  - The goal of the treatment is to decrease BPD symptoms by changing patients' mental representations of self and others to meaningfully improve overall functioning
- Systems training for emotional predictability and problem-solving (STEPPS), developed by Nancee Blum, is a group treatment that combines cognitive-behavioral elements and skills training with a systems component for individuals with whom a patient regularly interacts
- Besides the "big four," new evidence-based modalities for the treatment of BPD are emerging, such as dynamic deconstructive psychotherapy (DDP), developed by Robert Gregory
  - DDP is a year-long manualized treatment that encourages patients to assign their emotions and reflect on their experiences using translational neuroscience, object relations theory, and deconstruction philosophy elements

Two-minute tutorial

What are the neurobiological underpinnings in the development and treatment of BPD?

Genetics

- Familial and twin studies imply genetic vulnerability at the root of BPD, with an estimated heritability of approximately 40%
- Genome-wide association studies (GWAS) have shown that BPD genetically overlaps with BP, schizophrenia (SP), and major depressive disorder (MDD)
- So far, no single nucleotide polymorphism has reached significance at GWAS level; however, future studies with larger samples may identify some of the genetic risk factors that confer risk for BPD

Gene–environment interaction

- A safe, nurturing, and trusting environment is critical for the development of the neurological pathways underlying emotional regulation, internal reflection, and appraisal of danger during early childhood
- Early-life trauma, stress, and neglect can interrupt one of the major pathways that regulate emotional responses in BPD – the hypothalamic–pituitary–adrenal (HPA) axis
- Interruption of the HPA axis lends itself to prolonged cortical responses due to loss of negative feedback mechanisms and plays a major role in the clinical manifestation of BPD
- The hippocampus projects to the HPA axis to provide negative feedback during emotional stimulation or stress
- The experience of affection during the critical developmental period is essential in the regulation of glucocorticoid receptor density in the hippocampus
- Early-life experiences also may alter the transcription of the genes responsible for the expression of glucocorticoid receptors
  - In individuals with early trauma, heavy methylation can silence the transcription factors responsible for serotonin receptor genes and glucocorticoid receptors
    - In fact, methylation of these genes and consequent silencing were found to correlate with the severity of BPD
    - In comparison, affection during critical periods fosters major demethylation events that increase the transcription factors responsible for a robust glucocorticoid receptor density and a tightly regulated stress response
  - Post-mortem studies of patients with an early history of trauma showed a decreased density of glucocorticoid receptors

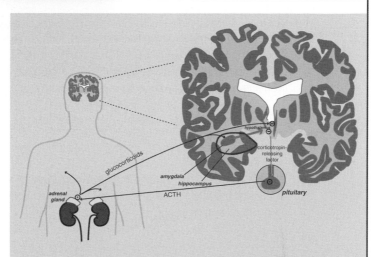

Figure 15.1 Hypothalamic–pituitary–adrenal (HPA) axis. The normal stress response involves activation of the hypothalamus and a resultant increase in corticotropin-releasing factor (CRF), which in turn stimulates the release of adrenocorticotropic hormone (ACTH) from the pituitary. ACTH causes glucocorticoid release from the adrenal gland, which feeds back to the hypothalamus and inhibits CRF release, terminating the stress response. The amygdala and hippocampus also provide input to the hypothalamus, to suppress activation of the HPA axis.

Neurobiological pathways

- The amygdala, also known as a regulator of emotional responses, is responsible for relaying messages to the DLPFC (responsible for executive function) and the VMPFC (responsible for reflection and contemplation)
- BPD patients have increased amygdala activity, causing them to experience emotions more intensely
- Compounding increased amygdala activity, patients with BPD have decreased relay of information from the amygdala to the DLPFC and VMPFC
  - This may reflect a loss of top-down control over visceral, primitive emotions
- Patients without BPD have a robust relay from the amygdala to these structures to address stressors, quantify them, and decide what to do next
  - In other words, non-BPD patients have a better chance to think through intense emotions and weigh the pros/cons of acting on these emotions

259

- Due to the aforementioned neurobiological pathways, patients with BPD experience emotions more intensely, possess decreased executive function during periods of stress, and undergo a prolonged stress response secondary to low-density glucocorticoid receptors and hypermethylation

Brain imaging in BPD

- Imaging studies have shown differences in the volume of and activity in brain structures related to emotion and impulsivity in individuals with BPD
- Structures with reduced volume in BPD have hypermetabolism due to postulated loss of inhibition resulting in impulsive behavior and overly negative attributions
- Imaging studies have certain limitations as many BPD patients have psychiatric comorbidities, hence the interpretation of results is additionally complicated

Pharmacotherapy

- BPD is characterized by affective dysregulation (affective lability, anger, and fear of abandonment), behavioral dysregulation (impulsivity and risky behaviors, suicidality and self-injurious behavior), and disturbances in relatedness (chronic emptiness, unstable relationships, and poor sense of self)
- So far, no medications have been approved by the FDA for BPD treatment but vafidemast, for example, is currently in regulatory trials
- However, certain medications such as antidepressants, mood stabilizers, and antipsychotics are being used routinely in clinical practice to target specific BPD symptoms
- Studies have shown that 90–99% of patients with BPD are on psychotropic medications, and frequently there is concomitant use of several medications (polypharmacy)
- Clinical practice guidelines are inconsistent regarding medication use in BPD
- The American Psychiatric Association has recommended the use of pharmacotherapy as a second-line treatment for affective dysregulation in patients with BPD, with therapy being the first-line treatment
- Mood stabilizers have been proven effective in diminishing impulsivity, suicidal ideation, and positive symptoms of psychiatric conditions such as BP. Their role in treating symptoms that overlap with BPD is an ongoing subject of investigation

- The role of lithium (Eskalith) in placebo-controlled studies initially illustrated improvement in global functioning and mood in patients with BPD; however, these results could not be replicated in future studies
- Similarly, the role of carbamazepine (Equetro) in placebo-controlled studies has not shown consistent or reliable results
- Studies have shown that topiramate (Topamax) and lamotrigine (Lamictal) can improve symptoms of anger and aggression in BPD
- Topiramate (Topamax) has illustrated improved anxiety and interpersonal sensitivity in smaller sample studies
- Lamotrigine (Lamictal), topiramate (Topamax), and aripiprazole (Abilify) reduced impulsivity in studies
- Divalproex (Depakote), lamotrigine (Lamitcal), topiramate (Topamax), haloperidol (Haldol), aripiprazole (Abilify), quetiapine (Seroquel), olanzapine (Zyprexa), omega-3 fatty acids, and amitriptyline (Elavil) can improve symptoms of affective dysregulation in BPD
- Aripiprazole (Abilify), quetiapine (Seroque), and olanzapine (Zyprexa) were recommended to manage psychotic symptoms in patients with BPD
- Atypical antipsychotics may be useful in targeting anxiety, anger, impulsivity, and paranoia / dissociative behavior in patients with BPD

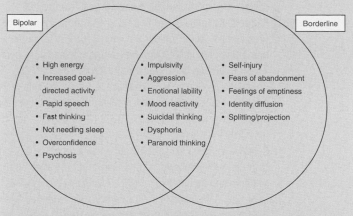

Figure 16.2 Phenomenological overlaps between bipolar and borderline personality disorders.

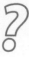

Post-test question

Which medication is least likely to precipitate a myasthenic crisis in a patient with MG?

A. Lithium (Eskalith)
B. Lamotrigine (Lamictal)
C. Carbamazepine (Equetro)
D. Quetiapine (Seroquel)

Answer: B

Lithium (Eskalith) can precipitate a myasthenic crisis. Although the mechanism is not entirely elucidated, it is believed that it causes dysfunction of the NMJ. Lamotrigine (Lamictal) is considered relatively safe to be prescribed in MG patients, and, so far, there are no reports of lamotrigine-induced adverse effects. Carbamazepine (Equetro) can impact the bioavailability of immunosuppressive treatment due to its effect on the CYP450 system. Quetiapine (Seroquel) has anti-adrenergic and anticholinergic properties that are thought to lead to the worsening of myasthenic symptoms.

References

1. Abualkhair, L, Almaghrabi, A, Al Edrees, N, et al. Unmasking of myasthenia gravis after introduction of oral risperidone in a schizophrenic Saudi male: a case report. *Cureus* 2021; 13:e20541
2. Blum, N, St John, D, Pfohl, B, et al. Systems Training for Emotional Predictability and Problem Solving (STEPPS) for outpatients with borderline personality disorder: a randomized controlled trial and 1-year follow-up. *Am J Psychiatry* 2008; 165:468–78
3. Bozzatello, P, Rocca, P, Baldassarri, L, et al. The role of trauma in early onset borderline personality disorder: a biopsychosocial perspective. *Front Psychiatry* 2021; 12; https://doi.org/10.3389/fpsyt.2021.721361
4. Cattane, N, Rossi, R, Lanfredi, M, et al. Borderline personality disorder and childhood trauma: exploring the affected biological systems and mechanisms. *BMC Psychiatry* 2017; 17:221
5. Choi-Kain, LW, Albert, EB, Gunderson, JG. Evidence-based treatments for borderline personality disorder: implementation, integration, and Stepped Care. *Harv Rev Psychiatry* 2016; 24:342–56
6. Choi-Kain, LW, Finch, EF, Masland, SR, et al. What works in the treatment of borderline personality disorder. *Curr Behav Neurosci Rep* 2017; 4:21–30

7. Crawford, MJ, MacLaren, T, Reilly, JG. Are mood stabilisers helpful in treatment of borderline personality disorder? *BMJ* 2014; 349:g5378

8. Goldberg, JF. *Personality Disorders and Traits*. Cambridge: Cambridge University Press, 2021.

9. Goodman, M, Carpenter, D, Tang, CY, et al. Dialectical behavior therapy alters emotion regulation and amygdala activity in patients with borderline personality disorder. *J Psychiatr Res* 2014; 57:108–16

10. Gregory, RJ, Remen, AL. A manual-based psychodynamic therapy for treatment-resistant borderline personality disorder. *Psychotherapy (Chic)* 2008; 45:15–27

11. Hancock-Johnson, E, Griffiths, C, Picchioni, M. A focused systematic review of pharmacological treatment for borderline personality disorder. *CNS Drugs* 2017; 31:345–56

12. Jordan, H, Ortiz, N. Management of insomnia and anxiety in myasthenia gravis. *J Neuropsychiatry Clin Neurosci* 2019; 31:386–91

13. Lis, E, Greenfield, B, Henry, M, et al. Neuroimaging and genetics of borderline personality disorder: a review. *J Psychiatry Neurosci* 2007; 32:162–73

14. Martín-Blanco, A, Ferrer, M, Soler, J, et al. Association between methylation of the glucocorticoid receptor gene, childhood maltreatment, and clinical severity in borderline personality disorder. *J Psychiatr Res* 2014; 57:34–40

15. McGowan, PO, Sasaki, A, D'Alessio, AC, et al. Epigenetic regulation of the glucocorticoid receptor in human brain associates with childhood abuse. *Nat Neurosci* 2009; 12:342–8

16. Oldham, JM, Glen Gabbard, CO, Goin, MK, et al. *Practice Guideline for the Treatment of Patients with Borderline Personality Disorder*. Washington, DC: American Psychiatric Association 2010

17. Paris, J. Suicidality in borderline personality disorder. *Medicina* 2019; 55:223

18. Perez-Rodriguez, MM, Bulbena-Cabré, A, Bassir Nia, A, et al. The neurobiology of borderline personality disorder. *Psychiatr Clin North Am* 2018; 41:633–50

19. Radtke, KM, Schauer, M, Gunter, HM, et al. Epigenetic modifications of the glucocorticoid receptor gene are associated with the vulnerability to psychopathology in childhood maltreatment. *Transl Psychiatry* 2015; 5:e571

20. Sheikh, S, Alvi, U, Soliven, B, et al. Drugs that induce or cause deterioration of myasthenia gravis: an update. *J Clin Med* 2021; 10:1537

21. Skoglund, C, Tiger, A, Rück, C, et al. Familial risk and heritability of diagnosed borderline personality disorder: a register study of the Swedish population. *Mol Psychiatry* 2021; 26:999–1008

22. Stahl, SM. *Mood Disorders and the Neurotransmitter Networks Norepinephrine and γ-Aminobutyric Acid (GABA)*, 5. Cambridge: Cambridge University Press, 2021, 244–82

23. Starcevic, V, Janca, A. Pharmacotherapy of borderline personality disorder: replacing confusion with prudent pragmatism. *Curr Opin Psychiatry* 2018; 31:69–73

24. Taubner, S, Volkert, J. Evidence-based psychodynamic therapies for the treatment of patients with borderline personality disorder. *Clin Psychol Eur* 2019; 1:1–20

25. Thomas, N, Gurvich, C, Kulkarni, J. Borderline personality disorder, trauma, and the hypothalamus–pituitary–adrenal axis. *Neuropsychiatr Dis Treat* 2019; 15:2601–12

26. Watanabe, Y, Hongo, S. Long-term efficacy and safety of lamotrigine for all types of bipolar disorder. *Neuropsychiatr Dis Treat* 2017; 13:843–54

27. Witt, SH, Streit, F, Jungkunz, M, et al. Genome-wide association study of borderline personality disorder reveals genetic overlap with bipolar disorder, major depression and schizophrenia. *Transl Psychiatry* 2017; 7:e1155

28. Yadav, D. Prescribing in borderline personality disorder – the clinical guidelines. *Prog Neurol Psychiatry* 2020; 24:25–30

29. Zhang, TY, Labonté, B, Wen, XL, et al. Epigenetic mechanisms for the early environmental regulation of hippocampal glucocorticoid receptor gene expression in rodents and humans. *Neuropsychopharmacology* 2013; 38:111–23

Case 16: Spending money does not make a bipolar diagnosis

The Question: When is activation in a depressive disorder anxious versus manic?

The Psychopharmacological Dilemma: It may be harder to treat anxiety in a bipolar patient as antidepressants should be avoided

Chris Damiani

Pretest self-assessment question

What is the typical rate of conversion from major depressive disorder (MDD) to bipolar I disorder (BP1) over time?

A. 1%
B. 2%
C. 8%
D. 50%

Patient evaluation on intake

- A 34-year-old female with a chief complaint of "years of depression and anxiety"
- Part-time case worker at a group home, with anxiety that impacts functioning both at work and in completing activities of daily living at home
- Fearful of potential side effects and hesitant to make medication changes or even engage in individual psychotherapy

Psychiatric history

- Both depressive and anxiety symptoms emerged as a teenager once her father passed away due to an unexpected cardiac event while she was present
- Began to experience insomnia beginning in her teens, as well as general restlessness
- Began to worry incessantly about numerous aspects of her daily life
- Previously diagnosed with bipolar II disorder (BP2); however, on evaluation, only endorses one short period with excessive spending with no financial ramifications and no other hypomanic symptoms
- Prescribed high-dose lamotrigine (Lamictal) 500 mg/d from previous provider given the presumptive diagnosis
- One psychiatric hospitalization due to feeling overwhelmed a year ago

- Has difficulty working part-time as a case worker and takes days off due to anxiety
  - Feeling easily fatigued
  - Difficulty sleeping
  - Incessant, uncontrollable worry
- States that most effective medication has been the benzodiazepine (BZ) anxiolytic, alprazolam (Xanax)
- Endorses increasing panic attacks several times per week
  - Reports abrupt tachycardia, shortness of breath, paresthesias, fear of impending doom, palpitations, and chest tightness with occasional glottis sensation
- Admits to depressive symptoms
  - Decreased sleep, amotivation, anhedonia, decreased energy, difficulty concentrating, and denies suicidal ideation

Social and personal history

- College graduate with a bachelor's in psychology
- Currently working as part-time case worker
- Spouse is employed full-time; no financial strain. Living in affluent suburb
- Has one child aged 9 who is doing well
- Does not use drugs or alcohol

Medical history

- Hashimoto's thyroiditis, currently prescribed levothyroxine (Synthroid)
  - Thyroid levels are normal
- Lower back pain and bilateral knee pain

Family history

- Denies any known mental illness in any family member

Medication history

- Trialed on olanzapine (Zyprexa), duloxetine (Cymbalta), buspirone (BuSpar), lurasidone (Latuda), citalopram (Celexa), clonazepam (Klonopin), venlafaxine (Effexor XR)
- Reports that she does not know the length of treatment or doses
- Feels that she is sensitive to medications and that these may not have been full trials due to unwanted side effects

Current medications

- Lamotrigine (Lamictal) 500 mg/d, an antiepileptic mood stabilizer
- Alprazolam (Xanax) 2 mg/d, a GABA-A positive allosteric modulator, BZ anxiolytic

Psychotherapy history

- Patient met with a therapist in her teens, as well as her 20s, but currently is not interested in any kind of psychotherapy

Patient evaluation on initial visit

- Onset of depressive and anxiety symptoms began at the age of 13 when she witnessed her father pass away
- Reports that symptoms have intensified throughout her teens and 20s and are now unmanageable
- Has seen numerous psychiatrists since she was 13 years old and is currently being prescribed medications by her primary care clinician, who urged her to now see a psychiatrist
- States compliance with medications but reports side effects that often cause her to quit treatments early
- Currently tolerating lamotrigine (Lamictal) and alprazolam (Xanax) compliantly but still has significant psychiatric symptoms
- Reports 25% improvement from alprazolam (Xanax) at most
- Hesitant to begin new medications

Question

Is there anything else that you would like to know about the patient?

Does she have post-traumatic stress disorder (PTSD)?

- Psychiatric review of systems screening suggested no other disorders
- She specifically witnessed her father's death but denied any reliving events after
- Reports it was traumatic and difficult as a result growing up, but does not seemingly meet full PTSD criteria

Does she have panic disorder (PD)?

- Psychiatric review of systems screening suggested no other disorders
- She develops acute somatic and psychological symptoms consistent with panic attacks lasting 10–20 minutes each time
- They are not triggered by social or traumatic cues

- She does not have any 1-month period where she feared implications of these attacks, nor did her behavior change (avoidance, agoraphobia) due to these attacks
- They happen only when she is depressed and feeling overwhelmed, perhaps exhibiting anxious distress

Attending physician's mental notes: initial psychiatric evaluation

- Patient not prescribed selective serotonin reuptake inhibitor (SSRI), serotonin–norepinephrine reuptake inhibitor (SNRI), or a serotonin partial agonist / reuptake inhibitor (SPARI) currently, which have better outcomes for MDD and for generalized anxiety disorder (GAD), which are her likely diagnoses
- Suspect that her father's death was a clear trauma and precipitating event, but she does not have PTSD now
  - This type of trauma may predispose to worse psychopharmacological outcomes
  - This likely predisposes her to the MDD and GAD symptoms she has now
- Panic attacks are likely driven by her MDD and might be considered psychomotor agitation or anxious distress
- Reports history of BP2 and is maintained on the mood stabilizer and antiepileptic, lamotrigine (Lamictal), higher than normal dose
  - This medication has not alleviated her anxiety or MDD
  - She has no rashes or other significant side effects, which is fortunate
- Might benefit from an SSRI or SNRI antidepressant, but worry about escalating her possible bipolarity into mixed features or hypomania
- Mixed features include the presence of both depressive and manic/hypomanic symptoms. This poses a challenge diagnostically
- The presence of mixed features can indicate that the patient may have bipolar disorder (BP) or possibly convert to BP in the future

Further investigation

Is there anything else that you would like to know about the patient?

How legitimate was the hypomania event?

- When asked about any 4-day periods meeting typical hypomania criteria, she responds negatively
- When anxious, she will speak fast and think fast due to worry, but is never feeling euphoric or mood-elevated

- She had one period of excessive spending, but seemingly did not meet other criteria for hypomania then, at least retrospectively while taking her history
- She always has thoughts that race due to worry but they are never incomplete
- She sleeps poorly, also due to worry, and never awakens with extra energy but rather has fatigue

Attending physician's mental notes: initial psychiatric evaluation (continued)

- After further thought and evaluation, she does not have BP2
- She was also re-screened for PTSD and denies flashbacks, nightmares, etc., now
- Regardless, her anxiety is very high and disruptive to her wellbeing
- This could be MDD with anxious distress, but she seems to have GAD symptoms regardless of MDD level and severity
- She recollects times of euthymia but still being immensely anxious, suggesting she has MDD and GAD comorbidly

Question

If this patient is BP2, and we have erroneously removed this diagnosis, what is likely to happen if an SSRI/SNRI antidepressant is added to help her anxiety now?

- She may develop mixed features or rapid cycling
- She could be pushed into hypomania or mania
- She could convert from BP2 to BP1, which is more severe in nature

What is the difference between MDD with anxious distress and MDD with GAD?

- Anxious distress is defined as the presence of at least two of the following symptoms during the majority of the day in a major depressive episode (MDE):
  - Feeling keyed-up or tense
  - Feeling unusually restless
  - Difficulty with concentration because of worry
  - Fear that something awful might happen
  - Feeling that the individual might lose control of himself or herself
- If the MDD is premorbid and the anxiety symptoms only occur while depressed then the patient meets criteria for MDD with anxious distress
- If the patient's GAD was premorbid to the depressive disorder then the patient carries two diagnoses: GAD and MDD

Case outcome: first interim follow-up at week 4

- SSRI escitalopram (Lexapro) started at low dose of 5 mg/d to avoid side effects, using an initially subtherapeutic dose, and to build patient confidence in the medication being used
- Decreased alprazolam (Xanax) 1 mg/d and 0.5 mg at bed as patient felt confident with the addition of an SSRI she would improve
- Lamotrigine (Lamictal) 500 mg/d continued with goal of decreasing dose in the future once anxiety is better managed
- Denies any initial side effects and reports 20–30% less anxiety and depression
- Ambivalent about starting psychotherapy still

Question

What would you do next?

- Increase escitalopram (Lexapro) to 10 mg/d which is a therapeutic dose
- Obtain pharmacogenetic testing to see why she is prone to side effects
- Increase escitalopram (Lexapro) to better treat BP2 depression
- Keep escitalopram (Lexapro) low to avoid side effects and see whether it will work despite being a lower than normal dose

Case outcome: second interim follow-up visit at 2 months

- Escitalopram (Lexapro) continued at 5 mg/d, lamotrigine (Lamictal) 500 mg/day, and alprazolam (Xanax) at 0.5 mg in the morning and 1 mg at night, based on patient preference and fear of side effects
- Continues to remain ambivalent about psychotherapy
  - Suggested she try cognitive behavioral therapy (CBT)
    - It is a 1-hour commitment over 12–15 weeks only
    - Continued to use motivational approach to foster better medication acceptance as well
- Chief complaint now is her report of non-restful sleep and fatigue during the day
- Started on melatonin 3 mg at night
- Discussed sleep hygiene approaches

Attending physician's mental notes: second interim follow-up visit (month 2)

- Feel more confident that she suffers from MDD and GAD, and not BP2 now
  - No evidence of any hypomania symptoms when low-dose SSRI added

- ○ Certainly need to monitor for any treatment-emergent activations (TEAs) or mixed features, as this would indicate a possible conversion to BP
- Will need to be patient and not fall into the same trap as previous providers by pushing her too fast to increase medication dosing
  - ○ Could develop real side effects and quit the SSRI, thwarting her outcomes
  - ○ Could develop nocebo psychological side effects as well

Case outcome: interim follow-up visits through 5 months

- Patient reported 20% fewer depressive and anxiety symptoms compared to previous visit but still symptomatic, perhaps having a response now and 50% better overall
- Escitalopram (Lexapro) increased to 10 mg/d and subsequently to 15 mg/d
  - ○ At 15 mg/d, reported night sweats and vivid dreams
- As anxiety symptoms were lessened, patient agreed to taper alprazolam (Xanax) to 0.5 mg now only twice per day
  - ○ Once tapered, reported increase in non-restful sleep with more initial insomnia
- Developed increased panic/agitation attacks with symptoms including shortness of breath, palpitations, tachycardia, fear of impending doom, parasthesias

Question

What would you do next?

- Increase the benzodiazepine (BZ) anxiolytic back again to her usual dose
- Add an antihypertensive α_2 receptor agonist (guanfacine [Tenex] or clonidine [Catapres]) for agitation, instead of re-escalating the BZ
- Add a sedating norepinephrine antagonist / selective serotonin antagonist (NaSSA) such as mirtazapine (Remeron)
- Add a sedating serotonin antagonist / reuptake inhibitor (SARI) antidepressant such as trazodone (Desyrel)
- Replace the SSRI with an SNRI or a serotonin partial agonist / reuptake inhibitor (SPARI) antidepressant such as vilazodone (Viibryd)
- Add an antihistamine H1 receptor antagonist (hydroxyzine [Vistaril]) to treat her agitation
- Add a 5-HT$_{1A}$ partial receptor agonist such as buspirone (BuSpar) to better treat the GAD

Attending physician's mental notes: second interim follow-up visit (month 5)

- Really do not want to re-escalate her alprazolam (Xanax) and would prefer to have her on more antidepressant-based approaches if possible
- Will need to see whether she will accept off-label use of sleep-inducing medications and anti-agitation medications outside of the BZ family while we work on her basic antidepressants
- May require rational polypharmacy while we try to obtain global symptom improvement
- Will need to streamline and taper some medications once this is achieved

Case outcome: interim follow-up visits through 6 months (continued)

- Patient was not willing to take hydroxyzine (Vistaril) due to fear of cardiac complications
- Agreed to be prescribed clonidine (Catapres) 0.1 mg/d and titrated to 0.1 mg twice per day for breakthrough anxiety-related symptoms
- Trazodone (Desyrel) 25 mg/d for sleep was started, but patient stated this caused premature ventricular contractions and ectopic heart beats and it was stopped
- Melatonin was next increased to 10 mg/d and alleviated her insomnia
- The above medications were added to treat her more palpable symptoms of insomnia and agitation, but her underlying MDD and GAD were only partially responding
- After further education and support, agreed to lower escitalopram (Lexapro) down to 10 mg/d, where it was partially effective and also side-effect free
- A buspirone (Buspar) combination strategy was allowed after discussing its mechanism of action as a 5-HT$_{1A}$ receptor partial agonist and its FDA approval for GAD, and its now proposed off-label use for MDD at 15 mg/d
- Remains uninterested in CBT

Attending physician's mental notes: second interim follow-up visit (month 6)

- Ideally, agitation and insomnia are lowered, which is likely key to keeping her distress low and allowing her to accept goal of using an SSRI plus the combined 5-HT$_{1A}$ partial agonist over the longer term, to reach a remission of GAD and MDD

- If this works, will streamline her medications, ideally to just these two
- She is 50% better which is her best success yet, which is promising

Case outcome: interim follow-up visits through 9 months

- Escitalopram (Lexapro) continued at 10 mg/d with good tolerability
- Gradually, buspirone (BuSpar) is increased and tolerated at 45 mg/d without issue
- MDD symptoms remit
- Panic attacks resolve
- GAD symptoms are minimal but present
- Insomnia is minimal

Question

What would you do now?

- As she is nearly remitted in all symptom areas, make no changes for several years
- Continue to streamline away from the insomnia and agitation medications
- Refer for CBT

What are her risks if she has residual MDD symptoms of insomnia and psychomotor agitation?

- No additional risks
- Greater risk of MDD relapse or recurrence

What are her risks if she has residual GAD symptoms of insomnia and psychomotor agitation?

- No additional risks
- Greater risk of MDD relapse or recurrence

Case outcome: interim follow-up visits through 12 months

- Goal was to continue streamlining medications and to gain remission in all areas
- Escitalopram (Lexapro) continued at 10 mg/d and buspirone (BuSpar) at 45 mg/d
- Attempts made to taper off other medications
  - Lamotrigine (Lamictal) is tapered off as the patient not considered to be BP2 and it was ineffective at controlling MDD and GAD
  - Clonidine (Catapres) initially removed without issue

- ◦ Alprazolam (Xanax) removed gradually but insomnia returned, despite ongoing melatonin 10 mg/d being used at bed
  - ▪ Eventually alprazolam (Xanax) used at only 0.25 mg at bed
  - ▪ Fully effective for ongoing insomnia management
  - ▪ Melatonin is no longer needed
- ◦ Patient is in full remission of MDD and GAD by using an SSRI, a 5-HT$_{1A}$ partial agonist, and low-dose BZ

Case debrief

- Patient presented with anxiety and depressive symptoms that have intensified since teenage years
- Through accurate history-taking, accurate diagnoses were made and, by not having BP2, allowed a greater variety of pharmacologic treatments to be tried for her MDD and GAD symptoms
- Furthermore, her PTSD and PD-like symptoms were most suggestive of GAD plus MDD comorbidity
- Her initial medications were both ineffective and likely not warranted, given that she was felt not to have BP2
- Going back to basics of treating MDD and GAD with an antidepressant was warranted, albeit using an empathic validated approach was needed to escalate dosing to a therapeutic level
- Used several medication approaches, with good informed consent and empiric and validating support to treat symptoms gradually into a full MDD and GAD remission

Take-home points

- Always screen MDD patients for bipolarity
  - ◦ If bipolar, antidepressants risk worsening of BP
- Always screen MDD patients for PTSD
  - ◦ If PTSD present, risk of less robust antidepressant outcomes
- Accurate history-taking always required, especially if you are the second, third, etc., psychopharmacologist involved in a patient's care
  - ◦ Do not trust historical diagnoses, and do your own evaluation
- Must treat anxiety disorders to remission to prevent MDD relapse
- In patients who report sensitivity to medication, consider starting at lower doses than are usually therapeutic, in order to build alliance and minimize potential side effects

Performance in practice

What could have been done better here?

- A more accurate history-taking and appropriate rating scales could have been completed during her initial presentation
- Further attempts could have been made in order to have the patient engage in therapy for a more robust response in combination with medication
- Could have attempted to use quetiapine XR (Seroquel XR) at a low dose both to target anxiety and augment antidepressant and attempt to taper alprazolam (Xanax) completely

What are possible action items for improvement in practice?

- Investigate patient-driven screening tests that might better delineate BP1 or BP2 from MDD
    - Altman Mania Rating Scale (AMRS)
    - Mood Disorders Questionnaire (MDQ)
    - Rapid Mood Screener (RMS)

Tips and pearls

- Take your time in an interview and obtain an accurate history
- If possible, also interview a collateral source if BP is suspected
- Use rating scales to help diagnosis
- Don't forget about psychotherapy

Two-minute tutorial

Treating agitation in depression and anxiety

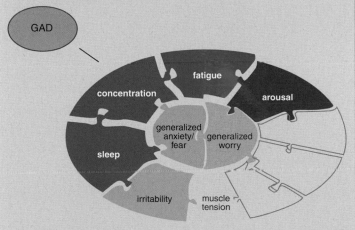

Figure 16.1 Notice the symptoms that comprise GAD. Arousal is a hallmark symptom.

Symptom-Based Algorithm for Treating Depression Part One:
Deconstructing Most Common Residual Diagnostic Symptoms

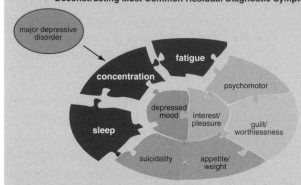

Figure 16.2 Notice the symptoms that comprise MDD. Presented in this diagram is 'psychomotor', which in MDD can be seen as psychomotor retardation or as psychomotor agitation. The latter can be indistinguishable from that seen above in GAD.

Associate Symptoms With Brain Regions, Circuits, and Neurotransmitters That Regulate Them

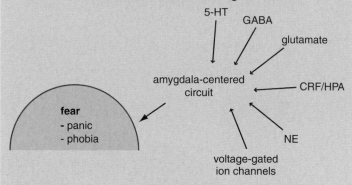

Figure 16.3 Regarding the development of fear and anxiety, many systems may be involved, creating elevations of noradrenergic tone, losses of GABAergic tone, etc.

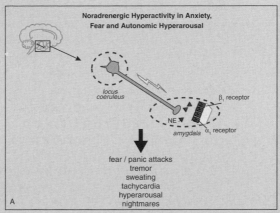

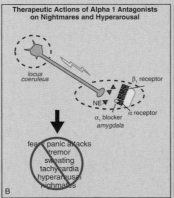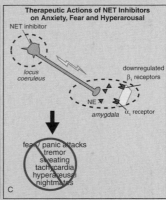

Figure 16.4 (A) Norepinephrine provides input not only to the amygdala fight-or-flight center but also to many regions to which the amygdala projects; thus, it plays an important role in the fear response. Noradrenergic hyperactivation can lead to anxiety, panic attacks, tremors, sweating, tachycardia, hyperarousal, and nightmares. Alpha₁ and β₁-adrenergic receptors may be specifically involved in these reactions. (B) Noradrenergic hyperactivity may be blocked by the administration of α_1-adrenergic antagonists, which can lead to the alleviation of anxiety and other stress-related symptoms. (C) Noradrenergic hyperactivity may also be blocked by the administration of a norepinephrine transporter (NET) inhibitor, which can have the downstream effect of downregulating β_1-adrenergic receptors. Reduced stimulation via β_1-adrenergic receptors could therefore lead to the alleviation of anxiety and stress-related symptoms. Theoretically, α_2 receptor antagonists centrally in the CNS may decrease noradrenergic output downstream, also leading to less adrenergic activity and less anxiety and agitation.

The following medications are known to mechanistically lower norepinephrine neurocircuitry firing, and may be used clinically in lieu of BZ anxiolytics, SSRI/SNRI antidepressants, atypical antipsychotics, or calcium channel blocking antiepileptics as an off-label approach to treat agitation and anxiety in certain cases

- Dexmedetomidine sublingual (Igalmi)
  - Alpha$_2$ receptor agonist recently FDA-approved for agitation in bipolar and schizophrenia (SP) patients
  - Typically dosed 120–180 mcg sublingual and can be repeated at 2 hours with lower dosing as needed
  - Common side effects can include oral hypoesthesia, dry mouth, hypotension, lightheadedness, and dizziness, as well as drowsiness
- Clonidine (Catapres)
  - Alpha-2 receptor agonist
  - It is primarily used as an anti-hypertensive, but commonly used off-label for anxiety-related symptoms
  - Clonidine (Catapres) is often used off-label to treat agitation associated with opioid withdrawal, as an augmentation strategy
  - Clonidine ER (Kapvay) was initially used to offset agitating and activating side effects in children treated with stimulants but now is also recognized as a stand-alone effective Attention-Deficit/Hyperactivity Disorder (ADHD) treatment
  - Typically, clonidine (Catapres) is dosed from 0.1 mg to 0.4 mg/d in divided doses
  - Common side effects include hypotension, lightheadedness, dizziness, drowsiness, xerostomia, and sometimes GI upset
- Guanfacine (Tenex)
  - Alpha-2 receptor agonist
  - Like clonidine (Catapres), this medication is also an anti-hypertensive
  - Typically dosed 1 mg to 3 mg at bed
  - Common side effects can include hypotension, lightheadedness, and dizziness, as well as drowsiness
  - Just like slow-release clonidine ER (Kapvay), which is approved to treat kids with ADHD, a slow-release guanfacine (Intuniv) is also approved for childhood ADHD
- Propranolol (Inderal)
  - A non-selective β_1 and β_2 receptor antagonist
  - Commonly used as an antihypertensive, but also used in anxiety-related disorders – most commonly specific phobia, situational (performance) type

- Can be dosed 10 mg to 60 mg/d as needed, or in a divided standing dose
- Side effects can include low heart rate, hypotension, drowsiness, lightheadedness
- Use with caution in patients with lung pathology such as asthma as non-selective beta blockers (BBs) may cause bronchospasm due to β_2 receptor antagonism
- Additionally, use with caution in patients with diabetes mellitus as BBs have the potential to mask the symptoms of hypoglycemia
- Prazosin (Minipress)
  - An α_1 receptor antagonist
  - Also used as an anti-hypertensive
  - Commonly used off-label for PTSD-related nightmares, as well as treating sleep disruption phenomena
  - Typically dosed 1–15 mg at bed
  - Side effects may include hypotension, dizziness, lightheadedness, drowsiness

Rating scale rant

How to determine if a patient presenting with depressive symptoms may have BP?

- BP1 and BP2 patients spend more time in the depressed phase than in a manic or hypomanic phase
- Over a third of unipolar patients are re-diagnosed as bipolar, and as many as 60% of patients with BP2 are diagnosed initially as unipolar
- Useful rating scales include:
  - Mood Disorders Questionnaire (MDQ): a cut-off score of 7 or higher indicates likelihood of bipolarity, and a further assessment for BP is needed
  - Rapid Mood Screener (RMS): a cut-off score of 4 indicates likelihood of bipolarity, and a further assessment for BP is needed
  - Altman Mania Rating Scale (AMRS): a cut-off score of 6 or higher indicates a high probability of a manic or hypomanic condition presently
- Features suggestive of BP include:
  - Depression at younger ages
  - Psychotic features
  - Mixed features

- Atypical features
- Post-partum onset
- Greater comorbid anxiety
- Family history of BP1
- Faster onset and diminution of depressive symptoms
- Robust, fast responses to antidepressants

Post-test question

What is the typical rate of conversion from major depressive disorder (MDD) to bipolar I disorder (BP1) over time?

A. 1%

B. 2%

C. 8%

D. 50%

Answer: C

A large cohort study of 90,000 individuals initially diagnosed with unipolar MDD were followed over time and 7–8% converted to BP, where the strongest predictor was a bona fide family history of BP1 diagnosis. Of note is that other studies have found rates from 20% to 30% as well.

References

1. American Psychiatric Association. *Diagnostic and Statistical Manual of Mental Disorders: DSM-5*, 5th edn. Arlington, VA: American Psychiatric Publishing, Inc., 2013
2. Altman, EG, Hedeker, D, Peterson, JL, et al. The Altman Self-Rating Mania Scale. *Biol Psychiatry* 1997; 42:948–55
3. Hirschfeld, RM, Williams, JB, Spitzer, RL, et al. Development and validation of a screening instrument for bipolar spectrum disorder: the Mood Disorder Questionnaire. *Am J Psychiatry* 2000; 157: 1873–5
4. Judd, LL, Akiskal, HS, Schettler, PJ, et al. A prospective investigation of the natural history of the long-term weekly symptomatic status of bipolar II disorder. *Arch Gen Psychiatry* 2003; 60:261–9
5. McGlashan, TH. Adolescent versus adult onset of mania. *Am J Psychiatry* 1988; 145:221–3
6. McIntyre, RS, Patel, MD, Masand, PS, et al. The Rapid Mood Screener (RMS): a novel and pragmatic screener for bipolar I disorder. *Curr Med Res Opin* 2021; 37:135–44

7. Musliner, KL, Østergaard, SD. Patterns and predictors of conversion to bipolar disorder in 91 587 individuals diagnosed with unipolar depression. *Acta Psychiatr Scand* 2018; 137:422–32

8. Schwartz, T. *Practical Psychopharmacology: Basic to Advanced Principles*, 1st edn. New York: Routledge, 2017

9. Tsai, SY, Lee, JC, Chen, CC. Characteristics and psychosocial problems of patients with bipolar disorder at high risk for suicide attempt. *J Affect Disord* 1999; 52:145–52

Case 17: Pain makes me anxious, and anxiety gives me pain

The Question: What are the treatment options for fibromyalgia (FM) when comorbid with other psychiatric disorders?

The Psychopharmacological Dilemma: What to do when the first-line treatments do not work in complex anxious patients?

Daniel Jackson and Sutanaya Pal

Pretest self-assessment question

What are the most common, evidence-based treatments for FM with comorbid psychiatric conditions?

A. Non-pharmacological: patient education, graded exercise, cognitive behavioral therapy (CBT)
B. Antidepressants: tricyclic antidepressants (TCAs), selective serotonin–norepinephrine reuptake inhibitors (SNRIs)
C. Gabapentinoids: gabapentin (Neurontin), pregabalin (Lyrica)
D. Analgesics: nonsteroidal anti-inflammatory drugs (NSAIDs), opioids
E. A, B, and C are correct

Patient evaluation on intake

- A 45-year-old female with chief complaint of significant pain that alternates from aching to sharp to dull quality that affects mostly her back and legs at baseline, with flare-ups of pain triggering significant worry and panic attacks
- Major depressive disorder (MDD), generalized anxiety disorder (GAD), and panic disorder (PD) diagnosed at age 23
  - Now endorses symptoms of depressed mood, anhedonia, trouble sleeping, decreased appetite, fatigue, trouble concentrating, and feelings of worthlessness
    - This has worsened over the last 2 months
  - Also reports significant anxiety about multiple matters, such as work, family, and finances, along with feeling restless, tired, having trouble concentrating, non-restful sleep, and muscle tension
    - These symptoms have persisted for years
  - She initially started having panic attacks that were unprovoked, about 2–3 times/week, from the age of 23
    - She currently reports that about half of her panic attacks are now precipitated by flare-ups of pain, and she is preoccupied about when next painful symptoms will occur
- History of postpartum depression after the birth of her two children

Psychiatric history

- No history of suicide attempts or self-injurious behaviors
- No mania, psychosis, or personality disorders
- No history of inpatient hospitalizations
- Received 6 months of CBT at the age of 23 for GAD, MDD, and PD with modest effect
- Received 2 months of supportive psychotherapy for postpartum depression after birth of first child with modest effect

Social and personal history

- Married with three children
- Education: high school graduate
- Occupation: works in retail part-time
- No history of abuse or trauma
- No substance use history

Medical history

- FM and asthma
- No history of treatment with opioids for chronic pain
- Hypertension (HTN) resolved with purposeful weight loss

Family history

- Mother and multiple cousins have a history of MDD
- Maternal uncle had bipolar disorder (BP)
- Mother's grandfather had alcohol use disorder (AUD)

Medication history

- Selective serotonin reuptake inhibitor (SSRI) citalopram (Celexa) 20 mg/d without improvement
- Sertraline (Zoloft) 150 mg/d without improvement (SSRI)
- Atypical antipsychotic augmentation with aripiprazole (Abilify) 10 mg/d used as adjunctive therapy for MDD
    - All were used with therapeutic timeframes
    - They would work briefly for 2–3 weeks, then efficacy was lost
- Alprazolam (Xanax), a benzodiazepine (BZ) anxiolytic 0.75 mg/d as needed
    - Has been useful for PD, decreasing panic attacks from every other day to every other month

Current medications

- Duloxetine (Cymbalta) 60 mg/d, an SNRI
- Alprazolam (Xanax) 1.5 mg/d, a BZ anxiolytic

Question

Based on what you know of this patient, should she be seen by a psychiatrist?

- Yes, she has MDD
- Yes, she has MDD with pain, and psychopharmacologists use medications that can treat both
- No, pain should be treated by another specialty

Patient evaluation on initial visit (continued)

- For the last 6–10 years, she has had significant pain that alternates from aching to sharp to dull quality that affects mostly her back and legs at baseline
    - The pain is both right- and-left-sided and occurs above and below the waist
- Flare-ups of pain in these areas trigger significant anxiety and panic attacks. She often worries and ruminates when the next pain exacerbation will occur
- She noted that her MDD was in remission with duloxetine (Cymbalta), with low-to-moderate effect on baseline anxiety and pain, with little effect on the pain exacerbation events
- On examination, 14 trigger points were positive, based upon typical FM mapping
    - The FM map shows the location of 31 tender points, with the presence of 13 or more tender points required for a diagnosis of fibromyalgia. The self-report survey also asks the patient for the severity of pain, along with the presence of other symptoms
- FACES pain scale was 4/10
    - The Wong–Baker FACES pain scale is an easy instrument to administer. It was originally developed as a tool for subjective assessment of pain in infants and children. Patients mark out the face/score which correlates best with the intensity of pain that they are experiencing. Scores are even numbers that range from 0 to 10, with 10 being the worst pain ever felt
- Her pain was also measured with the cold pressor time (CPT), an objective measure of pain with good test–retest reliability
    - Her initial CPT was 3 seconds, which is considered to be low pain tolerance compared to normal. Notably, her response to the stimulus was severe enough to make her cry

Widespread Pain Index (WPI) for Diagnosis of Fibromyalgia

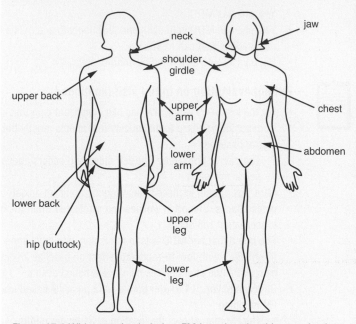

Figure 17.1 Widespread pain index. FM is a chronic widespread pain syndrome, formerly diagnosed based on the number of body areas in which the patient experiences pain (widespread pain index, or WPI), combined with the severity of associated symptoms (fatigue, waking unrefreshed, cognitive symptoms, and other somatic symptoms). This patient admitted to pain in most of these trigger point areas upon superficial or deep palpation.

Attending physician's mental notes: initial psychiatric evaluation

- Treatment with duloxetine (Cymbalta) 60 mg/d for 5 months constitutes a therapeutic time frame, as statistically significant pain relief compared to placebo has been demonstrated within 12 weeks in studies
- A less clear option would be to increase the dose of duloxetine (Cymbalta), as there may be some evidence that doses higher than 60 mg produce more pain relief, though carrying increased side effects
- Another option may be adding adjunctive treatment with gabapentin (Neurontin) or pregabalin (Lyrica) rather than replacing duloxetine

(Cymbalta) with another treatment altogether, as the duloxetine (Cymbalta) has already provided some benefit for pain and anxiety, and even more so for her MDD
- ○ Pregabalin (Lyrica) is approved for FM and has compelling off-label data for GAD use
- While there has not been as much research published about combination therapy with $\alpha_2\delta$ ligands such as gabapentin/pregabalin and SNRIs, their clinical benefit may have additive effects, theoretically
- Pain and symptoms of anxiety and depression have a complex relationship in FM. Studies have shown interactions among pain and mood symptoms; however, it is unclear from which direction these interactions occur
  - ○ For instance, studies have shown that improvements in mood may account for improvements in pain, and vice versa as well

Further investigation

Is there anything else that you would like to know about the patient?

Does she have previous physical trauma?

- No.

Does she have previous emotional trauma or neglect?

- No.

Based on what you know about this patient's history and comorbid FM symptoms, what would you do next?

- Continue duloxetine (Cymbalta) as the treatment course has not reached a therapeutic time frame
- Augment with gabapentin (Neurontin) off-label
- Switch to gabapentin (Neurontin) monotherapy
- Add a tricyclic antidepressant (TCA) off-label
- Add an NSAID
- Add an opioid analgesic

Case outcome: interim follow up at 8 weeks

- Continued duloxetine (Cymbalta) and started on gabapentin (Neurontin) at 300 mg/d and titrated eventually to 1800 mg/d in divided doses over 8 weeks
  - ○ Pain remained unchanged
- She reported modest improvements in GAD with a decreased frequency of PD attacks precipitated by pain
- Alprazolam (Xanax) use remained the same

Question

Considering her medication regimen and previous response, what are your treatment options at this point?

- Add low-dose naltrexone (ReVia)
- Add amitriptyline (Elavil), a TCA
- Switch to gabapentinoid monotherapy with pregabalin (Lyrica)
- Switch to tramadol (Ultram), a synthetic opioid (off-label)
- Switch to another SNRI
- Maximize any of the current medications – duloxetine (Cymbalta), alprazolam (Xanax), or gabapentin (Neurontin)

Attending physician's mental notes: subsequent visits (weeks 8–16)

- Among the TCAs, amitriptyline (Elavil) has the most evidence for efficacy and is frequently listed as first-line treatment in FM
  ○ It is part of the subgroup of TCAs that has more pronounced serotonin reuptake inhibitor (SRI) properties, which is useful given the patient's comorbid anxiety and panic attacks
  ○ Its metabolite, nortriptyline (Pamelor), is also a TCA but with norepinephrine reuptake inhibitor (NRI) activity
  ○ NRIs seem to be more effective for pain management in animal models
  ○ However, increased anticholinergic muscarinic, anti-alpha adrenergic, and antihistaminergic effects often produce difficulty with side effects
- Among the opioid analgesics, those with weaker opioid activity are preferred. While there is some evidence for tramadol (Ultram) in the relief of pain in FM, the risks (addiction) inherent in their use generally do not lead them to be recommended as first-line treatment
  ○ This medication has purported SNRI properties as well
- Data suggests that duloxetine has clinically relevant benefits for pain relief of 30% or greater, as well as global improvement in patients. However, support is lacking for improvements in pain of 50% or greater for doses ranging from 30 mg to 120 mg

Case outcome: 12 to 16 weeks

- At 12 weeks, her duloxetine (Cymbalta) was cross-titrated with amitriptyline (Elavil) while monitoring for adverse effects
- She was seen again at 16 weeks (4 weeks after the cross-titration was complete) to examine her response to amitriptyline (Elavil)
- 75 mg/d was given with modest effect on lowering pain

- However, she developed significant urinary retention, dry mouth, and constipation
- Elected to discontinue this TCA and asked for alternative therapies for her pain and other symptoms of FM

Question

Given her history and response, what are your treatment options at this point?

- Switch to desipramine (Norpramin), which is the least anticholinergic of the TCAs
- Switch to pregabalin (Lyrica)
- Switch to low-dose naltrexone (ReVia)
- Restart duloxetine (Cymbalta), an SNRI, and titrate higher
- Add tramadol (Ultram), a synthetic opioid
- Switch to milnacipran (Savella), a more adrenergic SNRI

Attending physician's mental notes: subsequent visit (week 20)

- Low-dose naltrexone has slowly gained recognition as an alternative treatment for FM, but reports are limited in number
- Two small randomized controlled trials (RCTs) have shown efficacy in FM
- Her duloxetine (Cymbalta) was restarted as it was effective for her MDD, GAD, and PD, and titrated to 60 mg/d again
- Of note, weaker opioids such as tramadol (Ultram) have shown to produce some improvement in pain, with no improvement in function. Further, there is considerable risk of dependence and adverse effects (such as sedation, tolerance, opioid-induced hyperalgesia)
- There is no compelling evidence for the use of stronger opioids for the treatment of FM

Case outcome: interim follow-up at 20 weeks

- Low-dose naltrexone (ReVia) was started at 0.1 mg twice a day, which was gradually increased to 9 mg/d in divided doses
- Duloxetine (Cymbalta) was continued
- Alprazolam (Xanax) use is now rare
- Significant improvement noted
  - Less subjective reporting of pain
  - Significant improvement of CPTs: 34 seconds at 2 weeks of treatment, and 87 seconds at 4 weeks of treatment (initial time of 3 seconds)

Case debrief

- FM is frequently comorbid with other psychiatric disorders, most commonly depression and anxiety which increase the impairment caused by FM
- FM typically makes MDD/GAD worse
- MDD appears to make FM patients feel more pain
- Patient was initially treated with antidepressants, which seemed to help with her MDD, GAD, PD, but without any effect on her FM pain
  - ○ SSRIs tend not to help neuropathic pain symptoms
- Next was tried on gabapentin (Neurontin), which improved her GAD but unfortunately not her FM pain
- Next was placed on the TCA amitriptyline (Elavil) instead of the SNRI duloxetine (Cymbalta), but she could not tolerate it
- The greatest FM pain benefit came from augmentation with low-dose naltrexone (ReVia) while maintaining her original SNRI duloxetine (Cymbalta). In this manner, her MDD and both anxiety disorders were treated and maintained in remission, while her pain symptoms were secondarily addressed and mitigated as well

Take-home points

- FM is hard to treat as it involves chronic, likely neuropathic pain (which is difficult to treat in itself), but it is also accompanied by depression, anxiety, and other psychiatric symptoms
- The origins of FM may include sleep deprivation due to alpha wave intrusion, loss of restorative sleep and hormones, segmental or central neuronal sensitization, etc., where it may require multiple types of medications to address each etiology
- The treatment option selected is often based on the patient's symptoms and the side-effect profile of the drugs

Performance in practice: confessions of a psychopharmacologist

What could have been done better here?

- Concern for side effects may prevent raising the dose of duloxetine (Cymbalta) to provide additional pain relief. There is some evidence to suggest that doses higher than 60 mg may provide additional pain benefit. In this case, the side effects from a duloxetine (Cymbalta) increase may likely have been less than those from adding the TCA in its place
- Pregabalin (Lyrica) is FDA-approved for FM and may be better tolerated at higher doses than gabapentin (Neurontin), but it comes

with a low-level risk of addiction and drug likeability. It could have been utilized as it has greater data concerning FM

- Nortriptyline (Pamelor) and desipramine (Norpramin) have greater NRI activity than amitriptyline (Elavil) and have anticholinergic, antihistaminergic, and less anti-alpha adrenergic effects. Therefore, they may have been a more viable alternative to amitriptyline
- Along with nortriptyline (Pamelor) and desipramine (Norpramin), the SNRI milnacipran (Savella) has significant NRI activity and certainly would have fewer side effects than a TCA
- Levomilnacipran (Fetzima) is an active enantiomer of milnacipran, which has greater noradrenergic activity than the original molecule. It is an SNRI approved for use only in MDD, but it could have the same efficacy as its parent drug on pain and the other symptoms of FM
- While SSRIs do not carry the hypothesized benefits of NRI activity on dampening pain signaling, there is some mild evidence that supports their efficacy in FM

Tips and pearls

- FM is a complex condition which usually requires non-pharmacological and multimodal treatments
- It is important to remember that non-pharmacological methods of treatment are first-line, effective, and safe options, such as:
  - Graded exercise
  - CBTs
  - Complementary and alternative therapies (CAM) like yoga, Tai chi, etc.
  - One essential non-pharmacological intervention is patient education to explain the condition, set treatment expectations, and inform them about multimodal approaches. This simple intervention has been shown to improve symptoms and reduce disability claims
- Beyond non-pharmacological interventions, drug combinations are often required to treat the various symptoms of the disease

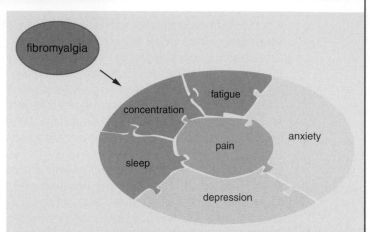

Figure 17.2 Symptoms of FM. In addition to pain as a central feature of FM, many patients experience fatigue, anxiety, depression, disturbed sleep, and problems concentrating.

Two-minute tutorial

Part I: FM diagnosis

- The American College of Rheumatology suggested in 2016 that FM must include generalized pain in 4 out of 5 body regions for 3 months
- A WPI of greater than 6 and Symptom Severity Score (SSS) greater than 4

Part II: FM psychopharmacology

- In the US, duloxetine (Cymbalta) and milnacipran (Savella) are approved SNRIs for FM treatment
- Pregabalin (Lyrica) is approved as well. It blocks calcium channels in pain fiber pathways to dampen pain signaling into the CNS
- Other agents below are off-label and offer several different mechanisms that theoretically may reduce FM pain

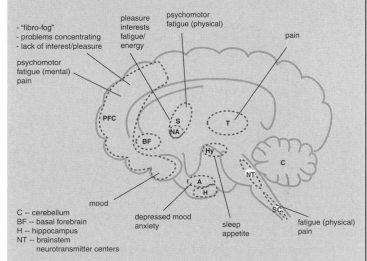

**Match Each Symptom of Fibromyalgia
to Hypothetically Malfunctioning Brain Circuits**

Figure 17.3 Symptom-based algorithm for FM. A symptom-based approach to treatment selection for FM follows the theory that each of a patient's symptoms can be matched with malfunctioning brain circuits and neurotransmitters that hypothetically mediate those symptoms; this information is then used to select a corresponding pharmacological mechanism for treatment. Pain is linked to transmission of information via the thalamus (T), while physical fatigue is linked to the striatum (S) and spinal cord (SC). Problems concentrating and lack of interest (termed "fibro-fog") as well as mental fatigue are linked to the prefrontal cortex (PFC), specifically the dorsolateral PFC. Fatigue, low energy, and lack of interest may all also be related to the nucleus accumbens (NA). Disturbances in sleep and appetite are associated with the hypothalamus (Hy), depressed mood with the amygdala (A) and orbital frontal cortex, and anxiety with the amygdala. For example, blocking sodium or calcium channels will dampen pain fibers from sending signals up the spinal cord and may lower firing in the central nervous system (CNS) if pain sensitization has occurred. Increasing noradrenergic tone in the descending spinal cord pathways will increase GABAergic interneuronal activity, also decreasing pain signaling toward the brain. Use of opioids may lower limbic firing, dampening the fear response regarding pain, amongst other mechanisms.

Naltrexone

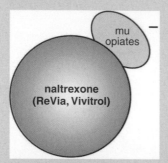

Figure 17.4 Naltrexone (ReVia/Vivitrol) on the left is approved to treat alcohol use disorder (AUD) but is used at times to treat self-injurious behavior and chronic pain syndromes. It antagonizes μ-opioid receptors and may block pleasurable responses to addictive or repetitive activities.

- Naltrexone comes in two forms – oral (ReVia) and injectable (Vivitrol)
  - It antagonizes *μ*-opioid receptors
- FDA-approved for alcohol dependence and blockade of exogenously administered opioids
  - Prevents the euphoric or rewarding effect of alcohol and opioids
  - Reduces craving for and, hence, consumption of alcohol and opioids
  - Reduces days of heavy drinking
- Usual dose: oral – 50 mg/d, injection – 380 mg every 4 weeks. Must ensure that the patient is opioid free for 7–10 days. A urine drug screen or a naloxone challenge test is used to ensure that they are opioid free, to prevent precipitating severe withdrawal
- Naltrexone has been used in low doses (1–5 mg/d), whereby it behaves like a glial modulator and mitigates the effect of pro-inflammatory effects of Toll-like receptor 4
  - These doses also cause transient blockade of opioid receptors resulting in upregulation of the endogenous opioid system
  - At the neuroimmunological level, it may be of more relevance in treating FM than for its upregulation of the endogenous opioid system
- Baseline liver function testing (LFT) may be useful when treating AUD
- Common side effects include nausea, vomiting, decreased appetite, and dizziness. Injection site reactions can occur including redness, swelling, tenderness, etc.

- Severe side effects include eosinophilic pneumonia, hepatocellular damage, and severe injection site reactions
- If a patient is dependent on opioids, or in acute opioid withdrawal, has a failed naloxone challenge test, or is allergic to naltrexone or a component of the injection diluent, then use is contraindicated
- Low-dose naltrexone has been used to treat FM, multiple sclerosis (MS), Crohn's disease, cancers, and complex regional pain syndrome (CRPS)
- Preliminary randomized controlled trials have shown that low-dose naltrexone may be effective in FM

Milnacipran (Savella)

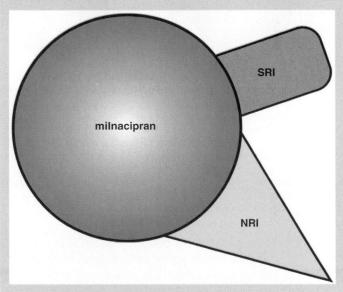

Figure 17.5 Milnacipran (Savella) is somewhat different than other SNRIs in that it has the strongest relative actions at NET compared to SERT among the four approved SNRIs. Some data even suggests that its actions at NET are stronger than those at SERT, while the other SNRIs are generally the opposite. Data suggests that milnacipran may have efficacy for both pain and cognitive symptoms in FM. Milnacipran is approved for the treatment of depression in several countries outside the US, and approval for FM is pending worldwide. Milnacipran (Savella) may be more energizing and activating than some other SNRIs due to its relatively potent noradrenergic actions, and may cause more sweating and urinary hesitancy. Milnacipran (Savella) is generally given twice daily due to its short half-life.

- Milnacipran (Savella) is FDA-approved for FM
- Dosed at 12.5–200 mg/d in two divided doses
- Has greater NRI activity than most SNRIs
- At high doses, may antagonize N-methyl-D-aspartate (NMDA) glutamate receptors, which may contribute to actions in lowering chronic pain

Pregabalin (Lyrica)

gabapentin   **pregabalin**

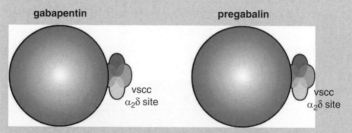

Figure 17.6 Gabapentin (Neurontin) and pregabalin (Lyrica) are anticonvulsants also approved for neuropathic pain (both), FM (pregabalin [Lyrica]), and anxiety (pregabalin [Lyrica], in Europe). They may also enhance slow-wave sleep, and are not approved for BP. These agents have a mechanism of action different from other known mood stabilizers: they bind to the $\alpha_2 c$ subunit of VSCCs. Thus, they are also called $\alpha_2 \delta$ ligands. This action reduces neurotransmitter release (e.g., glutamate). Alpha 2δ ligands may be helpful in treating ancillary symptoms of BP such as sleep disturbances and anxiety, but most studies fail to show robust mood-stabilizing actions on either mania or depression.

- FDA-approved for FM, diabetic peripheral neuropathy, postherpetic neuralgia, and neuropathic pain secondary to spinal cord injury
- The therapeutic effects on pain are thought to be due to activity as an $\alpha_2 \delta$ ligand
  - When bound to an $\alpha_2 \delta$, this mechanism allows blockade of calcium influx into neuronal pain fibers, thus lowering their ability to fire and pain to be perceived in the CNS
- Regulatory studies have shown benefit in FM when using doses in the 300–550 mg range

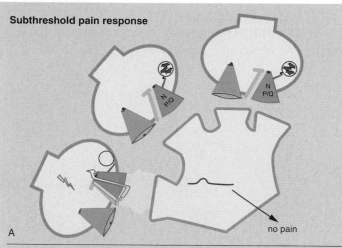

Subthreshold pain response

A   no pain

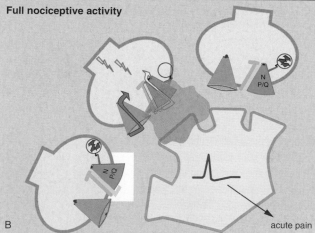

Full nociceptive activity

B   acute pain

Figure 17.7 Pain transmission and inhibition of pain signals via gabapentin (Neuontin) or pregabalin (Lyrica). Notice in (A) that minimal to no amount of pain fiber activation is occurring as there is minimal sodium (Na) channel opening and resultant depolarization of the secondary pain fiber. P/Q-type calcium channels are high-voltage gated calcium channels contributing to vesicle release at synaptic terminals. N-type calcium channels are essential for the release of neurotransmitters from nociceptors in neurons of the dorsal horn of the spinal cord. In (B), there is a greater amount of pain fiber activation, and some acute pain is noticed. This may happen in an acute injury.

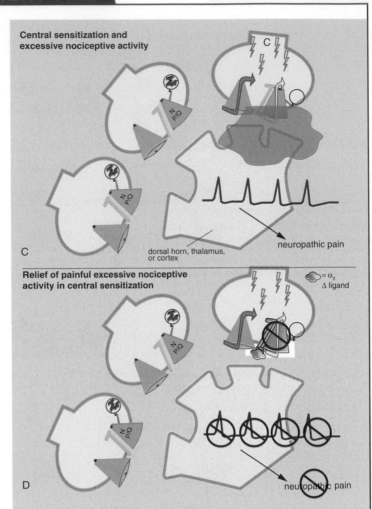

Central sensitization and excessive nociceptive activity

C

dorsal horn, thalamus, or cortex

neuropathic pain

Relief of painful excessive nociceptive activity in central sensitization

= α₂
Δ ligand

D

neuropathic pain

Figure 17.7 In (C), there is much more neuronal activation as calcium (Ca) channels are also activated, allowing further activation of pain fibers and possibly even causing a repetitive action in the spinal cord, thalamus, or sensory cortex in the CNS. In (D), a neuronal calcium channel blocking agent such as gabapentin (Neurontin) or pregabalin (Lyrica) is introduced, diminishing the amount of pain that can register in the sensory cortex, and much less pain is experienced by the patient.

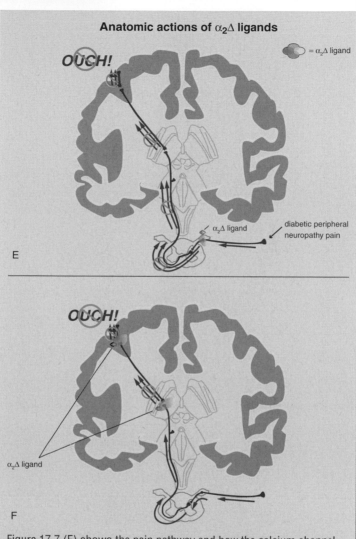

Figure 17.7 (E) shows the pain pathway and how the calcium channel blocking ($\alpha_2\delta$ ligand) agents may block and intercept peripheral pain signals.

Tricyclic antidepressants (TCAs)

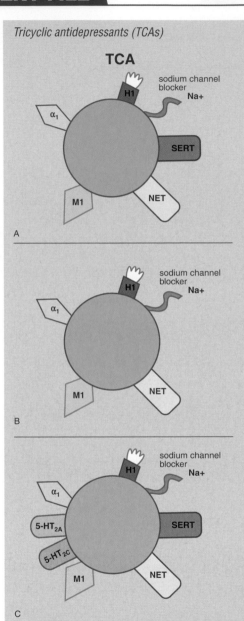

Figure 17.8 TCAs. All TCAs block reuptake of norepinephrine and are antagonists at histamine 1 (H_1), α_1-adrenergic, and muscarinic cholinergic receptors; they also block voltage-sensitive sodium channels (A, B, and C). Some TCAs are also potent inhibitors of the serotonin reuptake pump (A, C), and some may additionally be antagonists at serotonin (5-HT) 2A and 2C receptors (C).

- None of the TCAs is FDA-approved for FM. Nonetheless, amitriptyline (Elavil) remains a first-line treatment in most guidelines, and it is the most commonly used TCA for FM
  - In fact, it is frequently used as a comparison group for efficacy in studies with other potential FM medications
- Nortriptyline (Pamelor) and desipramine (Norpramin) are TCAs with greater NRI activity than amitriptyline (Elavil) and may be effective options for patients who cannot tolerate amitriptyline (Elavil) due to anticholinergic, antihistaminergic, and anti-alpha adrenergic effects
- Lower doses of TCAs, relative to doses needed to treat MDD, may be beneficial in FM
  - This may be due to the TCA's ability to block sodium channels in pain fibers even at lower doses, as seen in Figure 17.8

Tramadol (Ultram)

Endogenous opioid neurotransmitters

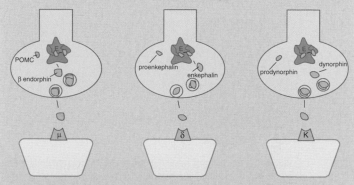

Figure 17.9 Endogenous opioid neurotransmitters. Endogenous opioids are peptides derived from precursor proteins called POMC (pro-opiomelanocortin), proenkephalin, and prodynorphin. Parts of these precursor proteins are cleaved off to form endorphins, enkephalins, or dynorphin, which are then stored in opioid neurons and released during neurotransmission to mediate reinforcement and pleasure. Neurons that release endorphin synapse with sites containing μ-opioid receptors, those that release enkephalin synapse with sites containing δ-opioid receptors, and those that release dynorphin synapse with sites containing κ-opioid receptors. Opioids and synthetic opiates have the ability to activate similar pathways to reduce pain.

- Typically, opioids are avoided in treating FM and other neuropathic pain conditions and are reserved for short-term use for acute injury and in palliative care
- Tramadol (Ultram) is a synthetic opiate and may be considered in the treatment of FM due to its lower abuse potential relative to other opioids, as well as having properties that could decrease central sensitization of pain, namely serotonin- and norepinephrine-reuptake inhibition and glutamate inhibition
- While there is some clinical research to support its use, most studies have been characterized as smaller in size and of lower quality compared to phase III regulatory studies
- Potential limitation as combination therapy with TCAs or SNRIs due to increased risk of serotonin syndrome and seizures

Sodium oxybate (Xyrem)

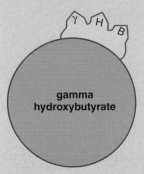

Figure 17.10 Sodium oxybate (Xyrem). Sodium oxybate (Xyrem), also known as γ-hydroxybutyrate (GHB), acts as a full agonist at GHB receptors and as a partial agonist at $GABA_B$ receptors. It is approved for use both in cataplexy and for excessive sleepiness and appears to enhance slow-wave sleep. This latter property may help treat FM, which often shows alpha wave intrusions into deep sleep cycles preventing restorative sleep. Here, FM may be thought of as a result of a sleep disorder, rather than as a pain condition.

- Sodium oxybate (Xyrem) is a CNS depressant and $GABA_B$ receptor partial agonist that is FDA-approved for narcolepsy
- It increases slow-wave sleep, and thus can ameliorate sleep difficulties in FM; however, it did not gain FDA approval due to safety concerns of respiratory suppression, addiction, and its potential misuse as a date rape drug
- There is evidence of significant improvement of pain, but studies vary regarding rates of discontinuation due to adverse effects

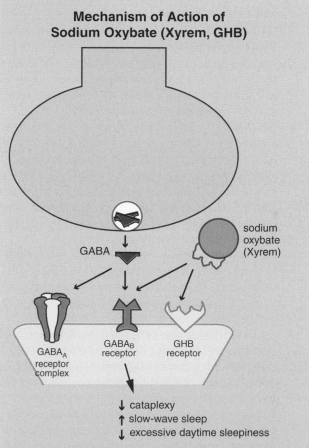

Mechanism of Action of Sodium Oxybate (Xyrem, GHB)

GABA

sodium oxybate (Xyrem)

GABA$_A$ receptor complex

GABA$_B$ receptor

GHB receptor

↓ cataplexy
↑ slow-wave sleep
↓ excessive daytime sleepiness

Figure 17.11 Mechanism of action of sodium oxybate (Xyrem). Sodium oxybate (Xyrem) binds as a full agonist to GHB receptors and as a partial agonist at GABA$_B$ receptors. Its actions at GABA$_B$ receptors are presumed to be responsible for its clinical effects of improving slow-wave sleep and reducing cataplexy. As a partial agonist, sodium oxybate causes less stimulation of GABA$_B$ receptors than GABA itself but more than in the absence of GABA. Thus, it can reduce GABA$_B$ stimulation when GABA levels are high and increase it when GABA levels are low.

- A lower-salt version of this medication and possibly a slow-release preparation are available and being investigated for narcolepsy and idiopathic hypersomnia

Part III: FM conclusion

- FM involves 6 symptom clusters, which can be remembered using this helpful mnemonic: "FIBRO" for "Fatigue and Fog (cognitive dysfunction), Insomnia (difficulties with all aspects of sleep including initiation, maintenance, and restorative), Blues (depression and anxiety), Rigidity (stiffness in muscles and joints), and Ow! (widespread pain and tenderness)"

- The American College of Rheumatology's older criteria for diagnosing FM include widespread pain and tenderness in at least 11 out of the 18 specific tender points, which typically occur bilaterally and above and below the waist, whereas their newer criteria suggest 4 out of 5 areas and use of validated rating scales

- The 2011 modification of the American College of Rheumatology's criteria for diagnosing FM includes various other symptoms common in this condition as well

- Patients can fill out a self-report survey that includes precise locations of the pain, along with the presence and severity of several other symptoms such as mood disturbances, memory, fatigue, sleep, headache, and bowel problems, to aid in diagnosis and monitoring

- Central sensitization or amplification of pain is the most common description of FM's etiology, although the exact mechanism of its pathophysiology is controversial. The blockade of voltage-sensitive calcium channels by $\alpha_2\delta$ ligands (gabapentinoids) is one theorized means of reducing pain amplification at the level of the dorsal horn, thalamus, and cortex. SNRIs may enhance the serotonergic and noradrenergic inhibition of nociceptive transmission at the level of the dorsal horn, thus preventing pain signals from moving toward the CNS

- Researchers have hypothesized whether the modulation of opioid tone has implications for treatment of FM, considering the similarities between opioid withdrawal and FM. Additionally, many FM patients' endogenous opioid receptors are occupied at baseline, which is abnormal compared to controls

- Both FM and opioid withdrawal conditions have chronic musculoskeletal pain, fatigue, sleep problems, diaphoresis, cognitive problems ("fibro-fog"), diarrhea, depression, and anxiety
  - A single-blind, crossover study followed by a small, randomized, controlled, double-blind study has demonstrated the reduction of pain in FM utilizing low-dose naltrexone (ReVia)
  - Given that inflammatory markers predicted treatment response in these studies, the therapeutic effect of low-dose naltrexone (ReVia) may have relevance at the neuroimmunological level as well

Post-test question

What are the most common, evidence-based treatments for FM with comorbid psychiatric conditions?

A. Non-pharmacological: patient education, graded exercise, cognitive behavioral therapy (CBT)

B. Antidepressants: tricyclic antidepressants (TCAs), selective serotonin–norepinephrine reuptake inhibitors (SNRIs)

C. Gabapentinoids: gabapentin (Neurontin), pregabalin (Lyrica)

D. Analgesics: nonsteroidal anti-inflammatory drugs (NSAIDs), opioids

E. A, B, and C are correct

Answer: E

Non-pharmacological options have the highest level of evidence in support of their efficacy. Patient education has been proven to be invaluable in helping patients understand the condition and to set treatment expectations. Graded exercise (including aerobic and strengthening) has proven to be very effective. Even increasing activity is helpful for many patients. Pain-based CBT is effective, and there are many internet-based programs. Finally, complementary and alternative methods such as Tai chi, yoga, and acupuncture are safe and effective.

TCAs and SNRIs are among the first-line pharmacotherapy options. They have the most evidence in support of their efficacy. TCAs are used off-label but still recommended as a first-line therapy. They improve pain along with several other symptoms such as sleep, bowel, and bladder problems. They are usually not effective antidepressants at lower doses but are effective for FM. Another good way to decide which drugs to choose would be to target comorbid conditions, such as depression and sleep. SNRIs can be used for people with depression and anxiety; duloxetine (Cymbalta) and milnacipran (Savella) are FDA-approved for FM.

NSAIDs and opioids: There is little evidence of efficacy for NSAIDs or opioids. Opioids are generally not effective for treating chronic FM pain and have a propensity for adverse effects and dependence.

Gabapentinoids: Gabapentin (Neurontin) and pregabalin (Lyrica) are among the first-line pharmacotherapy options, with the latter being FDA-approved for FM. These $\alpha_2\delta$ ligands can be used initially with those with sleep disturbances as well as anxiety (both off-label).

References

1. Arnold, LM, Hess, EV, Hudson, JI, et al. A randomized, placebo-controlled, double-blind, flexible-dose study of fluoxetine in the treatment of women with fibromyalgia. *Am J Med* 2002; 112:191–7

2. Arnold, LM, Rosen, A, Pritchett, YL, et al. A randomized, double-blind, placebo-controlled trial of duloxetine in the treatment of women with fibromyalgia with or without major depressive disorder. *Pain* 2005; 119:5–15

3. Beakley, B, Kaye, A, Kaye, A. Tramadol, pharmacology, side effects, and serotonin syndrome: a review. *Pain Physician* 2015; 18:395–400

4. Bennett, RM, Kamin, M, Karim, R, et al. Tramadol and acetaminophen combination tablets in the treatment of fibromyalgia pain: a double-blind, randomized, placebo-controlled study. *Am J Med* 2003; 114:537–45

5. Boomershine, CS. Fibromyalgia: the prototypical central sensitivity syndrome. *Curr Rheumatol Rev* 2015; 11:131–45

6. Borchers, AT, Gershwin, ME. Fibromyalgia: a critical and comprehensive review. *Clin Rev Allergy Immunol* 2015; 49:100–51

7. Carville, SF, Arendt-Nielsen, L, Bliddal, H, et al. EULAR evidence-based recommendations for the management of fibromyalgia syndrome. *Ann Rheum Dis* 2008; 67:536–41

8. Clauw, DJ. Fibromyalgia: a clinical review. *JAMA* 2014; 311:1547–55

9. da Rocha, AP, Mizzaci, CC, Nunes Pinto, ACP, et al. Tramadol for management of fibromyalgia pain and symptoms: systematic review. *Int J Clin Pract* 2020; 74:e13455

10. Derry, S, Cording, M, Wiffen, PJ, et al. Pregabalin for pain in fibromyalgia in adults. *Cochrane Database Syst Rev* 2016; 9:CD011790

11. Gilron, I, Chaparro, LE, Tu, D, et al. Combination of pregabalin with duloxetine for fibromyalgia: a randomized controlled trial. *Pain* 2016; 157:1532–40

12. Jackson, D, Singh, S, Zhang-James, Y, et al. The effects of low dose naltrexone on opioid induced hyperalgesia and fibromyalgia. *Front Psychiatry* 2021; 12:593842

13. Johnson, B, Ulberg, S, Shivale, S, et al. Fibromyalgia, autism, and opioid addiction as natural and induced disorders of the endogenous opioid hormonal system. *Discov Med* 2014; 18:209–20

14. Koenig, J, Jarczok, MN, Ellis, RJ, et al. Two-week test–retest stability of the cold pressor task procedure at two different

temperatures as a measure of pain threshold and tolerance. *Pain Pract* 2014; 14:E126–35

15. Marangell, LB, Clauw, DJ, Choy, E, et al. Comparative pain and mood effects in patients with comorbid fibromyalgia and major depressive disorder: secondary analyses of four pooled randomized controlled trials of duloxetine. *Pain* 2011; 152:31–7

16. Moore, AR, Straube, S, Paine, J, et al. Fibromyalgia: moderate and substantial pain intensity reduction predicts improvement in other outcomes and substantial quality of life gain. *Pain* 2010; 149:360–4

17. Ramanathan, S, Panksepp, J, Johnson, B. Is fibromyalgia an endocrine/endorphin deficit disorder? Is low dose naltrexone a new treatment option? *Psychosomatics* 2012; 53:591–4

18. Rico-Villademoros, F, Slim, M, Calandre, E. Amitriptyline for the treatment of fibromyalgia: a comprehensive review. *Expert Rev Neurother* 2015; 15:1–28

19. Russell, IJ, Kamin, M, Bennett, RM, et al. Efficacy of tramadol in treatment of pain in fibromyalgia. *J Clin Rheumatol* 2000; 6:250–7

20. Russell, IJ, Perkins, AT, Michalek, JE. Sodium oxybate relieves pain and improves function in fibromyalgia syndrome: a randomized, double-blind, placebo-controlled, multicenter clinical trial. *Arthritis Rheum* 2009; 60:299–309

21. Russell, JI, Mease, PJ, Smith, TR, et al. Efficacy and safety of duloxetine for treatment of fibromyalgia in patients with or without major depressive disorder: results from a 6-month, randomized, double-blind, placebo-controlled, fixed-dose trial. *Pain* 2008; 136:432–44

22. Schwartz, T. *Practical Psychopharmacology: Basic to Advanced Principles*, 1st edn. New York: Routledge, 2017

23. Spaeth, M, Bennett, RM, Benson, BA, et al. Sodium oxybate therapy provides multidimensional improvement in fibromyalgia: results of an international phase 3 trial. *Ann Rheum Dis* 2012; 71:935–42

24. Stahl, SM. *Stahl's Essential Psychopharmacology: Neuroscientific Basis and Practical Applications*, 5. Cambridge: Cambridge University Press, 2021

25. Thorpe, J, Shum, B, Moore, RA, et al. Combination pharmacotherapy for the treatment of fibromyalgia in adults. *Cochrane Database Syst Rev* 2018; 2:CD010585

26. Toljan, K, Vrooman, B. Low-dose naltrexone (LDN) – review of therapeutic utilization. *Med Sci (Basel)* 2018; 6:82

27. Tzadok, R, Ablin, JN. Current and emerging pharmacotherapy for fibromyalgia. *Pain Res Manag* 2020; 2020:6541798

28. Walsh, NE, Schoenfeld, L, Ramamurthy, S, et al. Normative model for cold pressor test. *Am J Phys Med Rehabil* 1989; 68:6–11

29. Welsch, P, Üçeyler, N, Klose, P, et al. Serotonin and noradrenaline reuptake inhibitors (SNRIs) for fibromyalgia. *Cochrane Database Syst Rev* 2018; 2:CD010292

30. Wolfe, F. How to use the new American College of Rheumatology fibromyalgia diagnostic criteria. *Arthritis Care Res (Hoboken)* 2011; 63:1073–4

31. Wolfe, F, Clauw, DJ, Fitzcharles, MA, et al. Fibromyalgia criteria and severity scales for clinical and epidemiological studies: a modification of the ACR preliminary diagnostic criteria for fibromyalgia. *J Rheumatol* 2011; 38:1113–22

32. Wolfe, F, Clauw, DJ, Fitzcharles, MA, et al. The American College of Rheumatology preliminary diagnostic criteria for fibromyalgia and measurement of symptom severity. *Arthritis Care Res (Hoboken)* 2010; 62:600–10

33. Wolfe, F, Smythe, HA, Yunus, MB, et al. The American College of Rheumatology 1990 criteria for the classification of fibromyalgia. Report of the Multicenter Criteria Committee. *Arthritis Rheum* 1990; 33:160–72

34. Younger, J, Mackey, S. Fibromyalgia symptoms are reduced by low-dose naltrexone: a pilot study. *Pain Med* 2009; 10:663–72

35. Younger, J, Noor, N, McCue, R, et al. Low-dose naltrexone for the treatment of fibromyalgia: findings of a small, randomized, double-blind, placebo-controlled, counterbalanced, crossover trial assessing daily pain levels. *Arthritis Rheum* 2013; 65:529–38

Case 18: The woman who couldn't focus

The Question: How do you treat a patient with symptoms of overlapping psychiatric diagnoses?

The Psychopharmacological Dilemma: Polypharmacy versus diagnostic confusion

Brian Coringrato and Melissa Abbuhl

Pretest self-assessment question

The ADHD symptom of poor attention/concentration may be found in which other DSM-5 diagnoses?
A. Major depressive disorder (MDD)
B. Bipolar disorder (BP), manic episode
C. Generalized anxiety disorder (GAD)
D. Delirium
E. All of the above

Patient evaluation on intake

- A 45-year-old woman with a chief complaint of depressed mood, anxiousness, difficulty concentrating, with a suicide attempt 1 month prior
- Endorses several months with multiple stressors that led to a suicide attempt
- Stressors included losing her job, coping with the suicide of a close friend, financial difficulties, and ongoing conflict with her boyfriend that led to her moving out
- These stressors have exacerbated her chronic feelings of depression, hopelessness, anxiety, and poor concentration
- She was discharged 2 days ago from an inpatient psychiatric unit following her now third lifetime suicide attempt

Psychiatric history

- Has experienced symptoms of depression and anxiety since she was in early adolescence, in the context of difficult family dynamics
- For depressive symptoms, she has the following: months of depressed mood, poor sleep, anhedonia, feelings of guilt, low energy, poor concentration, and daily suicidal thoughts without current plan or intent
- For anxiety, she has the following symptoms: worrying primarily about finances, her own mental health, and relationships; restlessness, fatigue, irritability, poor concentration, poor sleep

- Has been in and out of psychotherapy for many years and has had multiple medication trials, with limited success
- Evaluated by a psychiatrist at age 30 years old and diagnosed with adult ADHD
- First suicide attempt at age 22 via overdose after a friend died unexpectedly in a car accident, and she did not seek medical treatment
- Second suicide attempt at age 36 via overdose, followed with her first inpatient psychiatric admission
- She had a third suicide attempt 1 month ago via cutting, resulting in her second inpatient admission
- She was discharged with follow-up for further medication management and presented for this appointment
- Reports full DSM-5 MDD symptoms
  - Hopelessness, low mood, decreased motivation, poor sleep, anhedonia, decreased energy, feelings of guilt, and poor appetite
  - Endorses chronic passive suicidal ideation for many years
  - Last active suicidal ideation during the suicide attempt leading to the most recent admission, but denies active suicidal thinking at this time
- Worries frequently about a variety of issues, including many acute stressors
  - Unable to focus, increased irritability, muscle tension, and feelings of restlessness are noted
  - Even when stressors are less present, she still has this pattern of worrying
  - Unclear whether symptoms of hyperactivity and poor attention are due to an underlying anxiety diagnosis or due to her historical diagnosis of ADHD which is currently untreated
- Regarding ADHD, she reports often making careless mistakes, has difficulty sustaining attention, difficulty maintaining attention in conversations, poor adherence to instructions, poor organization, being easily distracted, fidgetiness, restlessness, and interrupting others often
- Significant alcohol and cannabis use are apparent, both daily, meeting criteria for cannabis use disorder (CUD) and alcohol use disorder (AUD)
  - Uses cannabis daily, 1.5 g/d
  - Uses alcohol primarily on the weekend nights, about 3–4 drinks each Friday and Saturday night with another 1–2 drinks on a single week night

- Was seeing a psychiatrist and therapist at another clinic prior to inpatient admission, however was not satisfied with her treatment there and requested a new referral to this clinic upon discharge
- Diagnosed with MDD, unspecified anxiety disorder, and borderline personality disorder (BPD) during her inpatient psychiatric admission

Social and personal history

- Father is a retired firefighter; mother is a retired store clerk
- Has two older brothers
- Graduated community college with an associate's degree
- Current relationship conflict with her boyfriend, now moved in with her friend instead and feels isolated despite this
- Has two sons, ages 22 and 18, who no longer live with her
- Unemployed, used to work as a waitress
- Friend died by suicide 3 months ago
- Consumes around 3–4 drinks each Friday and Saturday night with another 1–2 drinks on a single week night, and has no history of alcohol use treatment
  - Reports this negatively affected relationship with ex-boyfriend
- Daily cannabis use (1.5 g/d) from her own marijuana plants
  - Reports this aids her sleep and anxiety
  - Reports this increases her appetite and alcohol use
  - Reports better work performance when she does not use before/ during work

Medical history

- Arthritis and back pain
- Gastroesophageal reflux disease (GERD)

Family history

- Father has a history of GAD, treated with a benzodiazepine (BZ) anxiolytic
- Brother has a history of AUD and CUD

Medication history

- Selective serotonin reuptake inhibitors (SSRIs): sertraline (Zoloft), fluoxetine (Prozac)
- Stimulants: mixed amphetamine salts (Adderall), IR and ER
- BZ anxiolytic: alprazolam (Xanax)
- Serotonin–norepinephrine reuptake inhibitor (SNRI): duloxetine (Cymbalta)

- Norepinephrine–dopamine reuptake inhibitor (NDRI): bupropion XL (Wellbutrin XL)
- Serotonin partial agonist / reuptake inhibitor (SPARI): vortioxetine (Trintellix)

Current medications

- Quetiapine (Seroquel) 100 mg/d for sleep (atypical antipsychotic)

Psychotherapy history

- A 10-year history of intermittent psychotherapy with limited benefit
  - This included supportive psychotherapy and cognitive behavioral therapy (CBT)

Patient evaluation on initial visit

- Historical diagnosis of MDD, AUD, CUD, and ADHD (diagnosed in adulthood)
- Most recent diagnosis of BPD from inpatient team
- Persistent symptoms of depression, generalized anxiety, and poor attention with acute exacerbation of all symptoms due to recent psychosocial stressors
- She reports that her symptoms became overwhelming and led to the recent suicide attempt and her inpatient psychiatric admission
- Has been compliant with medication and psychotherapy, with little benefit apart from some improvement in sleep with the atypical antipsychotic quetiapine (Seroquel)
- Reports routine cannabis use is very helpful, but still presents here with a myriad of impairing symptoms
- Reports no current medication side effects
- Has good insight into the severity of her symptoms and is motivated to start treatment at a new clinic
- She is particularly interested in starting weekly dialectical behavioral therapy (DBT)
- Chronic passive suicidal ideation tends to be persistent, with no active intent or plan now

Question

Based on your clinical experience, would you expect a patient such as this to recover?

- Yes, she is educated, has family support, and is therapy-minded
- No, she has been resistant to multiple medications, has active substance use, chronic passive suicidal ideation, two psychiatric admissions, and multiple suicide attempts when stressed

Attending physician's mental notes: initial psychiatric evaluation

- The patient has had recurrent major depressive episodes (MDEs) since adolescence, with multiple medication trials with limited improvement overall: sertraline (Zoloft), fluoxetine (Prozac), duloxetine (Cymbalta), bupropion (Wellbutrin), vortioxetine (Trintellix)
- Diagnosis of BPD may be playing a role in her depressive treatment resistance and creates some diagnostic uncertainty given her overlapping symptoms
  - BPD is acutely exacerbated at this time given her psychosocial stressors and feelings of abandonment
- She also has a history of a persistent anxiety disorder, with severity directly correlated with acute stressors as well
  - Unclear whether this is BPD with recurrent adjustment disorders vs. GAD
  - Or possibly MDD with anxious distress
- The patient carries a historical diagnosis of ADHD, which was diagnosed when she was 35 years old by her previous psychiatrist
  - This is currently untreated and may be contributing to her current presentation, given her difficulties with navigating multiple stressors and her losing her job
  - Unclear whether ADHD presented before age 12
- Her overall symptoms are significantly impacting her daily functioning, given that she is having financial difficulties, trouble maintaining a job and advancing her career, and relationship distress, ultimately leading to her most recent psychiatric admission
- Cannabis use may lower agitation or frankly increase it and may cause impairment with concentration and create fatigue
- This may overlap with MDD symptoms
- It is unclear at this time why her previous medication trials have failed and whether this was due to side effects or lack of benefit
- It is also unclear whether these were fully therapeutic trials
- Her short course of CBT was unhelpful
- Psychotherapy has been intermittent
  - Recently started CBT with a new therapist and she does not feel this has been beneficial as of yet
  - She is interested in DBT given her introduction to and use of this modality during recent inpatient stay
- There have been inconsistencies in her treatment course as there have been multiple providers over the years
- She is currently only on the atypical antipsychotic quetiapine (Seroquel) 100 mg nightly for insomnia, and it is working well in this capacity

Question

Which of the following would be your next step?

- Discontinue the quetiapine (Seroquel) due to lack of total benefit and possible future adverse effects such as movement disorder or metabolic syndrome
- Start a medication for treatment of the historical ADHD diagnosis
- Start a new antidepressant for treatment of MDD and GAD
- Continue current medication and initiate weekly DBT with a new provider as the main long-term intervention

Attending physician's mental notes: initial psychiatric evaluation (continued)

- Patient seems to have had some previous therapeutic trials with first-line MDD treatments
  - First, the patient was trialed on sertraline (Zoloft) 200 mg/d and then fluoxetine (Prozac) 40 mg/d, both SSRIs without any benefit
  - She was then initiated on alternative treatment options in different antidepressant classes
    - NDRI, bupropion (Wellbutrin) at 300 mg/d
    - SPARI, vortioxetine (Trintellix) at 20 mg/d
    - SNRI, duloxetine (Cymbalta) at 60 mg/d
  - Previous medications were stopped for a variety of reasons
    - Sertraline (Zoloft) and fluoxetine(Prozac) both caused disrupted sleep
    - She reported some improvement with concentration on mixed amphetamine salts (Adderall) but describes inconsistent use due to overwhelming depression and hopelessness that caused poor medication adherence at that time; and ultimately discontinued upon first inpatient admission
    - Recalls some anxiety relief with the BZ anxiolytic alprazolam (Xanax), but prescriber changed and this was not restarted
    - Duloxetine (Cymbalta) caused GI upset
    - Bupropion XL (Wellbutrin XL) may have caused worsened anxiety
    - Vortioxetine (Trintellix) was an inadequate trial cut short when patient had a lapse in care and changed providers
    - Multiple medication trials and provider changes may be consistent with patient's diagnosis of BPD
  - There is uncertainty over her diagnosis and what should be the next treatment

- She also has a history of being prescribed mixed amphetamine salts (Adderall) several years ago after being diagnosed with ADHD at 35 years old
  - It appears this was discontinued during her first hospitalization and had never been restarted when she saw new providers
  - She noted some benefit; however, she was not consistent with treatment and there were concerns over her ongoing cannabis use
- There is also concern over the patient's chronic suicidal thoughts, with a recent suicide attempt
- She was willing to engage in detailed safety planning and should be placed on the clinic's "High-Risk List" for closer safety monitoring
- She appears discouraged and hopeless about her prognosis, given that these symptoms have persisted for several years and have been largely treatment resistant
- Does meet criteria for MDD, GAD, and CUD formally now
- It is unclear at this time whether she meets criteria for BPD or ADHD, but as more time is spent with patient will further evaluate
- It is also unclear whether the above diagnoses are truly comorbid, or whether they are contributing to each other
  - For example, CUD and BPD can both lead to MDD, GAD, and ADHD symptoms

Further investigation

Is there anything else that you would like to know about the patient?

- What about the impact of substance use on the patient's mood and medication compliance?
- Substance use history regarding alcohol and cannabis
  - Consumes around 7–10 drinks weekly, does not "get drunk," this does not interfere with daily functioning, and CAGE screening is negative
  - She has smoked approximately 1.5 grams of cannabis daily for several years and is unsure of the impact that this has on her mood or anxiety
  - Resistant to stopping, given that it "calms" her and helps her sleep

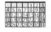

Case outcome: first interim follow-up visit 4 weeks later

- Patient has been doing weekly individual DBT with some initial benefit
  - Confirmed diagnosis of BPD by speaking with therapist and comparing findings

- ○ Key BPD symptoms include intense relationships with alternating idealization and devaluation, unstable self-image, impulsivity in substance use and reckless driving, recurrent suicidal behavior and threats, chronic feelings of emptiness, affective instability, intense and difficult to control anger
- No improvement for her anxiety, depression, or difficulty with attention, unfortunately
- Was continued on quetiapine (Seroquel) 100 mg/d due to benefit for insomnia
- Given possible adverse risks of continuing an antipsychotic, including metabolic changes and movement disorders, discussed possibly discontinuing this medication or, oppositely, increasing it for better effectiveness

Question

What changes would you have made to the patient's current medications?

- Continue quetiapine (Seroquel) given reported benefit with sleep
- Increase quetiapine (Seroquel) as larger doses may help with MDD, GAD, and BPD
- Initiate an alternative medication for sleep with a lower risk profile
- Initiate a new medication for depression and anxiety with a lower risk profile
- Start a medication for her untreated ADHD

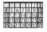

Case outcome: second interim follow-up visit at 2 months

- Patient agreeable to starting trazodone (Desyrel) 50 mg at bedtime, with plan to titrate up for treatment of insomnia and MDD
- Quetiapine (Seroquel) was discontinued
- Patient then experienced side effects from trazodone (Desyrel) including GI upset and self-discontinued it
- Is continuing with weekly DBT, however has some difficulty fully engaging in treatment sessions given active symptom of poor concentration
- Discussed possible medication options with patient and reviewed previous trials to discuss her adherence issues and any side effects she would like to avoid if possible
- Decided to start the SNRI venlafaxine (Effexor XR) 37.5 mg/d given patient's depression, anxiety, and chronic pain related to arthritis of knees
- Plan to increase it to 75 mg/d after 7 days if well tolerated, to achieve an initial therapeutic dose
- Eventually, the NRI properties may help purported ADHD symptoms

Attending physician's mental notes: second interim follow-up visit (month 2)

- The patient continues to be experiencing persistent symptoms of anxiety, depression, poor attention, and passive suicidality
- She was initially resistant to starting a new medication due to history of multiple failed trials
- However, now she feels it is time to start a new medication given persistence of symptoms and its interference with her therapy engagement
- Venlafaxine (Effexor XR) seems like a good option given her pain component and no previous trials with this medication
  - May need a higher dose to gain better norepinephrine-reuptake inhibition which has been linked to reducing pain signaling
  - She previously disliked duloxetine (Cymbalta) but seems willing to try a full dose of this SNRI instead
- The key is to manage her adherence and use the full dose range
- If this SNRI fails, she may need an augmentation or combination strategy

Question

What would you do next?

- Maximize this SNRI
- Combine with a mood-stabilizing atypical antipsychotic or epilepsy medication
- Add a stimulant
- Continue DBT

Case outcome: interim follow-up visits through 4 months

- Patient has been titrated up to venlafaxine (Effexor XR) 75 mg/d
- She has been tolerating the medication well, with some complaints of constipation relieved with over-the-counter (OTC) fiber supplements
- Reports mild improvement now in mood; however, persistent anxiety and difficulty with concentration continue
- Some improvement in sleep as well, without quetiapine (Seroquel) or trazodone (Desyrel) use
- Continues to endorse passive suicidal ideation, remains on High-Risk List at clinic

Attending physician's mental notes: interim follow-up visits through 4 months

- Given improvements on venlafaxine (Effexor XR), will increase dose to 150 mg/d and monitor for constipation worsening, hypertension, and other side effects
- Question remains whether the patient truly has ADHD or whether her difficulty with concentration and restlessness are instead due to her underlying depression, anxiety, BPD, and/or CUD comorbidities
  - Perhaps increased SNRI dose will potentiate more norepinephrine signaling and allow for better attention regardless of etiology
- Will continue monotherapy escalation with the SNRI and continue to evaluate patient's attention and hyperactivity
- If there is improvement, then this adds weight to the suspicion that these symptoms are related to her depressive and anxiety disorders rather than her BPD, CUD, and possible ADHD
- If not, will need to better address and treat the BPD and CUD

Case outcome: interim follow-up visits through 6 months

- The patient's venlafaxine (Effexor XR) has been titrated up to 225 mg/d
- Reported 30% improvement in mood and anxiety; however, persistent difficulties with concentration continue
- She now endorses decreased libido and more constipation, no longer easily relieved with fiber supplements
- Patient does not feel as though the side effects of venlafaxine (Effexor XR) are tolerable any longer and requests a medication change
- Some improvement in passive suicidal ideation is now seen
- Pain may be mildly improved
- She continues to follow up with DBT psychotherapy and has been implementing these skills with moderate success when she is feeling stressed

Question

What would you do next?

- Use different medication to treat constipation and continue SNRI
- Change to an atypical antipsychotic or mood-stabilizing epilepsy medication
- Add a stimulant for her ADHD

Attending physician's mental notes: interim follow-up visits through 6 months

- The patient has reported 50% improvement in mood and anxiety since starting an SNRI
- Side effects are intolerable to patient
- Discussed possibly using a lower dose while hoping to maintain effectiveness or initiating a different antidepressant to avoid current side effects
- Patient is not interested in adding an additional medication and does not wish to continue with venlafaxine (Effexor XR) but rather would prefer a monotherapy approach
- She has now failed two SNRIs, two SSRIs, a SPARI, and NDRI
- Discussed the possibility of pharmacogenetic testing to improve future medication selection and patient expressed interest
  - May increase patient confidence in next medication and enhance placebo effect and lower nocebo effects
- Will order pharmacogenetic test and taper patient off of venlafaxine (Effexor XR) slowly, with close monitoring for any symptom exacerbation or discontinuation side effects
- Will continue with DBT given some improvement with BPD symptoms and stress management
- Concern remains over the impact that cannabis and alcohol use are having on the patient's treatment-resistant symptoms
- She notes that she has decreased alcohol consumption to one drink every 4–5 nights; however, continues full daily cannabis use

Case outcome: interim follow-up visits through 9 months

- Pharmacogenetic testing results
  - Antidepressants
    - Significant gene–drug interaction: venlafaxine (Effexor), where she likely cannot process venlafaxine into desvenlafaxine (Pristiq) due to poor CYP2D6 hepatic metabolism
    - CYP2D6 poor metabolizer
    - CYP2D6*3 allele enzyme activity: none
    - CYP2D6*4 allele enzyme activity: none
  - Stimulants
    - Moderate gene–drug interaction: methylphenidate (Concerta)
    - Genotype may impact drug mechanism of action and result in moderately reduced efficacy
    - CES1A1 normal (both alleles normal)

- ADRA2A C/C alleles
- Moderately reduced response
- Some patients will have a reduced response to ADHD medications
- Patient was started on desvenlafaxine (Pristiq) given it may demonstrate better tolerability for her and we can ensure that an active drug is available in her system as CYP2D6 not required to be metabolized
- Titrated from 25 mg/d up to 150 mg/d with good tolerability, and no side effects
- The patient noted 60% improvement in symptoms of depression and anxiety
- Has much improvement in her chronic passive suicidal ideation, stating that this now is a fleeting thought at most a few times per week
- Patient is more future oriented, continues to participate in weekly DBT with a plan to terminate appropriately
- Vitals show an increase in the patient's blood pressure to 140/90, which is a possible adverse effect of her desvenlafaxine (Pristiq) as the increased norepinephrine results in greater vasoconstriction and a resultant pressure increase
- However, a closer look at the patient's years of documented blood pressure readings at various appointments shows that she does fluctuate between 110/70 and 140/90 often
- Patient saw her primary care clinician and, given the reported benefit of desvenlafaxine (Pristiq), it was decided that she would be started on hydrochlorothiazide (Microzide) to lower her blood pressure
  - Blood pressure subsequently normalized to 120/80
- Patient started a new full-time job with possibility of career advancement
- Despite improvement in mood and anxiety, patient continues to endorse significant impairment in attention
  - She fails to pay close attention to details, has difficulty sustaining attention, trouble with organization, and is easily distracted by external stimuli
- Adult ADHD Self-Report Scale (ASRS) v1.1 score was elevated at 45

Attending physician's mental notes: interim follow-up visits through 9 months

- Persistence of patient's inattentive symptoms, despite symptomatic resolution of depression and anxiety, gives further support to a possible diagnosis of ADHD

- These symptoms are disruptive to the patient's daily functioning and are limiting her progress at work
- Alternatively, CUD may be causing her cognitive issues
- At this time, it seems reasonable to start a medication for ADHD while using harm reduction to improve her CUD
- Given patient's history of substance use, including alcohol and cannabis, there is some concern about starting an addictive stimulant given their abuse potential
- She has no history of stimulant abuse, including cocaine or methamphetamines, and she did note some improvement when on mixed amphetamine salts (Adderall) in the past
- Entered into a safety contract regarding appropriate stimulant use if she agrees to lower cannabis use as well
- Ultimately elected to start lisdexamfetamine (Vyvanse) up to 30 mg every morning
- Continue to monitor patient's blood pressure, with close follow-up with primary care provider
- Continue to monitor patient's cannabis use
  - Obtain a quantitative urine level for cannabinoids
- The benefits appear to outweigh the risks at this time, as we need to improve her cognition and preserve her gainful employment

Case outcome: interim follow up visits through 12 months

- The patient endorses 80% improvement in depression and anxiety while on her SNRI desvenlafaxine (Pristiq) 150 mg/d
- However, difficulties with attention remained a clear problem for the patient
  - ADHD ratings (ASRS v1.1) score of 33 suggests clear problems
- Lisdexamfetamine (Vyvanse) titrated up to 60 mg/d with report of increased "jitteriness" and restlessness
- This was discontinued and next was started on a different stimulant, methylphenidate (Concerta) 18 mg/d, hoping for better effectiveness with fewer side effects
  - Methylphenidate (Concerta) titrated up to 54 mg/d
  - Tolerated well, with no side effects and noted significant improvement in attention ability
  - ASRS v1.1 demonstrated more than 50% reduction
  - This translated to improved functioning at her new job where she received ongoing positive feedback from supervisor
- Continues monthly maintenance DBT which has been stabilizing in regard to her clinical gains

- Ultimately feels as though symptoms are well controlled on current regimen and is happy with results
- Cannabis use decreased to minimal use before bed on work nights and on weekends, approximately 7 grams weekly (vs. 10.5 previously)

Case debrief

- A 45-year-old woman with a chief complaint of depressed mood, anxiousness, difficulty concentrating, and a suicide attempt 1 month prior
- Recent exacerbation of chronic feelings of depression, hopelessness, anxiety, and poor concentration
- Had been smoking cannabis heavily and daily
- Was discharged 2 days prior from inpatient psychiatric unit following her third suicide attempt
- Mood symptoms were ultimately stabilized on desvenlafaxine (Pristiq) following genetic testing
- However, despite improvement in depression and anxiety, her difficulties with inattentiveness remained with a positive correlation to ASRS scores
- Diagnosis of ADHD, inattentive type became more clear
- Patient was ultimately started on methylphenidate (Concerta), with subsequent improvement in attention and a decrease in ASRS score
- She reported an improvement in presenting symptoms, correlated with improved performance reports at work and better social interactions
- Cannabis use also decreased after patient was started on a stimulant, with patient feeling as though her hyperactivity was now managed and she did not need cannabis to relax her

Take-home points

- Some psychiatric symptoms are common across different disorders
- These include: poor concentration, decreased energy, restlessness, irritability, difficulty sleeping, etc.
- Use FDA-approved medications to treat the disorder first
- Consider off-label approaches if needed to treat target residual symptoms
  - Use pharmacodynamic knowledge to treat target symptoms
    - For example, increasing norepinephrine should help attention regardless of the disorder at hand
- It is important to remember that substance use can contribute to presenting symptoms and make achieving full remission difficult

Performance in practice: confessions of a psychopharmacologist

What could have been done better here?

- Insist on cannabis sobriety earlier, with patient education and motivational interviewing
- Insist on getting collateral ADHD historical information from parents or school system to confirm
- Consider repeat formal diagnostic ADHD testing
- Keep an open mind and always re-evaluate your initial diagnosis if the patient is not getting better
- Frequently check in with patient about their primary goals of treatment in order to focus on their chief symptom concerns

What are possible action items for improvement in practice?

- Alternative treatments for ADHD include non-stimulant agents that are not controlled substances, and which were not utilized in this case
- Agents known to treat ADHD that are not controlled substances include atomoxetine (Strattera), viloxazine (Qelbree), guanfacine ER (Intuniv), and clonidine ER (Kapvay)
- These agents have reduced abuse potential and therefore may provide particular benefit to patients with substance use disorders
- These are generally not considered first line except in specific cases in which a stimulant would be contraindicated

Tips and pearls

- The diagnosis of ADHD has diagnostic symptom overlap with the diagnoses of both MDD and GAD
- The diagnosis of ADHD, predominantly hyperactive type, should include 6 or more months of restlessness
- The diagnosis of ADHD, predominantly inattentive type, should include 6 or more months of difficulty sustaining attention and/ or lack of attention, both of which could be considered issues with concentration
- The diagnosis of MDD can include impaired concentration during at least a 2-week period of depressed mood
- The diagnosis of GAD can include difficulty concentrating and/or restlessness during at least a 6-month period of uncontrollable and excessive worrying
- Nonetheless, the symptoms of ADHD must be present prior to age 12 years old, and there is no specification for the age of symptom onset for MDD and GAD, so long as they are present for the designated amount of time

Mechanism of action moment

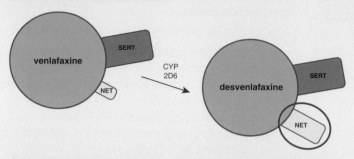

Figure 18.1 Venlafaxine and desvenlafaxine. Venlafaxine inhibits both the serotonin transporter (SERT) and the norepinephrine transporter (NET), thus combining two therapeutic mechanisms in one agent. Venlafaxine's serotonergic actions are present at low doses, while its noradrenergic actions are progressively enhanced as dose increases. Venlafaxine is converted to its active metabolite, desvenlafaxine, by CYP450 2D6. Like venlafaxine, desvenlafaxine inhibits reuptake of serotonin and norepinephrine, but its NET actions are greater relative to its SERT actions compared to venlafaxine. Venlafaxine administration usually results in plasma levels of venlafaxine that are about half those of desvenlafaxine; however, this can vary depending on genetic polymorphisms of CYP450 2D6 and whether patients are taking drugs that are inhibitors or inducers of CYP450 2D6. Thus, the degree of NET inhibition with venlafaxine administration may be unpredictable. Desvenlafaxine (Pristiq) has now been developed as a separate drug. It has relatively greater norepinephrine-reuptake inhibition than venlafaxine but is still more potent at the SERT.

- Comparison of venlafaxine (Effexor) and desvenlafaxine (Pristiq)
  - Venlafaxine inhibits both the serotonin transporter and the norepinephrine transporter
    - Serotonergic actions are present at low doses, whereas its noradrenergic actions are progressively enhanced as dose increases
    - Venlafaxine is converted to its active metabolite, desvenlafaxine, by CYP450 2D6
  - Desvenlafaxine is the active metabolite of venlafaxine
    - It also inhibits reuptake of serotonin and norepinephrine
    - However, it has relatively greater norepinephrine-reuptake inhibition than venlafaxine
    - It will have decreased interaction with other drugs that affect the CYP system
    - Therefore it may have a lower side-effect profile than venlafaxine

Two-minute tutorial

What is adult onset ADHD?

- According to DSM-5, ADHD symptoms must be present before 12 years old
- Previous versions of the DSM required earlier age of symptom onset, and by increasing the age to 12 years, more cases are sufficiently captured
- Early age of symptom onset may improve early diagnosis and therefore earlier intervention thereby avoiding the downstream detrimental side effects of untreated ADHD, such as increased substance use and accidental deaths
- The current age requirement may be designed to avoid over-diagnosing ADHD in adults who may be more likely to have alternative diagnoses to account for their symptomatology
- Further, symptoms of hyperactivity and impulsivity naturally improve (although not necessarily completely) as people age and the prefrontal cortex continues to develop
- However, patients will often present with symptoms consistent with ADHD that were not present or formally diagnosed before age 12
- What could be the cause?
    - Decline in cognitive function with age
    - Untreated medical condition, e.g., sleep apnea
    - Decline with multitasking that increases with age
    - Development of anxiety or depression, causing difficulties with concentration
    - Increase in substance use, such as cannabis, which can impact cognition
    - Possibly undiagnosed inattentive ADHD which has become more apparent with age and the related increase in tasks/responsibilities that need to be balanced (having children, full-time job, etc.)
- Determining the exact cause can be difficult and thus truly defining adult-onset ADHD is challenging
- Therefore, a detailed work-up and treatment of other disorders are important prior to starting an adult with poor concentration on a stimulant

Post-test question

The ADHD symptom of poor attention/concentration may be found in which other DSM-5 diagnoses?

A. Major depressive disorder (MDD)
B. Bipolar disorder (BP), manic episode
C. Generalized anxiety disorder (GAD)
D. Delirium
E. All of the above

Answer: E

Note that MDD and GAD specifically state that poor concentration are key symptoms. Manic patients experience distractibility, and delirious patients experience changes in alertness and poor attention. There is great DSM symptom overlap regarding the cognitive symptoms of attention and concentration.

References

1. American Psychiatric Association. *Diagnostic and Statistical Manual of Mental Disorders*, 5th edn., text rev. Arlington, VA: American Psychiatric Publishing, Inc., 2013
2. Paris, J, Bhat, V, Thombs, B. Is adult attention-deficit hyperactivity disorder being overdiagnosed? *Can J Psychiatry* 2015; 60:324–8
3. Stahl, SM. *Stahl's Essential Psychopharmacology: Neuroscientific Basis and Practical Applications*, 5. Cambridge: Cambridge University Press, 2021.

Case 19: The gentleman with sudden onset of akathisia on clozapine (Clozaril)

The Question: How does COVID-19 impact patients on clozapine?

The Psychopharmacological Dilemma: Treatment of akathisia

Nevena Radonjić

Pretest self-assessment question

What is the main metabolic pathway in the metabolism of clozapine (Clozaril)?
A. CYP1A2
B. CYP2C9
C. CYP2C19
D. CYP2D6
E. CYP3A4

Patient evaluation on intake

- A 41-year-old male with a long history of schizophrenia (SP) presents with a chief complaint of sudden onset of restlessness

Psychiatric history

- Onset of SP in his early 20s
- Usually experiences intermittent ideas of reference, and has prominent negative and cognitive symptoms
- One previous hospitalization 6 years ago for suicidal ideation and akathisia while taking paliperidone (Invega)
- Since then has been stable on clozapine (Clozaril), with difficulty in executive functioning and affective flattening, with occasional and brief ideas of reference
- Besides SP, has a history of obsessive–compulsive disorder (OCD) with repetitive checking behavior
- Reports experiencing in the past 2 weeks new onset of restlessness, with anxious distress, usually worse in the morning
- Stepfather contacted the clinic reporting that patient has been very anxious and not himself

Social and personal history

- Single, living with his stepfather
- Dropped out of school in 12th grade, unemployed, receiving social security disability insurance

- Used to smoke two packs of cigarettes daily, underwent successful smoking cessation on an outpatient basis with an adjustment in the dose of clozapine a year ago
- No history of alcohol use
- No use of any other illicit substances
- Drinks several cups of coffee during the day

Medical history

- Hyperlipidemia (HLD)
- Obesity

Family history

- Biological father has AUD

Medication history

- Atypical antipsychotics: paliperidone (Invega), lurasidone (Latuda), quetiapine XR (Seroquel XR)
- Typical antipsychotics: loxapine (Loxitane)
- Selective serotonin reuptake inhibitors (SSRIs): escitalopram (Lexapro)
- Serotonin receptor partial agonist: Buspirone (Buspar)

Current medications

- Clozapine (Clozaril) 350 mg/d
- Docusate (Colace) 200 mg/d
- Metformin (Glucophage) 1000 mg/d
- Vitamin D 50,000 IU/weekly

Psychotherapy history

- Attending monthly psychotherapy, mainly for support, well known to clinic

Patient evaluation on initial visit

- Sudden onset of morning anxiety and restlessness in the past 2 weeks
- Has an urge to move and is pacing
- This improves as the day evolves
- Reports being very stressed out as his car recently broke down and does not know how to go about fixing it

Question

This patient has been stable on clozapine (Clozaril) for many years. What do you predict will happen in the long term?

- Patients with SP on continuous clozapine (Clozaril) treatment have significantly lower long-term all-cause mortality rates compared to other antipsychotic use
- Treatment with clozapine (Clozaril) is associated with lower hospitalization risk, but higher cardiometabolic-related negative outcomes compared to other atypical antipsychotics
- Given reduced symptom burden, patients on clozapine (Clozaril) have enhanced quality of life

Attending physician's mental notes: initial psychiatric evaluation

- Patient is presenting for an urgent appointment with an acute change in mental status exam
- Noticeable psychomotor activation, differential diagnosis of agitation vs. akathisia
- Intact reality testing
- Patient's stepfather reports an extreme level of distress in the morning time and expressed concern given the sudden change

Further investigation

Is there anything else that you would like to know about the patient?

- *Is he compliant and safe on clozapine (Clozaril)?*
  - Patient's last clozapine/norclozapine levels from 6 months ago were 514/402 mcg/L which are in the therapeutic range
  - Blood work for a new clozapine level was drawn but results are still pending
  - Most recent absolute neutrophil count (ANC) is within normal limits
  - Last annual blood work for long-term monitoring of antipsychotic treatment showed elevated low-density lipoproteins (LDL) and triglycerides (TGA) while fasting glucose and hemoglobin A1c (HbA1c) were within the normal range
  - Noted elevated body mass index (BMI) of 31.8, and normal blood pressure 122/80
  - Last-administered Abnormal Involuntary Movement Scale (AIMS) 3 months ago was negative on all items
- *What about the potential drug interaction impact on clozapine metabolism and its levels?*

- Although several cytochrome (CYP) P450 isoenzymes participate in the biotransformation of clozapine (Clozaril), CYP1A2 is considered its main metabolic pathway
- The mean contribution of CYP1A2 depends on the dose of clozapine (Clozaril), and at lower concentrations CYP1A2 is responsible for 40–55% of biotransformation
- The patient denies any changes in medication regimen or use of any over-the-counter (OTC) medications
- Reports still abstaining from smoking, which is of importance as aryl hydrocarbons from cigarettes are a strong CYP1A2 **inducer** and could significantly **decrease** clozapine levels
- Reports an increase in caffeine intake in the past week as he was feeling very tired in the mornings and now taking six 12 oz cups of coffee compared to the previous two cups
- Caffeine is a moderate CYP1A2 inhibitor and could potentially lead to an increase in clozapine levels
- Denies eating grapefruit or starfruit that can **inhibit** CYP3A4 and potentially **increase** clozapine levels secondarily as well

- *How about COVID-19 status?*
  - COVID-19 infection and vaccination have been associated with an increase in cytokine levels, which may inhibit the activity of CYP1A2 resulting in the sudden increase in clozapine plasma levels
  - Several cases of clozapine toxicity have been reported with acute COVID-19 infection
  - Patient reports that 2 weeks ago he had received the second dose of mRNA COVID-19 vaccine
  - It is possible that a recent vaccination induced an immune response that affected his clozapine levels

- *How about OCD?*
  - Many studies have reported that OCD can be a comorbid diagnosis with SP, or that patients with SP can have OCD-like symptoms
  - Additionally, new onset of obsessive–compulsive symptoms can occur with clozapine (Clozaril) use
  - Patient reports having OCD tendencies all his life, but compulsions and repetitive behavior becoming worse with the initiation of clozapine (Clozaril)
  - Reports that most of the time his checking behavior is manageable and denies any recent worsening

Question

Based on what you know about this patient's history and current psychotropic regimen, is akathisia likely?

- Yes, as the patient is on an antipsychotic, hence extrapyramidal symptoms (EPS) are possible
- No, as clozapine (Clozaril) is usually not associated with significant EPS

Attending physician's mental notes: initial psychiatric evaluation

- In contrast to first-generation typical antipsychotics such as haloperidol (Haldol) and chlorpromazine (Thorazine), clozapine (Clozaril), due to its low affinity for dopamine-2 receptors (D_2s), tends to transiently occupy D_2s in the striatum, resulting in far fewer EPS than traditional antipsychotics
- Reported rates of akathisia in patients on clozapine (Clozaril) are between 3% and 6%
- On mental status examination, noticeable new onset of anxiety and perseveration
- Patient is restless, fidgeting in chair, often getting up
- Scored 4 on Barnes Akathisia Rating Scale (BARS), implying marked akathisia
- Could treat the akathisia with benzodiazepines (BZs) or beta blockers (BBs)
- Typically, anticholinergics are less effective for akathisia
- Patient could benefit from a decrease in the dose of clozapine (Clozaril) to 325 mg/d to see whether the akathisia will improve, but there is a concern about the loss of efficacy
- Given that patient is also feeling very anxious and distressed, may need BZ anxiolytic therapy

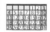

Case outcome: interim follow-up at 7 days

- Initiated BZ lorazepam (Ativan) 1.5 mg/d to target anxiety and akathisia
- Unfortunately, reports further worsening in the level of anxiety and distress
- Mornings are the most difficult and lorazepam (Ativan) only helps temporarily
- Endorsed acute suicidal ideation as he finds restlessness now unbearable
- Last time he felt this unwell was 6 years ago when he was hospitalized due to akathisia while taking paliperidone (Invega)
- Reports that he is feeling unsafe going home

Attending physician's mental notes: interim follow-up (day 7)

- Visible worsening, patient on exam is restless, pacing, with perseverative thought process
- Clozapine/norclozapine levels from a week ago were 559/373 mcg/L, not far from his baseline
- Given that patient has endorsed suicidal ideation and appears very distressed, warrants a psychiatric hospitalization for stabilization of symptoms

Case outcome: interim follow-up at 21 days

- Patient was hospitalized for 7 days
- Clozapine (Clozaril) dose was gradually decreased during the hospital stay from 350 mg/d to 250 mg/d and the patient was started on an anticholinergic, benztropine (Cogentin) 2 mg/d, for his akathisia instead
- Lorazepam (Ativan) was stopped
- Hydroxyzine (Vistaril), an antihistamine and anticholinergic anxiolytic, was started for morning anxiety 50 mg/d, and the patient found it helpful
- After discharge, reports that he is still experiencing some restlessness
- Says that suicidal ideation resolved but that morning anxiety and restlessness are not really any better
- He is now consistently having only two cups of coffee during the day as he is aware of the potential impact of the increase in caffeine intake on clozapine levels

Attending physician's mental notes: interim follow-up (day 21)

- Patient appears less distressed, but still restless in the chair and positive now for abnormal truncal movements such as pelvic tilts
- Latest clozapine/norclozapine levels 482/301 mcg/L
- Administered BARS and patient again scored 4
- Patient is now on, in addition to clozapine (Clozaril), benztropine (Cogentin) and hydroxyzine (Vistaril), which further add to the anticholinergic burden and increase risks of adverse effects

Question

Is benztropine (Cogentin) indicated in the treatment of akathisia?

- Although frequently used in clinical practice for the treatment of akathisia, the evidence to support the use of anticholinergic medications is very limited and at high risk of bias, with inconsistent efficacy findings in clinical trials

- Given these limitations and the high risk for cognitive and anticholinergic adverse effects, benztropine (Cogentin) is not recommended for routine use in akathisia treatment
- Benztropine (Cogentin) can be quite effective in the treatment of other EPS, such as dystonia and parkinsonism

Question

What about the anticholinergic burden of clozapine (Clozaril)?

- Clozapine (Clozaril) has a high affinity for muscarinic cholinergic receptors and is considered to have receptor antagonist activity at M1 and M3 receptors and agonist activity at M1–M5
  - Clozapine's M1 agonist activity is rather weak and the net result of clozapine on M1 receptor is its antagonism
- Antagonism of M1 and M3 receptors is considered to cause high rates of constipation, and other peripheral anticholinergic adverse effects have been seen
- Muscarinic agonist activity via M1 receptor is responsible for frequently observed sialorrhea in patients taking clozapine (Clozaril)

Question

Does hydroxyzine (Vistaril) have anticholinergic effect?

- Although many first-generation antihistamines such as diphenhydramine (Benadryl) have anticholinergic properties and are being used in the treatment of dystonia, hydroxyzine (Vistaril) has a much lower affinity for the muscarinic acetylcholine (ACh) receptors, and accordingly much lower – but still present – risk of anticholinergic side effects
- That means that this medication, if helpful, could be used for the treatment of anxiety in patients on clozapine (Clozaril) without adding as much to the cholinergic burden compared to benztropine (Cogentin)

Question

What would you do next?

- Taper off benztropine (Cogentin) and re-evaluate
- Start the BB propranolol (Inderal) to target akathisia symptoms better
- Further decrease the dose of clozapine (Clozaril)
- Re-start BZs to lower EPS

Case outcome: interim follow-up at 3 months

- Agrees to benztropine (Cogentin) taper and initiation of propranolol (Inderal) instead
  - Benztropine (Cogentin) dose was decreased by 25% weekly then discontinued
  - The propranolol (Inderal) dose was titrated up from 40 mg/d to 120 mg/d over the course of 4 weeks
- The sense of restlessness resolved but the patient was still very tired in the mornings
- Current clozapine/norclozapine levels 549/236 mcg/L

Attending physician's mental notes: interim follow-up (month 3)

- Patient at his baseline, more comfortable, not distressed, no observable EPS, with chronic SP symptoms continuing
- On exam, negative for restlessness, able to sit through an interview with a BARS equalling 0 now
- However, still feels quite tired in the mornings and it takes him a few hours to leave the bed due to sedation
- Noted that, although no change in the dose of clozapine (Clozaril), free clozapine levels increased
- Patient aware of food and medications that could potentially impact clozapine (Clozaril) metabolism and adhering to the treatment plan
- Unclear what is precipitating the observed increase in the clozapine level and it is possible that higher clozapine levels are the cause of morning fatigue/drowsiness/sedation

Question

Considering his current regimen and its risk/benefit profile, what would you do next?

- Keep the regimen as akathisia appears well controlled
- Further decrease the dose of clozapine (Clozaril) to see whether the dose reduction will improve morning-time fatigue/drowsiness/sedation
- Add a wakefulness agent such as modafinil (Provigil)

Case outcome: interim follow-up at 6 months

- Patient tolerated well further gradual clozapine (Clozaril) dose reduction from 250 mg/d to 200 mg/d without worsening of symptoms of SP and denies any suicidal ideation
- Morning sedation improved notably and the patient reports feeling at his baseline

- Reports that anxiety resolved as well and rarely needs hydroxyzine (Vistaril)

Case debrief

- Patient developed acute onset of akathisia possibly due to increase in clozapine levels
- In the absence of other changes, it is possible that COVID-19 vaccination resulted in an inflammatory response that transitorily impacted CYP1A2 metabolism leading to an increase in the level of clozapine and onset of akathisia, as we could not find other typical causes
- Although clozapine (Clozaril) is not associated with high rates of akathisia due to its low D_2 affinity, it is still possible for the patient to develop it, and it appears in this case possibly to be related to the increase in plasma level of clozapine
- Akathisia can result in significant distress and suicidal ideation and the patient experienced both
- Patient responded well ultimately to initiation of BB for treatment of akathisia, not an anticholinergic nor a BZ
- As the patient was still feeling drowsy in the mornings, most likely due to M1 receptor antagonism, the dose of clozapine (Clozaril) was further decreased and the clozapine level returned to the pre-hospitalization range
- Patient reports after the above-taken measures that he is feeling better and that restlessness resolved

Take-home points

- Neuroleptic-induced EPS include akathisia, dystonia, parkinsonism, and dyskinesias
- EPS occur in approximately 50–75% of patients on antipsychotics, with a higher incidence with typical vs. atypical antipsychotics
- Some atypical antipsychotics such as risperidone (Risperdal) and olanzapine (Zyprexa) have a dose-dependent risk for EPS, while that is not the case with other atypicals such as clozapine (Clozaril), iloperidone (Fanapt), lumateperone (Caplyta), and quetiapine (Seroquel)
- EPS often remain unrecognized, impact adherence to treatment, and significantly affect life quality
- Although the precipitating factor can be the same, D_2 blockade, treatment of EPS differs based on presenting symptoms
- Clinicians should routinely screen for EPS and have a good understanding of potential treatment options

- Administration of AIMS for assessment of dyskinesias is considered standard of care and the recommendation is to screen:
  - Every patient for movement disorder before starting either a typical or atypical antipsychotic
  - For typicals, AIMS should be administered every 6 months
  - For atypicals, AIMS should be administered every 12 months
  - For at-risk patients (elderly patients; patients with a history of dystonia, parkinsonism, or akathisia), every 3 months

Performance in practice: confessions of psychopharmacologist

What could have been done better here?

- Given limited evidence on the benefit of benztropine (Cogentin) use in the treatment of akathisia, different therapeutics such as BBs, serotonin 2A receptor (5-HT$_{2A}$) antagonists, or BZs could have been considered prior to initiating benztropine (Cogentin)
- Besides SP, the patient has OCD, which could potentially be treated by an SSRI rather than a higher dose of an antipsychotic
  - When considering the concomitant use of SSRIs with clozapine (Clozaril), the clinician needs to be mindful of potential drug–drug interactions
    - Fluvoxamine (Luvox) is a CYP1A2 inhibitor that could lead to an increase in plasma clozapine levels
    - Use of CYP2D6 inhibitors paroxetine (Paxil) and fluoxetine (Prozac) could also lead to an increase in plasma levels of clozapine
    - Although there are two case reports on the increase in plasma levels of clozapine (Clozaril) with concomitant sertraline (Zoloft) use, these data were not reproduced and generally it is considered that sertraline (Zoloft) minimally affects clozapine levels
    - Citalopram (Celexa), like sertraline (Zoloft), does not significantly affect plasma levels of clozapine

What are possible action items for improvement in practice?

- Physicians should be aware that patients on clozapine (Clozaril) have a higher risk of COVID-19 infection compared to those on other antipsychotics, and that inflammatory response in COVID-19 can inhibit the CYP1A2 metabolic pathway and increase levels of clozapine (Clozaril)
- Although this patient has a history of hyperlipidemia, he is currently not on any lipid-lowering agents and this could be further discussed with the patient's primary provider

Tips and pearls

- Clinicians should be aware of the pharmacodynamic and pharmacokinetic properties of clozapine (Clozaril)
- Clozapine (Clozaril) has a complex binding profile: besides 5-HT$_{2A}$/D$_2$ dual receptor antagonism, numerous other binding properties have been identified, most of which are more potent than its binding at the D$_2$ – α_1A, α 1B, 5-HT$_{2B}$, M1, H1, and many others
- Clozapine (Clozaril) has a half-life between 4 and 66 hours, with Tmax at 2.5 hours
- Plasma levels should be monitored 7 days after a dose adjustment, and every 6–12 months once a stable dose is achieved
- Clozapine (Clozaril) is metabolized to an active metabolite, norclozapine, and the inactive metabolite clozapine-N-oxide
- Although in clinical practice both clozapine and norclozapine plasma levels are determined, the consensus is that plasma clozapine levels correlate with medication efficacy
- The metabolic ratio of clozapine to norclozapine plasma levels is 1.32 in patients who are extensive metabolizers at all relevant CYP isoenzymes
- The primary use of norclozapine levels is in the monitoring of CYP1A2 activity, as a significant change in the metabolic ratio of clozapine and norclozapine implies the presence of an inducer or inhibitor

Mechanism of action moment

Psychotropic medications with anticholinergic properties

- Many psychotropic medications have high anticholinergic potency
  - Typical antipsychotics: chlorpromazine (Thorazine), fluphenazine (Prolixin), perphenazine (Trilafon), loxapine (Loxitane), thioridazine (Mellaril)
  - Atypical antipsychotics: clozapine (Clozaril), olanzapine (Zyprexa), quetiapine (Seroquel)
  - Antiparkinson medications: benztropine (Cogentin), trihexyphenidyl (Artane)
  - Antihistamines: diphenhydramine (Benadryl)
  - Tricyclic antidepressants: amitriptyline (Elavil), clomipramine (Anafranil), desipramine (Norpramin), doxepin (Silenor), imipramine (Tofranil), nortriptyline (Pamelor)
- Often anticholinergic medications such as benztropine (Cogentin), trihexyphenidyl (Artane), and diphenhydramine (Benadryl) are used for treatment of antipsychotic-induced EPS

- Use of medications with anticholinergic properties can result in central and peripheral side efffects

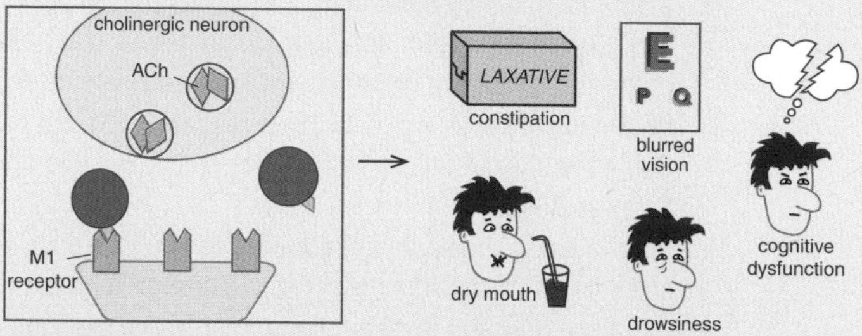

M1 Inserted

Figure 19.1 Side effects of muscarinic cholinergic receptor blockade. When psychotropics are introduced and have an affinity to antagonize and block M1 ACh receptors (represented with blue circle in synapse), it is often associated with central (drowsiness and cognitive dysfunction) and peripheral (constipation, blurred vision, dry mouth) side effects.

Two-minute tutorial

What is akathisia?

- Akathisia is a movement disorder characterized by subjective feelings of internal restlessness or jitteriness, with a compelling urge to move externally
- Although characterized as a movement disorder, akathisia is primarily a psychological symptom that manifests externally
- Akathisia most commonly occurs with the use of D_2 antagonists (antipsychotics and antiemetics) but has also been observed with lithium use and some SSRIs, possibly in a dose-related manner, as well as with vesicular monoamine transporter 2 (VMAT2) inhibitors for the treatment of tardive dyskinesia (TD)
- Akathisia can be acute and occur with the initiation of medication, or be tardive and emerge later during the treatment, usually months or years after taking a medication
- For akathisia to be considered tardive, the patient usually needs to be on the medication for at least 3 months
- A decrease in D_2 stimulation is a proposed mechanism underlying akathisia, although this theory is controversial
- SSRI-induced akathisia is proposed to be mediated by the activation of 5-HT_{2A} receptors, which results in a downstream inhibition of dopamine (DA) release

How to assess akathisia?

- Akathisia is diagnosed based on patients' subjective reports and a physical exam
- BARS is one of the most widely used rating scales that can aid in akathisia assessment
- BARS measures both subjective and objective symptoms
- When administering BARS, the patient is asked about awareness and distress related to restlessness, and the clinician assesses objective findings while observing patient sitting down and standing up
- The rating scale (Figure 19.2) is easy to administer and score, and its reliability, validity, and clinical utility have been well established

How to treat akathisia?

- Treatment of akathisia can be clinically challenging
- The clinician may consider lowering the dose of the offending medication or treating with centrally acting BBs, 5-HT$_{2A}$ receptor antagonists or BZs
- Although anticholinergic medications are often used in clinical practice for the treatment of akathisia, there is no compelling evidence to justify their use

Barnes Akathisia Rating Scale (BARS)

Instructions: Patient should be observed while they are seated, and then standing while engaged in neutral conversation (for a minimum of two minutes in each position). Symptoms observed in other situations, for example while engaged in activity on the ward, may also be rated. Subsequently, the subjective phenomena should be elicited by direct questioning.

Objective

0   Normal, occasional fidgety movements of the limbs
1   Presence of characteristic restless movements: shuffling or tramping movements of the legs/feet, or swinging of one leg while sitting, *and/or* rocking from foot to foot or "walking on the spot" when standing, but movements present for less than half the time observed
2   Observed phenomena, as described in (1) above, which are present for at least half the observation period
3   Patient is constantly engaged in characteristic restless movements, *and/or* has the inability to remain seated or standing without walking or pacing, during the time observed

Subjective

Awareness of restlessness
0   Absence of inner restlessness
1   Non-specific sense of inner restlessness
2   The patient is aware of an inability to keep the legs still, or a desire to move the legs, *and/or* complains of inner restlessness aggravated specifically by being required to stand still
3   Awareness of intense compulsion to move most of the time *and/or* reports strong desire to walk or pace most of the time

Distress related to restlessness

0   No distress
1   Mild
2   Moderate
3   Severe

Global Clinical Assessment of Akathisia

0   *Absent.* No evidence of awareness of restlessness. Observation of characteristic movements of akathisia in the absence of a subjective report of inner restlessness or compulsive desire to move the legs should be classified as pseudoakathisia.
1   *Questionable.* Non-specific inner tension and fidgety movements
2   *Mild akathisia.* Awareness of restlessness in the legs *and/or* inner restlessness worse when required to stand still. Fidgety movements present, but characteristic restless movements of akathisia not necessarily observed. Condition causes little or no distress.
3   *Moderate akathisia.* Awareness of restlessness as described for mild akathisia above, combined with characteristic restless movements such as rocking from foot to foot when standing. Patient finds the condition distressing.
4   *Marked akathisia.* Subjective experience of restlessness includes a compulsive desire to walk or pace. However, the patient is able to remain seated for at least five minutes. The condition is obviously distressing.
5   *Severe akathisia.* The patient reports a strong compulsion to pace up and down most of the time. Unable to sit or lie down for more than a few minutes. Constant restlessness which is associated with intense distress and insomnia.

Figure 19.2 Barnes Akathisia Rating Scale (BARS) – instructions, assessments, and scoring (Barnes, TRE. A rating scale for drug-induced akathisia. *Br J Psychiatry* 1989; 154:672–6).

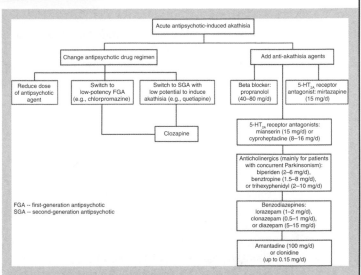

Figure 19.3 Proposed treatment guidelines for acute antipsychotic-induced akathisia (Poyurovsky, M. Acute antipsychotic-induced akathisia revisited. *Br J Psychiatry* 2010; 196:89–91).

Post-test question

What is the main metabolic pathway in the metabolism of clozapine (Clozaril)?

A. CYP1A2

B. CYP2C9

C. CYP2C19

D. CYP2D6

E. CYP3A4

Answer: A

Although all the above-mentioned cytochrome (CYP) P450 isoenzymes participate in the biotransformation of clozapine (Clozaril), CYP1A2 is considered the main metabolic pathway, particularly at low concentrations. The mean contributions of CYPs 1A2, 2C19, 3A4, 2C9, and 2D6 are 30%, 24%, 22%, 12%, and 6%, respectively.

References

1. Barnes, TRE. A rating scale for drug-induced akathisia. *Br J Psychiatry* 1989; 154:672–6
2. Bayraktar, İ, Yalçın, N, Demirkan, K. The potential interaction between COVID-19 vaccines and clozapine: a novel approach for clinical trials. *Int J Clin Pract* 2021; 75(8):e14441
3. Cranshaw, T, Harikumar, T. COVID-19 infection may cause clozapine intoxication: case report and discussion. *Schizophr Bull* 2020; 46:751
4. Edinoff, AN, Fort, JM, Woo, JJ, et al. Selective serotonin reuptake inhibitors and clozapine: clinically relevant interactions and considerations. *Neurol Int* 2021; 13:445–63
5. Gerlach, J, Lublin, H, Peacock, L. Extrapyramidal symptoms during long-term treatment with antipsychotics: special focus on clozapine and D1 and D_2 dopamine antagonists. *Neuropsychopharmacology* 1996; 14 Suppl.:35S–39S
6. Jeong, SH, Kim, YS. Challenges in prescribing clozapine in the era of COVID-19: a review focused on immunological implications. *Clin Psychopharmacol Neurosci* 2021; 19:411–22
7. Loonen, AJM, Stahl, SM. The mechanism of drug-induced akathisia. *CNS Spectrums* 2011; 16:7–10
8. Marder, SR, Essock, SM, Miller, AL, et al. Physical health monitoring of patients with schizophrenia. *Am J Psychiatry* 2004; 161:1334–49
9. Masuda, T, Misawa, F, Takase, M, et al. Association with hospitalization and all-cause discontinuation among patients with schizophrenia on clozapine vs other oral second-generation antipsychotics: a systematic review and meta-analysis of cohort studies. *JAMA Psychiatry* 2019; 76:1052–62
10. Meyer, JM, Stahl, SM. *Binding Profile, Metabolism, Kinetics, Drug Interactions and Use of Plasma Levels.* Cambridge: Cambridge University Press, 2019, 90–113
11. Poyurovsky, M. Acute antipsychotic-induced akathisia revisited. *Br J Psychiatry* 2010; 196:89–91
12. Poyurovsky, M, Weizman, A. Treatment of antipsychotic-induced akathisia: role of serotonin 5-HT2a receptor antagonists. *Drugs* 2020; 80:871–82
13. Pringsheim, T, Gardner, D, Addington, D, et al. The assessment and treatment of antipsychotic-induced akathisia. *Can J Psychiatry* 2018; 63:719–29
14. Roiter, B, Pigato, G, Antonini, A. Prevalence of extrapyramidal symptoms in in-patients with severe mental illnesses: focus on Parkinsonism. *Front Neurol* 2020; 11:593143

15. Stahl, SM. *Targeting Dopamine and Serotonin Receptors for Psychosis, Mood, and Beyond: So-Called "Antipsychotics,"* 5. Cambridge: Cambridge University Press, 2021.

16. Tio, N, Schulte, PFJ, Martens, HJM. Clozapine intoxication in COVID-19. *Am J Psychiatry* 2021; 178:123–7

17. Vermeulen, JM, van Rooijen, G, van de Kerkhof, MPJ, et al. Clozapine and long-term mortality risk in patients with schizophrenia: a systematic review and meta-analysis of studies lasting 1.1–12.5 years. *Schizophr Bull* 2019; 45:315–29

Case 20: The pregnancy blues

The Question: How to balance risks of untreated perinatal mood and anxiety disorders (PMADs) vs. risks of taking psychotropic medications during pregnancy?

The Psychopharmacological Dilemma: Finding a safe and effective treatment for PMADs during pregnancy

Nevena Radonjić

Pretest self-assessment question

Exposure to selective serotonin reuptake inhibitors (SSRIs) during pregnancy increases the risk of which of the following?

A. Spontaneous abortion (miscarriage)
B. Persistent pulmonary hypertension
C. Congenital malformations
D. Long-term behavioral effects
E. All of the above
F. None of the above

Patient evaluation on intake

- A 33-year-old female 5 months pregnant presenting with worsening major depressive disorder (MDD) and generalized anxiety disorder (GAD)
- Reports in past few months feeling profoundly depressed, difficulty functioning, oversleeping, and isolating at home
- Worries about the baby coming and not being able to take care of it

Psychiatric history

- Onset of depression and anxiety in early teen years with intermittent remission of symptoms
- Has been intermittently in individual therapy and has antidepressant medications managed by her primary care clinician (PCC) now
- Negative for inpatient hospitalizations and no history of suicide attempts

Social and personal history

- The patient is a college graduate and works for a legal firm
- She is married and describes her husband as supportive and their relationship stable
- This is her first and planned pregnancy

- Reports having a good relationship with her family, but that they are not living close by and that she feels uncomfortable asking for their help
- Negative for any substance use

Medical history

- Diabetes mellitus type 2 (DM2), stable
- Hypothyroidism, stable
- Tension headaches
- Hyperlipidemia (HLD)
- Hypertension (HTN), stable

Family history

- MDD in mother and father
- Attention-Deficit/Hyperactivity Disorder (ADHD) in sister and multiple cousins

Medication history

- Previous medication trials
  - SSRIs
    - Fluoxetine (Prozac) – up to 40 mg/d with partial effectiveness
    - Citalopram (Celexa) – up to 40 mg/d
  - Atypical antipsychotics: aripiprazole (Abilify) 2 mg/d
  - Other: buspirone (Buspar) 22.5 mg/d

Current medications

- Citalopram (Celexa) 40 mg/d, an SSRI
- Levothyroxine (Synthroid) 50 mg/d
- Labetalol (Trandate) 400 mg/d
- Metformin (Glucophage) 2000 mg/d
- Acetylsalicylic acid (ASA) 81 mg/d
- Prenatal vitamins
- Vitamin C

Attending physician's mental notes: initial psychiatric evaluation

- Patient reports worsening of mood in the past 3 months since aripiprazole (Abilify) was stopped by primary care physician in 8th gestational week (gw) due to PCC being worried about exposure to atypical antipsychotics during pregnancy

- Reports that prior to that she was on citalopram (Celexa) 20 mg/d and aripiprazole (Abilify) 2 mg/d with a good effect and that she was euthymic for past year
- Stated that the dose of citalopram (Celexa) was increased to 40 mg/d 2 months ago but that there was no improvement in mood and anxiety symptoms without aripiprazole (Abilify) present
- Reports a debilitating depression now affecting her ability to perform activities of daily living, such as taking a shower and getting dressed. She is also struggling to go to work and do household chores
- Expressed being worried about how she will take care of the baby given her current condition and that she plans to breastfeed
- On exam presents as dysphoric, with restricted and flat affect, denies any suicidal ideation, and endorsed being hopeful that she can feel better with medication adjustment
- Clinical presentation is consistent with MDD and GAD
- Appears that worsening of the mood symptoms temporally correlates with discontinuation of the aripiprazole (Abilify) more so than any new social stressors
- Patient is already on the maximum dose of SSRI, hence further increase in the dose of citalopram (Celexa) is not possible

Questions

Given that the patient had been on the combination of SSRI and atypical antipsychotic (aripiprazole [Abilify]) until the 8th gestational week of pregnancy, was the discontinuation of aripiprazole (Abilify) a justified step?

- Every pregnancy carries a background risk of 3–5% of having a birth defect
- Harmful exposures during the first trimester of pregnancy have the greatest chance of causing major birth defects
- Clinicians have to balance risks of untreated PMADs vs. risks of exposure to the medication itself
- In 2015, the FDA put into effect the Requirements for Pregnancy and Lactation Labeling, also known as the "Pregnancy and Lactation Labeling Rule" (PLLR), which replaced previous pregnancy risk categories (A, B, C, D, and X)
- The PLLR required changes to the content and format for the information presented in prescription drug labeling to assist healthcare providers in assessing benefit vs. risk and subsequent counseling of pregnant women and nursing mothers who need to take the medication, allowing them to make educated and informed decisions for themselves and their children

- Based on the available studies, there is no evidence that exposure to aripiprazole (Abilify) during the pregnancy increases background risk of birth defects per PLLR
- Additionally, the embryo was already exposed to aripiprazole until the 8th gestational week
- Given that the patient had been euthymic on the regimen, it would have been justified to continue the combination of SSRI and atypical antipsychotic as untreated PMADs can result in adverse effects on mother, baby, and mother–baby dyad

Based on what you know about this patient's history and current symptoms, what would you consider to be the next reasonable step?

- Increase the frequency of individual therapy
- Refer to evidence-based psychotherapy for MDD, such as cognitive behavioral therapy (CBT)
- Continue current regimen as the patient is pregnant and consider adjusting the medication after the delivery
- Switch to a different SSRI or serotonin–norepinephrine reuptake inhibitor (SNRI) antidepressant
- Restart aripiprazole (Abilify), an atypical antipsychotic, for augmentation of her current SSRI antidepressant as the patient is experiencing worsening of mood symptoms and previously did well on the combination of SSRI and this atypical antipsychotic

Attending physician's mental notes: initial psychiatric evaluation (continued)

- During the pregnancy, the goal for the patient is to be euthymic and for there to be stability in mood and anxiety symptoms
- Although switching to a different SSRI or SNRI would be a reasonable choice, during the pregnancy try to limit the exposure to different medications
- Interestingly, escitalopram (Lexapro) is an active S-enantiomer of citalopram and could be used instead as the dose can be increased without the risk of QTc prolongation
- The embryo was already exposed to citalopram (Celexa) and aripiprazole (Abilify) and switching to a third medication would result in another exposure with uncertain clinical benefits
- Discussed with the patient that both medications are compatible with breastfeeding and that they are found in small amounts in breast milk
- The patient agreed to restart aripiprazole (Abilify) 2 mg/d as she found it beneficial in the past

Case outcome: interim follow-ups through 1 month

- The patient reports tolerating aripiprazole (Abilify) well and endorsed improvement in mood symptoms within the first few weeks
- Reports that she is overall feeling 50% better, now able to leave her bed, take care of herself and the household
- Reports that she is now attending individual supportive therapy each week

Questions

What is the recommended dose of aripiprazole (Abilify) as an adjunct in the treatment of MDD?

- It has an approved initial dose of 2–5 mg/d, with a recommended target dose of 5–10 mg/d and a maximal dose of 15 mg/d
- Aripiprazole (Abilify) is mainly metabolized via CYP2D6 and CYP3A4 pathways and potential interactions with inhibitors of these metabolic pathways need to be considered when dosing the medication
- Aripiprazole (Abilify) dosing is halved if the patient is taking CYP2D6 inhibitors such as fluoxetine (Prozac), paroxetine (Paxil), and bupropion XL (Wellbutrin XL)
- If taken with strong inhibitors of both CYP2D6 and CYP3A4 the dose needs to be quartered
- In contrast, for patients on strong CYP3A4 inducers such as carbamazepine (Equetro), the dose needs to be doubled over the period of 1–2 weeks

What other atypical antipsychotics are FDA-approved for the treatment of MDD?

- Besides aripiprazole (Abilify), quetiapine XR (Seroquel XR), brexpiprazole (Rexulti), cariprazine (Vraylar), and a combination of fluoxetine + olanzapine (Symbiax) have been approved as adjuncts in the treatment of MDD
- Currently, lumateperone (Caplyta) is in phase 3 trials as an adjunctive therapy in the treatment of patients with MDD
- In clinical practice, risperidone (Risperdal) is used off-label as an adjunct in the treatment of MDD, as is lurasidone (Latuda), but risperidone (Risperdal) has one large positive randomized controlled trial (RCT) showing effectiveness

What baseline tests need to be completed if a patient is on an atypical antipsychotic?

- Every patient needs baseline fasting glucose, hemoglobin A1c (HbA1c), and lipid panel, which should be re-checked within 3 months, then annually
- Additionally, weight, body mass index (BMI), blood pressure, and waist circumference should be obtained prior to starting the medication and repeated after 3 months, then annually
- Abnormal Involuntary Movement Scale (AIMS) should be administered annually to monitor for the occurrence of tardive dyskinesia (TD) for patients on atypical antipsychotics

Attending physician's mental notes: interim follow-ups through 1 month

- Noticeable improvement in mood symptoms with the restart of aripiprazole (Abilify) and patient able to function better, but still not quite at her baseline and not in remission
- Given a history of DM2 and HLD, the patient is already on metformin (Glucophage) and the PCC is monitoring lipid panel and HbA1c
- Reviewed the most recent EKG performed by PCC and noted that QTc interval is within normal limits (less than 450 msec)
- Patient agreeable to further increase in the dose of aripiprazole (Abilify) and the dose has been adjusted up to 5 mg/d

Case outcome: interim follow-ups through 2 months

- The patient is now 7 months pregnant, presents with a brighter affect, reports overall improvement in mood symptoms, ability to experience joy, is taking care of self as usual, and is back to work
- Appears that patient has achieved remission of MDD
- Reports tolerating well the combination of current medications and denies any adverse effects
- Stated however that she has been getting more anxious in the past weeks and that sleep has been impaired
- Shared being worried about upcoming delivery and getting everything ready for baby's arrival
- Although finds family supportive, does not feel comfortable asking for help

Attending physician's mental notes: interim follow-ups through 2 months

- Appears that the patient has responded well to an increase in the dose of aripiprazole (Abilify)
- Given that the patient is 7 months pregnant, insomnia is expected due to overall discomfort, increase in urinary frequency, fetal movements, and leg discomfort associated with the third trimester of pregnancy
- Although insomnia often occurs in third trimester, if untreated it can lead to worsening of mood and anxiety symptoms
- It is also possible that the anxiety the patient is experiencing is contributing to reported sleep disturbances and, vice versa, that she is more anxious due to poor sleep
- Patient would benefit from more active family involvement, and education related to upcoming delivery and breastfeeding

Questions

What is the first-line treatment for anxiety in pregnancy?

- Although there is no comprehensive algorithm for a treatment approach to perinatal anxiety, CBT is an effective strategy for mild anxiety disorders
- For moderate to severe perinatal anxiety, pharmacotherapy in combination with therapy is recommended

What is the first-line treatment for insomnia in pregnancy?

- CBT for insomnia is considered to be the first-line approach for the treatment of perinatal insomnia
- If pharmacotherapy is being considered, benzodiazepines (BZs), sedating antihistamines (doxylamine [Unisom], diphenhydramine [Benadryl], hydroxyzine [Vistaril], and trazodone [Desyrel]) are possible options
- Given the limited data on the reproductive safety of hypnotic benzodiazepine receptor agonists (BZRAs) such as zolpidem (Ambien), zaleplon (Sonata), and eszopiclone (Lunesta), short-term use of BZ might be the preferred option

Given the above-stated, what would you do next?

- Validate and normalize her symptoms as insomnia and anxiety are normal and expected prior to delivery
- Utilize CBT and relaxation techniques for reduction of symptoms of both anxiety and insomnia
- Start a short-term course of BZ lorazepam (Ativan), for treatment of anxiety and insomnia

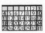

Case outcome: interim follow-ups through 6 months

- Patient was already on the maximum dose of SSRI and also on an atypical antipsychotic, and was uncomfortable with the idea of taking any additional medications such as BZ or antihistamines during pregnancy
- She has expressed interest in starting CBT with a therapist and responded well to relaxation techniques, with relief in anxiety symptoms
- With the help of the therapist, her family was more involved, which in turn further helped with a decrease in anxiety
- She also attended breastfeeding and birthing classes that were useful in preparation for delivery
- Patient's mood symptoms remained in remission after the delivery, with some fluctuations in anxiety only

Case debrief

- Patient has a long history of recurrent MDD and her mood symptoms worsened after the adjunctive atypical antipsychotic was stopped due to fear of teratogenicity
- Although the dose of citalopram (Celexa) was increased in its place, MDD symptoms were still present and worsened, and she sought the help of a specialist
- Patients with a history of more than two episodes of MDD in a lifetime will most likely experience worsening of mood symptoms if the treatment is stopped
- Patient responded well to re-initiation of aripiprazole (Abilify) but the dose of medication needed to be further adjusted to achieve remission
- Perinatal anxiety and insomnia are frequent comorbidities in depressed patients, but sometimes are treated as adjustment disorder
- CBT is an effective treatment strategy for both anxiety and insomnia and the patient responded well to incorporating relaxation techniques

Take-home points

- This case emphasizes the importance of good, well-informed mental healthcare during pregnancy
- The goal of the psychiatric treatment should be remission of symptoms, and many women are undertreated during pregnancy due to fear of medication use

- Here, the patient achieved mood stability and euthymia prior to conception, but experienced worsening of symptoms once the atypical antipsychotic was stopped
- This patient already had DM2, HLD, and HTN, and the use of an atypical antipsychotic could further worsen these conditions
- However, the severity of her MDD warranted treatment, and she responded well to re-initiation of aripiprazole (Abilify)
- In addition, the patient benefited from behavioral and family interventions

Performance in practice: confessions of a psychopharmacologist

What could have been done better here?

- Ideally, the clinician's goal would be for the patient's mood symptoms to be stable at the time of preconception as well as during the pregnancy
- Given that she was euthymic on a combination of SSRI and an atypical antipsychotic, discontinuation of the atypical antipsychotic aripiprazole (Abilify) late in the first semester was likely not warranted and led to the destabilization of symptoms
- First-trimester risk of exposure already occurred
- Better understanding of the risks of untreated PMADs vs. risks of taking psychotropics during the pregnancy could have been helpful in making medical decisions and counseling the patient

What are possible action items for improvement in practice?

- Psychiatrists should feel comfortable prescribing medications during different periods of the woman's reproductive life cycle, including pregnancy
- Psychiatrists should be aware of resources on medication safety during pregnancy and breastfeeding, and consider risks of untreated PMADs vs. risks of psychotropic medications by using PLLR

Tips and pearls

- If the patient is of childbearing age, birth control and family planning should be an integral part of usual treatment planning
- Clinicians should consider pregnancy and breastfeeding when discussing medications with patients
- It is recommended to actively include family in treatment planning and provide psychoeducation on perinatal depression and anxiety as well as medication risks

- Treating provider should coordinate care with the PCC and obstetrician, as well as other specialists included in the care of the patient
- Besides biological and psychological factors, treating provider should also take into account social determinants of mental health

Mechanism of action moment

How does aripiprazole (Abilify) augment antidepressants?

- Aripiprazole (Abilify) is a D_2/5-HT_{1A} partial dual receptor agonist approved for the treatment of schizophrenia and bipolar disorder, bipolar maintenance, and augmentation of antidepressants in the treatment of MDD
- Aripiprazole (Abilify) is one of the most commonly prescribed augmenting adjuncts to SSRI/SNRI in the treatment of MDD
- Its prominent partial 5-HT_{1A} agonist action most likely underlies antidepressant effects
- Secondary properties with potential antidepressant action may also be contributory, including D_3, 5-HT_7, 5-HT_{2C}, and α_2 antagonist actions

How does partial 5-HT_{1A} agonism help with affective symptoms?

- 5-HT_{1A} receptors are inhibitory and located both presynaptically on serotonergic neurons and postsynaptic on many neurons, including excitatory glutamatergic pyramidal cells
- 5-HT_{1A} partial agonism on glutamatergic pyramidal cells leads to disinhibition of dopamine (DA) release in the prefrontal cortex needed for improvement of negative, cognitive, and affective/depressive symptoms
- Besides its effect on affective symptoms, partial 5-HT_{1A} agonism also opposes D_2 antagonism / partial agonism in certain pathways, resulting in a reduction of many motor side effects, although akathisia can still commonly occur

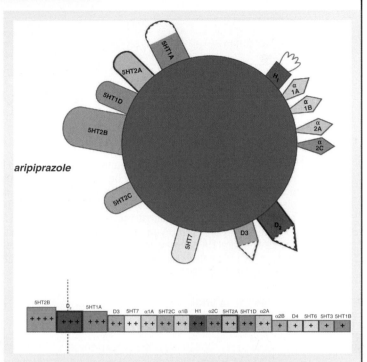

Figure 20.1 Aripiprazole's pharmacological and binding profile. This figure portrays a qualitative consensus of current thinking about the binding properties of aripiprazole. Aripiprazole is a partial agonist at D_2s rather than an antagonist. Additional important pharmacological properties that may contribute to its clinical profile include 5-HT$_{2A}$ antagonist actions, 5-HT$_{1A}$ partial agonist actions, 5-HT$_7$ antagonist actions, and 5-HT$_{2C}$ antagonist actions.

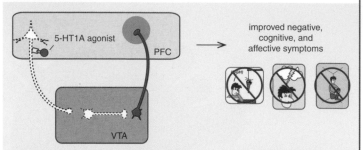

Figure 20.2 5-HT$_{1A}$ receptor partial agonism and downstream DA release. 5-HT$_{1A}$ receptors are located on descending glutamatergic pyramidal neurons that indirectly innervate mesocortical DA neurons via a GABAergic interneuron in the ventral tegmental area (VTA). 5-HT$_{1A}$ partial agonism reduces glutamatergic output in the VTA, leading to reduced activity of the GABA interneuron and therefore disinhibition of the mesocortical DA pathway. Increased DA release in the prefrontal cortex (PFC) can potentially reduce cognitive, negative, and affective symptoms of psychosis.

Two-minute tutorial

What are PMADs?

- The term perinatal mood and anxiety disorders (PMADs) refers to mood and anxiety disorders that occur during the pregnancy or postpartum period
- DSM-5 defines the postpartum period as "any time during the pregnancy and 4 weeks postpartum"
- In clinical practice, the term "postpartum" often refers to the first year after giving birth, as defined by the World Health Organization (WHO)
- PMADs encompass perinatal depression / MDD, GAD, obsessive–compulsive disorder (OCD), and post-traumatic stress disorder (PTSD)
- PMADs are common, with an estimated prevalence of 15–20% of the general population, and are considered to be the most common perinatal complication
- PMADs carry significant economic and public health burdens and profoundly affect the mother, child, and family
- The American College of Obstetricians and Gynecologists recommends that all pregnant and postpartum patients are at least once screened during the perinatal period for anxiety and depression symptoms
- The most commonly used screening tool is the Edinburgh Postnatal Depression Scale (EPDS) which captures depressive symptoms

with comorbid anxiety and contains 10 questions, with a maximum score of 30. The cut-off for screening to be considered positive is 10–13
- The main difference between the most commonly used self-rating scale for depression, Patient Health Questionnaire 9 (PHQ-9), and EPDS is that the latter does not address sleep and fatigue as these are presumed to be affected in the perinatal period due to childcare
- EPDS additionally addresses anxiety symptoms that are highly prevalent in patients during the perinatal period

Risks of untreated PMADs

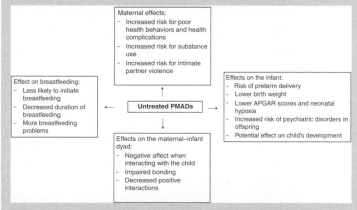

Figure 20.3 Untreated PMADs can have adverse effects on mother, infant, maternal–infant dyad, and breastfeeding

Non-pharmacological treatments for PMADs

- Psychological interventions are effective in the treatment of perinatal depression
- CBT and interpersonal therapy (IPT) have the most evidence for effectiveness in the treatment of perinatal depression
- Other studied psychological interventions with possible benefits in PMADs
  ○ Behavioral activation
  ○ Mindfulness
  ○ Psychological or social support
  ○ Psychoeducation or education-based interventions
- Complementary and alternative medicine (CAM) treatments
  ○ Often preferred by patients, hence clinicians need to be familiar with CAM therapies and systematically inquire about their use

- May be reasonable to consider for women in the perinatal period, but the safety and efficacy of these relative to standard treatments are still to be systematically determined
- Most commonly used CAM treatments
  - Omega-3 fatty acids
  - Folate
  - S-adenosyl-methionine (SAM)
  - St. John's wort
  - Bright light therapy
  - Exercise
  - Massage
  - Acupuncture

Risks of prescribing psychotropic medications during pregnancy

- Majority of psychotropic medications can be safely prescribed during pregnancy
- When prescribing medications during pregnancy, clinicians have to consider the risk and benefits of the medication and balance it with the risks of untreated PMADs
- There is no decision without risk and an individualized approach is recommended and should be well documented in the chart
- The potential effect of the medication on offspring differs depending on the gestational age at exposure
- The risk of teratogenicity is highest in the first trimester when organogenesis takes place
- Divalproex (Depakote) and carbamazepine (Equetro) carry the risk of neural tube closure defect and generally are not recommended to be prescribed to women of childbearing age
- Lithium (Eskalith) use during the first trimester carries the risk of cardiac malformations, including Ebstein's anomaly, but most recent studies demonstrate that the magnitude of this effect is smaller than previously established
- Clinicians need to be aware of whether the exposure to the medication can result in teratogenicity, have a long-term effect on the child's development, or have a direct effect that can lead to neonatal toxicity or withdrawals
- Clinicians also need to be aware of possible maternal risks of SSRIs and depression
  - Gestational hypertension and pre-eclampsia
  - Delivery – increased risk of:
    - placenta previa
    - placental abruption

- premature rupture of membranes
- the need for induction of labor and C-section
- Postpartum hemorrhage

SSRIs and SNRIs in the treatment of PMADs

- SSRIs and SNRIs are the main groups of medications used in the treatment of PMADs
- If the patient has never been on a medication, then a medication with a short half-life, and low concentration in the breast milk, should be recommended
  - Avoiding fluoxetine (Prozac), for example, as it has longer half-life
- If the patient has a history of previous medication trials, it is prudent to use medications that were helpful in the past and resulted in remission of symptoms
- The main limitation in the use of SSRIs and SNRIs during the pregnancy is lack of randomized controlled studies
- Additionally, previous studies compared outcomes of depressed women on SSRIs/SNRIs with healthy women, with no adjustment for confounding factors such as PMADs

Antidepressants and breastfeeding

- All psychotropic medications readily pass into breast milk
- The amount of medication secreted into breast milk is usually significantly lower compared to the amount that passed through the placenta
- Relative infant dose (RID) is a valuable and practical guide to indicate the extent of drug exposure to the infant while breastfeeding
- The RID calculates the weight-adjusted dose in an infant relative to the weight-adjusted dose in the mother
- The RID of most commonly prescribed antidepressants varies from 0.5 – 14%, with sertraline (Zoloft) and paroxetine (Paxil) being the medications with the lowest RID (0.5 – 3%), and fluoxetine up to 14%
- If the infant has been exposed to the medication during pregnancy, it is generally recommended to continue with the same medication while breastfeeding

Post-test question

Exposure to selective serotonin reuptake inhibitors (SSRIs) during pregnancy increases the risk of which of the following?

A. Spontaneous abortion (miscarriage)
B. Persistent pulmonary hypertension
C. Congenital malformations
D. Long-term behavioral effects
E. All of the above
F. None of the above

Answer: F

Large studies and meta-analyses showed that antidepressants do not add to the risk of spontaneous abortion. Although the FDA in 2006 issued an alert for a potential association between SSRIs and persistent pulmonary hypertension of the newborn, the most recent data showed no difference when adjusted for confounding factors. When it comes to congenital malformations, the best available evidence indicates that there is no additional risk of congenital malformations in women who used antidepressants. No cognitive and behavioral effects of antidepressant exposure during the pregnancy were found, and there is no evidence of associated IQ deficits or long-term behavioral problems

References

1. Branquinho, M, Rodriguez-Muñoz, MF, Maia, BR, et al. Effectiveness of psychological interventions in the treatment of perinatal depression: a systematic review of systematic reviews and meta-analyses. *J Affect Disord* 2021; 291:294–306
2. Brooks, E, Cox, E, Kimmel, M, et al. *Risk of Untreated Symptoms of PMADs in Pregnancy and Lactation.* Cham, Switzerland: Springer, 2021, 45–54
3. Byatt, N, Deligiannidis, KM, Freeman, MP. Antidepressant use in pregnancy: a critical review focused on risks and controversies. *Acta Psychiatr Scand* 2013; 127:94–114
4. Chad, L, Pupco, A, Bozzo, P, et al. Update on antidepressant use during breastfeeding. *Can Fam Physician* 2013; 59:633–4
5. Dean L, Kane, M. Aripiprazole therapy and CYP2D6 genotype. Sept. 22, 2016 [Updated Feb. 10, 2021]. In: Pratt VM, Scott SA, Pirmohamed M, et al. (eds.) *Medical Genetics Summaries* [internet]. Bethesda, MD): National Center for Biotechnology Information (US); 2012– ; www.ncbi.nlm.nih.gov/books/NBK385288
6. Deligiannidis, KM, Freeman, MP. Complementary and alternative medicine therapies for perinatal depression. *Best Pract Res Clin Obstet Gynaecol* 2014; 28:85–95

7. El Marroun, H, Jaddoe, VW, Hudziak, JJ, et al. Maternal use of selective serotonin reuptake inhibitors, fetal growth, and risk of adverse birth outcomes. *Arch Gen Psychiatry* 2012; 69:706–14

8. Eléfant, E, Hanin, C, Cohen, D. Pregnant women, prescription, and fetal risk. *Handb Clin Neurol* 2020; 173:377–89

9. Gadot, Y, Koren, G. The use of antidepressants in pregnancy: focus on maternal risks. *J Obstet Gynaecol Can* 2015; 37:56–63

10. Galbally, M, Lewis, AJ, Buist, A. Developmental outcomes of children exposed to antidepressants in pregnancy. *Aust N Z J Psychiatry* 2011; 45:393–9

11. Hashmi, AM, Bhatia, SK, Bhatia, SK, et al. Insomnia during pregnancy: diagnosis and rational interventions. *Pak J Med Sci* 2016; 32:1030–7

12. Huybrechts, KF, Bateman, BT, Palmsten, K, et al. Antidepressant use late in pregnancy and risk of persistent pulmonary hypertension of the newborn. *JAMA* 2015; 313:2142–51

13. Huybrechts, KF, Palmsten, K, Avorn, J, et al. Antidepressant use in pregnancy and the risk of cardiac defects. *N Engl J Med* 2014; 370:2397–407

14. Kjaersgaard, MIS, Parner, ET, Vestergaard, M, et al. Prenatal antidepressant exposure and risk of spontaneous abortion – a population-based study. *PLoS One* 2013; 8:e72095

15. Lee, HJ, Kim, SM, Kwon, JY. Repetitive transcranial magnetic stimulation treatment for peripartum depression: systematic review & meta-analysis. *BMC Pregnancy and Childbirth* 2021; 21:118

16. Levinson-Castiel, R, Merlob, P, Linder, N, et al. Neonatal abstinence syndrome after in utero exposure to selective serotonin reuptake inhibitors in term infants. *Arch Pediatr Adolesc Med* 2006; 160:173–6

17. Lomonaco-Haycraft, KC, Hyer, J, Tibbits, B, et al. Integrated perinatal mental health care: a national model of perinatal primary care in vulnerable populations. *Prim Health Care Res Dev* 2018; 20:e77

18. Malm, H, Brown, AS, Gissler, M, et al. Gestational exposure to selective serotonin reuptake inhibitors and offspring psychiatric disorders: a national register-based study. *J Am Acad Child Adolesc Psychiatry* 2016; 55:359–66

19. Nelson, JC, Pikalov, A, Berman, RM. Augmentation treatment in major depressive disorder: focus on aripiprazole. *Neuropsychiatr Dis Treat* 2008; 4:937–48

20. Osborne, L, Birndorf, C. *Depressive Disorders*. Arlington, VA: American Psychiatric Publishing, Inc., 2022.

21. Patorno, E, Huybrechts, KF, Bateman, BT, et al. Lithium use in pregnancy and the risk of cardiac malformations. *N Engl J Med* 2017; 376:2245–54. https://doi.org/10.1056/NEJMoa1612222

22. Payne, JL. Psychopharmacology in pregnancy and breastfeeding. *Psychiatr Clin North Am* 2017; 40:217–38

23. Payne, JL. Psychopharmacology in pregnancy and breastfeeding. *Med Clin North Am* 2019; 103:629–50

24. Rommel, AS, Momen, NC, Molenaar, NM, et al. Antidepressant use during pregnancy and risk of adverse neonatal outcomes: a comprehensive investigation of previously identified associations. *Acta Psychiatr Scand* 2022; 145:544–56

25. Ross, LE, Grigoriadis, S, Mamisashvili, L, et al. Selected pregnancy and delivery outcomes after exposure to antidepressant medication: a systematic review and meta-analysis. *JAMA Psychiatry* 2013; 70:436–43

26. Van den Bergh, BR, Van Calster, B, Smits, T, et al. Antenatal maternal anxiety is related to HPA-axis dysregulation and self-reported depressive symptoms in adolescence: a prospective study on the fetal origins of depressed mood. *Neuropsychopharmacology* 2008; 33:536–45

27. Ward, HB, Fromson, JA, Cooper, JJ, et al. Recommendations for the use of ECT in pregnancy: literature review and proposed clinical protocol. *Arch Womens Ment Health* 2018; 21:715–22

28. Wisner, KL, Bogen, DL, Sit, D, et al. Does fetal exposure to SSRIs or maternal depression impact infant growth? *Am J Psychiatry* 2013; 170:485–93

29. Yonkers, KA, Norwitz, ER, Smith, MV, et al. Depression and serotonin reuptake inhibitor treatment as risk factors for preterm birth. *Epidemiology* 2012; 23:677–85

Case 21: The menopause blues

The Question: How do you treat depression and vasomotor symptoms in menopause?

The Psychopharmacological Dilemma: Medications vs. supplements in the treatment of vasomotor and mood symptoms in perimenopause

Nevena Radonjić and Jaclyn Blaauboer

Pretest self-assessment question

What medication(s) has the most evidence in the treatment of both perimenopausal depression and vasomotor symptoms (VMS)?
A. Selective serotonin reuptake inhibitors (SSRIs)
B. Serotonin–norepinephrine reuptake inhibitors (SNRIs)
C. Gabapentin (Neurontin)
D. Clonidine (Catapres)
E. All of the above

Patient evaluation on intake

- A 52-year-old woman presenting for initial psychiatric evaluation with the chief complaint of not tolerating venlafaxine ER (Effexor XR)
- In the past year she has been struggling with depression, anxiety, weight gain, and impaired sleep, and hot flashes are significantly affecting her life quality

Psychiatric history

- History of major depressive disorder (MDD) with peripartum onset at age 26
- Reports that at that time she was treated by her obstetrician and had multiple antidepressant trials
- Reports that she later went for supportive counseling when she was going through a divorce, but only for a few sessions
- Since this, reports that she has been doing reasonably well until last year when her primary care clinician (PCC) started the SNRI venlafaxine ER (Effexor XR), to treat her low mood and increasing VMS
- Never required inpatient hospitalization, denies any history of suicidal ideation or self-injurious behavior (SIB)

Social and personal history

- College graduate, married, has a 26-year-old daughter
- Has owned an advertising firm for the past 20 years

- Reports that COVID-19 pandemic impacted her business, contributing to her high level of anxiety
- Currently living with her husband with whom she gets along well
- Her daughter helps with her business and is a great source of support

Medical history

- Hyperlipidemia (HLD)
- Breast cancer survivor

Family history

- Denies any significant psychiatric history in family members

Medication history

- Developed rashes from SSRIs such as sertraline (Zoloft), paroxetine (Paxil), and fluoxetine (Prozac), hence the trials were brief and subtherapeutic
- Reports that she also tried bupropion XL (Wellbutrin XL), a norepinephrine–dopamine reuptake inhibitor (NDRI), but developed a rash as well
- A brief tricyclic (TCA) amitriptyline (Elavil) trial was stopped due to constipation

Current medications

- Venlafaxine ER (Effexor XR) 37.5 mg/d, an SNRI
- Diphenhydramine (Benadryl) 25 mg/d, an antihistamine used for sleep
- Magnesium 500 mg/d over the counter (OTC)

Attending physician's mental notes: initial psychiatric evaluation

- The patient reports that she has been struggling in the past year with more MDD and generalized anxiety disorder (GAD)
- Reports that she gained 15 lb and finds weight gain very bothersome
  - Shared that weight gain is impacting self-image and self-confidence
- Reports further that in the past 2 years she has been getting very little sleep, as every 2 hours she is being awakened by VMS
- Noted increase in the level of anxiety due to impaired sleep and being irritable

- Stated that at times she has difficulty recognizing herself and that due to irritability she can be very unpleasant in daily interactions
- Shared not being interested in hormone replacement therapy (HRT) for the treatment of VMS as she is apprehensive about possible long-term hormonal adverse effects
- Reports that her PCC started her on venlafaxine ER (Effexor XR) 37.5 mg/d and that she wants to get off the medication as she attributes weight gain to it
- Stated that she often misses taking the medication in the morning as she has to take it with food and has no appetite, hence experiencing uncomfortable SNRI withdrawal symptoms
- Additionally, reports sexual dysfunction in the past year that she also attributes to venlafaxine ER (Effexor XR)
- Denies any suicidal ideations and is hopeful that she can go back to being her old self

Question

Is there anything else that you would like to know about the patient?

When was her last period?

- Reports that she used a progestin-based intrauterine device (IUD) for the past 10 years, which resulted in irregular and sporadic periods, hence unsure of the length and regularity of periods over the last decade
- Reports that the last time she had spotting was 2 years ago
- Stated that approximately at the same she started gaining weight, having hot flashes, and struggling with impaired sleep
- Finds hot flashes to be intolerable and barely getting a few hours of uninterrupted sleep

How do we determine whether the patient is in perimenopause or menopause?

- Large cohort studies such as The Study of Women Across the Nation (SWAN), Melbourne Women's Mental Health Study, and Penn Ovarian Aging Study demonstrated that menopausal transition lasts a median of 4 years, with the median age of onset at 47, progression to late menopausal transition at a median age of 49, and final menstrual period at age 51–2
- The assessment of perimenopause is a clinical assessment, based on the changes in the menstrual cycle and the appearance of other symptoms
- In perimenopause, menses start to vary in frequency, length, and amount of flow

- Early perimenopause is characterized by the persistent difference of 7 days or more in the length of consecutive cycles or skipped cycles
- Late phase of perimenopause is characterized by amenorrhea that lasts longer than 60 days
- A woman is considered to be in menopause 1 year after her final menstrual period
- Hormone testing is not necessary as the levels of estradiol, progesterone, luteinizing hormone (LH), and follicle-stimulating hormone (FSH) fluctuate even during the same day, hence obtaining their level may not be truly helpful
- This patient has been using IUD for the past 10 years which affected her regular cycle and she is not able to provide a detailed history regarding the frequency and length of her period
- Appears that the last observed spotting was over 2 years ago when she also started experiencing VMS and she is currently likely in menopause

What about her sexual function?

- Reports being sexually active but sexual drive almost completely diminished in the past year
- Complained of vaginal dryness and inability to achieve orgasm, which is very frustrating
- Reports that her weight gain is affecting her sexuality and that she is feeling uncomfortable with her body

What about lab work?

- The review of complete blood count (CBC), comprehensive metabolic panel (CMP), and thyroid panel was unremarkable

Attending physician's mental notes: initial psychiatric evaluation (continued)

- This patient has a history of postpartum depression and appears to have worsening of mood and anxiety symptoms that started in menopause
- Both postpartum period and menopause are characterized by fluctuations in the level of estrogen and appear to be contributing to her observed mood symptoms
- Many of the symptoms present in menopause, such as low mood, weight gain, impaired sleep, decreased sexual drive, and impaired concentration/memory are present as well in MDD
- Self-rating scales – the Patient Health Questionnaire (PHQ-9) and Generalized Anxiety Disorder Questionnaire (GAD7) – have been administered, and she scored 17 and 11 respectively, where both are elevated

- She is meeting the criteria for MDD, recurrent, moderate, and GAD
- She is already on low-dose SNRI which is a reasonable choice for treatment of both MDD and VMS, although on a very low dose and is intermittently compliant
- Given the low dose and sporadic intake, appears that she is only getting side effects of the medication and not seeing much benefit

Question

What is recommended dose of venlafaxine ER in the treatment of VMS?

- For patients with VMS without MDD, low doses of venlafaxine ER (Effexor XR) ranging from 37.5 mg/d to 75 mg/d are appropriate

- For patients who have VMS and meet the criteria for MDD, the dose of venlafaxine ER (Effexor XR) should be titrated according to the clinical presentation through the full MDD dosing range, 75–225 mg/d

Does she meet the criteria for hypoactive sexual desire disorder (HSDD)?

- HSDD is characterized by the presence of any of the below-listed symptoms for at least 6 months that results in personal distress, and is also not due to other psychiatric disorders or other medical conditions or medications
  - A lack of sexual motivation
  - Reduced or absent spontaneous desire to erotic cues and stimulation or inability to maintain desire or interest throughout sexual activity
  - Loss of desire to initiate or participate in sexual activity, including behavioral responses such as avoidance of situations that could lead to sexual activity, not secondary to a sexual pain disorder
- Patient is reporting almost completely absent sexual desire for over a year, which appears to correlate with the onset of menopause more than with her SNRI use
- Menopause is characterized by a decline in the levels of both estrogen and testosterone, which affect sexual functioning
- This patient has a decrease in sexual desire/motivation but is also currently in menopause and the clinician needs to differentiate whether HSDD is a primary disorder or a consequence of other conditions – in this case, menopause

What would you do next?

- Provide education on SNRIs and their potential benefit in the treatment of VMS and MDD and emphasize the need to take medication daily at the same time to prevent withdrawal symptoms
- Increase the dose of venlafaxine ER (Effexor XR) as the patient has been on a subtherapeutic dose for several months
- Taper off venlafaxine ER (Effexor XR) as she does not want to be on the medication any longer, and start alternative medication known for VMS effectiveness

Case outcome: interim follow-ups through 2 weeks

- The patient was adamant that she does not want to take venlafaxine ER (Effexor XR) due to withdrawal symptoms and sexual dysfunction
- She agreed to a very gentle taper, venlafaxine 25 mg/d for 5 days, then 12.5 mg/d for 5 days, then to be stopped
- Discussed the possibility of starting clonidine (Catapres) 0.1 mg/d to target VMS and she was agreeable to trying it
- Reports that she completed the venlafaxine taper 5 days ago and is still struggling with withdrawal symptoms such as "brain zaps" that she finds very uncomfortable
- Reports that she took clonidine (Catapres) 0.1 mg for a few nights only and stopped taking it as she did not see a clear benefit
- Reports that hot flashes and insomnia are again intolerable and asking for help with these
- Stated that all along she has been working with an integrative medicine specialist and that she is taking seven different supplements for various medical problems

Attending physician's mental notes: interim follow-ups through 2 weeks

- The patient again stopped taking the medication – clonidine (Catapres) – after an inadequate trial, even after in-depth psychoeducation on the medication, its dosing, and effects
- Additionally, appears that the patient feels more comfortable not taking the prescription medications and prefers taking supplements
- She agreed to bring into the office all supplements she is taking for the physician to review their active ingredients
- She agreed to start gabapentin (Neurontin), a calcium channel blocking antiepileptic, for treatment of VMS

PATIENT FILE

Question

Are natural supplements effective in the treatment of VMS?

- Although approximately 75% of women experience menopausal symptoms, many of them are reluctant to use HRT or other medications during the perimenopausal transition
- Majority of women using supplements do not disclose it to their mental health clinicians and clinicians often do not ask about it, most likely due to limited experience with alternative medical practices
- Black cohosh, soy products, and red clover are among the botanicals most often used for the relief of VMS
  - Black cohosh:
    - The exact mechanism is still not clearly understood
    - Based on available studies, it is postulated that it has a serotonergic effect
    - Effective in the treatment of VMS and depression with an overall positive safety profile for up to 6 months
    - The usual recommended dose is 40 mg/d
  - Phytoestrogen extracts:
    - Soy/isoflavones:
      - Proposed estrogenic mechanism of action
      - Minimal impact on menopausal symptoms, but there is a potential benefit for the cardiovascular system, bones, and cognition
      - Asian diet usually contains 40–80 mg/d of isoflavones, and women in these countries have fewer menopausal complaints
    - Red clover:
      - Contains isoflavonoid and coumestan that are proposed to mediate pro-estrogenic effects
      - The usual daily dose is 80 mg/d
- Behavioral modifications such as wearing loose clothes, sipping cold drinks, avoiding spicy food, and keeping a lower room temperature are often the first recommended step
- Currently, there is no evidence supporting the benefit of exercise or yoga on VMS

Case outcome: interim follow-ups through 6 months

- Although the patient agreed to a gabapentin (Neurontin) trial, she canceled subsequent appointments as she opted to continue with therapy and integrative medicine, but no prescription medications
- She continued with individual therapy, mostly on an as-needed basis
- Her VMS and mood symptoms persisted and she was not willing to take any psychiatric medications

Case debrief

- This patient had a history of MDD with peripartum onset and has again developed depressive symptoms when she entered perimenopause/menopause
- She tried several psychiatric medications in her lifetime that she would stop after only a brief low-dose trial due to perceived adverse effects
- Appears that being on a psychotropic medication was ego-dystonic to this patient and she was unwilling to continue medication trials
- She tried low-dose SNRI venlafaxine ER (Effexor XR) the longest, but due to her inability to tolerate withdrawal symptoms asked to see a psychiatrist to be tapered off the medication
- She was only willing to try the lowest possible dose of clonidine (Catapres) and gabapentin (Neurontin) and stopped both after a brief trial even after psychoeducation on both was provided
- She expressed a preference to be treated with "natural" supplements instead and stopped coming for psychiatric appointments
- She still continued seeing a therapist intermittently, mostly when in crisis and feeling overwhelmed

Take-home points

- Estrogen has an important role in the central nervous system and its fluctuations can impact mood
- Patients in perinatal and perimenopausal periods are at higher risk of depression due to pronounced variability in estrogen fluctuations or low estrogen states
- Some evidence suggests that, as the level of estrogen decreases, so does the density of 5-HT$_{2A}$ receptors and the activity of serotonin lowers
- There is symptom overlap between perimenopause and MDD symptoms
- Some perimenopausal symptoms, such as hot flashes and impaired sleep, can further worsen mood and increase anxiety
- Psychopharmacologists should be aware of hormonal fluctuations in their patients and screen regularly for mood symptoms
- Collaboration between PCC, gynecologist, and psychiatrist is needed for adequate care to be provided
- Patients with VMS only are candidates for HRT, usually in the first year of menopause
- Patients presenting with VMS and mood symptoms are candidates for SSRI/SNRI off-label treatment
- Many patients are not interested in medications and are more comfortable taking supplements and making behavioral modifications

Performance in practice: confessions of a psychopharmacologist

What could have been done better here?

- Some patients are reluctant to take psychotropic medications and feel more comfortable exploring behavioral modifications and supplements for treatment of VMS and mood symptoms
- Here, the patient was taking multiple supplements that the clinician did not address at the initial appointment
- This conversation early on could have potentially resulted in the strengthening of therapeutic alliance and the opportunity to work together long term
- Additionally, the patient complained of sexual dysfunction that could have been prioritized in the treatment plan

What are possible action items for improvement in practice?

- Clinicians should have a good understanding of physiological changes related to perimenopause/menopause, and available treatment options
- Review the latest evidence on alternative treatments of VMS

Tips and pearls

- Sexual function is often affected during the perimenopausal transition and can adversely affect mood, self-esteem, quality of life, and relationship with the partner
- It is important for the provider to discuss sexual dysfunction with their patients and address three main stages of sexual response – desire, arousal, and orgasm
- Sexual function is affected by numerous factors, such as psychological, social, and medical history, that should be included in the evaluation
- Physicians often feel uncomfortable addressing sexual dysfunction due to different barriers such as lack of research, knowledge, education, and treatment of sexual dysfunction in females
- Dopamine has a positive influence on all stages of sexual response, while serotonin has an adverse effect on sexual function, typically
- Given that many psychotropic medications can impact either dopamine or serotonin signaling, it is important for a physician to address possible adverse effects of medications on sexual function before starting them
- Patients experiencing sexual side effects from psychotropics are less likely to continue the treatment, and timely psychoeducation can be helpful in addressing and managing these sexual adverse effects

Mechanism of action moment: the neurobiology of VMS

- VMS are defined as an excessive heat dissipation response that occurs in about 75% of perimenopausal and postmenopausal women
- During VMS, patients can experience widespread cutaneous vasodilatation followed by profuse body sweating resulting in the sensation of heat, sweating, flushing, chills, clamminess, and anxiety
- Increased body mass index and cigarette smoking are major risk factors for menopausal VMS
- Besides a decrease in the level of estrogen, there is also increased sympathetic activation via α_2-adrenergic receptors that contribute to the initiation of hot flashes
- It is postulated that these changes narrow the thermoneutral zone in symptomatic women and, as a result, even small elevations in the core body temperature trigger full VMS
- Estrogen replacement is the most effective treatment of VMS, reducing them by 75% within the first year
- However, many women are not willing to take estrogen for VMS and many prescribers are not willing to treat long term with HRT due to concerns about adverse effects such as the increased risk for breast cancer
- SNRI antidepressants such as venlafaxine ER (Effexor XR) and desvenlafaxine (Pristiq) may be beneficial in the treatment of VMS
- Paroxetine, an SSRI, with a dose of 7.5 mg/d, is the only FDA-approved antidepressant for the treatment of VMS, and it is believed that it is helpful due to its weak theoretical noradrenergic activity
- Other SSRIs have shown inconsistent results in the treatment of VMS
- Clonidine (Catapres), an α_2 receptor agonist, might be useful in the treatment of VMS via its central α-adrenergic dampening activity, with the usual daily dose 0.1 mg/d
- Gabapentin (Neurontin) at the dose of 900 mg/d is also used off-label for the treatment of VMS, and some patients benefited from higher doses up to 2700 mg/d

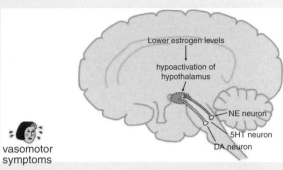

Figure 21.1 The neurobiology of vasomotor symptoms (VMS). In perimenopause, estrogen levels irregularly fluctuate, presumably leading to monoaminergic dysregulation of the hypothalamic thermoregulatory centers that clinically manifests as VMS. Estrogen replacement is the most effective treatment for VMS, but many women are unwilling to take HRT due to concerns of long-term adverse effects. SSRIs and SNRIs are available non-hormonal treatment options. Low-dose SSRI paroxetine (Brisdelle), 7.5 mg/d, is the only non-hormonal FDA-approved medication for the treatment of VMS, possibly due to its weak SNRI properties. Other SSRIs have shown inconsistent results in the treatment of VMS. SNRIs such as venlafaxine ER (Effexor XR) are considered beneficial in the treatment of VMS. Blue: DA (dopaminergic neurons); yellow: 5-HT (serotonergic neurons); purple: NE (noradrenergic neurons).

Two-minute tutorial

The role of estrogen in the brain

- Besides its role in reproductive function, estrogen has a complex effect on the brain
- Estrogen affects neurodevelopment, mood, behavior, and memory, and plays a role in neurodegenerative processes
- Estrogen exerts its effect via estrogen receptors (ERs) that are widely distributed in the brain
- Currently, three different classes of ERs are recognized (Table 21.1): nuclear receptors, ERβ, and membrane receptor coupled ER1 (GPER1)
- ERβ has been postulated as the main mediator of the antidepressant effects of estrogen

Table 21.1 Distribution of estrogen receptors in the brain

Nuclear receptors

ERα	ERβ	Membrane receptor
• Allocortex	• Allocortex	• Allocortex
• Amygdala	• Hippocampus	• Isocortex
• Bed nucleus of stria terminalis	• Amygdala	• Hippocampus
• Hypothalamus	• Bed nucleus of stria terminalis	• Hypothalamus
• Periaqueductal gray	• Raphe nuclei	• Anterior tegmental nucleus
• Preoptic area	• Substantia nigra	• Cerebellum
• Locus coeruleus	• Globus pallidus	• Locus coeruleus
	• Ventral tegmental area	• Preoptic area

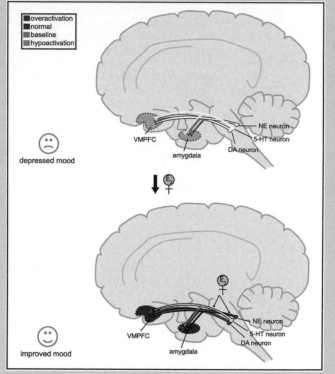

Figure 21.2 Estrogen as a trimonoamine modulator for depression. Unlike classic antidepressants that require several weeks to exert their therapeutic effects through several mechanisms, including desensitization of serotonin 5-HT$_{1A}$ receptors and α_2 adrenoreceptors, estrogens desensitize monoaminergic receptors within hours. Estrogen can presumably boost the actions of one or more monoamines (dopamine, norepinephrine, and serotonin) and is considered to be a trimonoamine modulator. Therefore, a decrease in estrogen levels observed in perimenopause can lower monoamine levels and its activity and increase the risk for the onset of depression.

Menopause and depression

- As previously stated, menopause, due to intense hormonal fluctuations, represents a period of increased vulnerability for the onset of depression
- Women with a history of depression are at the highest risk of exacerbation of disease during the perimenopausal transition
- Additionally, hormonal changes (lower estrogen) during menopause increase the risk of new onset of depression among women with no previous history
- There is symptom overlap between MDD and perimenopause as depicted below, as low energy, poor concentration, insomnia, weight gain, and decreased libido are present in both

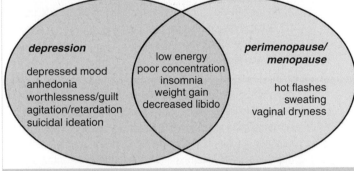

Figure 21.3 The symptom overlap between VMS of perimenopause/menopause and depression.

Menopause and bipolar disorder (BP)

- Women with BP are at high risk of worsening of mood during reproductive events
- Almost 60% of women with a history of BP report worsening of mood during menopause
- Women who experienced their first depressive, hypomanic, or manic episode at an earlier age were more likely to experience mood changes during reproductive events
- There is an association between earlier onset of the first episode of MDD and menopause-related mood symptoms
- The majority of women who have menopause-related mood symptoms and had given birth also experience more postnatal mood episodes
- Furthermore, the onset of bipolar I disorder (BP1) seems to have a bimodal distribution, with the first peak in the late teens to early 20s, and the second peak in the mid-40s to mid-50s

- This timeline suggests a possible association between reproductive events, such as estrogen loss, and the onset of BP
- There have been limited studies on the first onset of BP during the perimenopausal period
- Factors associated with increased risk of conversion from MDD to BP during the menopausal transition include alcohol use disorder (AUD), substance use disorder (SUD), and a variety of anxiety disorders

Post-test question

What medication(s) has the most evidence in the treatment of both perimenopausal depression and vasomotor symptoms (VMS)?

A. Selective serotonin reuptake inhibitors (SSRIs)

B. Serotonin–norepinephrine reuptake inhibitors (SNRIs)

C. Gabapentin (Neurontin)

D. Clonidine (Catapres)

E. All of the above

Answer: B

Although SSRIs are effective (Paroxetine [Paxil] may have the best data) in the treatment of mood symptoms, medications with both serotonergic and noradrenergic activity, such as SNRIs, may be superior in the treatment of mood symptoms accompanied with VMS. Both clonidine (Catapres) and gabapentin (Neurontin) are effective in the treatment of VMS; however, they typically are not used for the treatment of MDD.

References

1. Avis, NE, Brambilla, D, McKinlay, SM, et al. A longitudinal analysis of the association between menopause and depression results from the Massachusetts Women's Health Study. *Ann Epidemiol* 1994; 4:214–20

2. Chen, LC, Yang, AC, Su, TP, et al. Symptomatic menopausal transition and subsequent bipolar disorder among midlife women with major depression: a nationwide longitudinal study. *Arch Womens Ment Health* 2017; 20:463–8

3. Cohen, LS, Soares, CN, Joffe, H. Diagnosis and management of mood disorders during the menopausal transition. *Am J Med* 2005; 118:93–7

4. Davis, SR, Jane, F. Menopause, sex and perimenopause. *Aust Fam Physician* 2011; 40:274–8

5. Freedman, RR. Hot flashes: behavioral treatments, mechanisms, and relation to sleep. *Am J Med* 2005; 118 Suppl, 12B:124–30

6. Geller, SE, Studee, L. Botanical and dietary supplements for menopausal symptoms: what works, what does not. *J Women's Health (Larchmt)* 2005;14:634–49

7. Kingsberg, SA. Hypoactive Sexual Desire Disorder: understanding the impact on midlife women. *Female Patient* 2011; 36:1–4

8. Kroon, JS, Wohlfarth, TD, Dieleman, J, et al. Incidence rates and risk factors of bipolar disorder in the general population: a population-based cohort study. *Bipolar Disord* 2013; 15:306–13

9. Lee, JH, Lee, JE, Harsh, V, et al. Pharmacotherapy for sexual dysfunction in women. *Curr Psychiatry Rep* 2022; 24:99–109

10. Marsh, WK, Templeton, A, Ketter, TA, et al. Increased frequency of depressive episodes during the menopausal transition in women with bipolar disorder: preliminary report. *J Psychiatr Res* 2008; 42:247–51

11. Pachman, DR, Jones, JM, Loprinzi, CL. Management of menopause-associated vasomotor symptoms: current treatment options, challenges and future directions. *Int J Womens Health* 2010; 2:123–35

12. Parish, SJ, Hahn, SR, Goldstein, SW, et al. The International Society for the Study of Women's Sexual Health process of care for the identification of sexual concerns and problems in women. *Mayo Clin Proc* 2019; 94:842–56

13. Perich, TA, Roberts, G, Frankland, A, et al. Clinical characteristics of women with reproductive cycle–associated bipolar disorder symptoms. *Aust N Z J Psychiatry* 2017; 51:161–7

14. Saito, K, Cui, H. Emerging roles of estrogen-related receptors in the brain: potential interactions with estrogen signaling. *Int J Mol Sci* 2018; 19:1091

15. Stahl, SM, Muntner, N. *Depression in Women: Treating Symptoms throughout the Life Span.* Cambridge: Cambridge University Press, 2021, 129–42

16. Stubbs, C, Mattingly, L, Crawford, SA, et al. Do SSRIs and SNRIs reduce the frequency and/or severity of hot flashes in menopausal women: HHS public access summary of the issues. *J Okla State Med Assoc* 2017; 110:272–4

Case 22: The lady who felt "funny" on the medication

The Question: How do you manage tremors in psychiatric practice?

The Psychopharmacological Dilemma: Risks vs. benefits of long-term lithium (Eskalith) use

Nevena Radonjić

Pretest self-assessment question

Lithium-induced tremors can occur with which of the following?
A. Initiation of medication
B. Long-term use of medication
C. Toxicity due to high levels of lithium
D. Concomitant use with antipsychotic
E. All of the above

Patient evaluation on intake

- A 60-year-old woman with a sudden change in mental status and behavior

Psychiatric history

- Diagnosed with bipolar I disorder (BP1) in her early 20s
  - Has been maintained on lithium (Eskalith) but had a few brief psychotic episodes that responded well to a short course of a low dose of typical antipsychotic haloperidol (Haldol) 2 mg/d
  - Last psychotic episode 10 years ago
  - History of several emergency room (ER) evaluations for psychosis
  - However, no history of psychiatric admissions
  - No history of suicidality
  - In supportive therapy for many years, well known to the clinic where she attends compliantly
- Sudden worsening was seen over the last 3 weeks
  - Per family, patient not acting herself and went to neighbor's house in the middle of the night without any apparent reason; later was found by ambulance wandering the streets
  - Daughter reports that she took the patient to two different ERs for acute change in behavior, but after the evaluations she was cleared and discharged home instead
  - Patient's symptoms seem to wax and wane and unfortunately was lucid when was evaluated in ER
  - Family worried whether the patient is taking her medications consistently as they had found a full pillbox from last month

- ○ Daughter tearfully states that she has not seen her mother "this bad" for many years
- ○ Last time she was this unwell was when she was drinking alcohol and not engaged in mental health treatment
- ○ Patient oppositely reports that she is doing well and is upset with her children for wanting to "lock her up"
- States that she is taking her psychotropic medication as prescribed currently

Social and personal history

- Graduated high school and has been working since in retail
- Divorced, has two children from the first marriage
- Currently in a stable relationship for the past 20 years
- In the past used alcohol, but sober for over 20 years

Medical history

- History of breast cancer, in remission
- Hypertension (HTN)
- Tension headaches
- Allergic rhinitis

Family history

- Maternal grandfather has a history of unspecified mood disorder and, later in life, dementia
- Mother now has dementia as well
- Father had active alcohol use disorder (AUD) for many years, later in life sustained sobriety
- Daughter has a history of AUD, currently in stable remission as well, for more than 1 year
- Her son has active opioid use disorder (OUD)

Medication history

- Stable for many years on lithium (Eskalith)
- Brief period of requiring a low dose of haloperidol (Haldol) 2 mg/d for psychotic symptoms

Current medications

- Lithium (Eskalith) 900 mg/d, a mood stabilizer, and last lithium level 0.9 mEq/L
- Multivitamin
- Levocetirizine (Xyzal) 5 mg/d

Psychotherapy history

- In supportive monthly psychotherapy

Attending physician's mental notes: initial psychiatric evaluation

- Presents on exam as pleasant, alert, and oriented to person, place, and time
- Patient was initially guarded, but as the interview progressed was more comfortable and stated that she did get into a motor vehicle accident and that she remembers going to the neighbor but not having the best recollection of events before or afterward
- She has disclosed that she has been having paranoia related to her sister's behavior, which she is aware is unusual, and has some reality testing intact
- Sleep has been impaired and endorsed difficulty falling asleep and sustaining sleep
- 3 weeks ago, she had foot surgery and she has been taking medications for pain control

Question

Based on what you know about this patient's history and current symptoms, would you consider delirium as a possible diagnosis?

- Yes, as her mental status appears to fluctuate and she recently had a medical procedure where she was started on pain medications
- No, as the patient in the past has had a history of psychotic episodes and her lithium pillbox is full

Attending physician's mental notes: initial psychiatric evaluation (continued)

- On exam, the patient presents with intact sensorium, able to engage in the interview and maintain focus
- There is no waxing/waning of consciousness
- The thought process during the interview was organized and coherent
- The onset of symptoms correlates with the time of her medical procedure
- Differentially, could be drug intoxication, delirium, psychosis due to medical reasons, or acute manic episode
- The patient is on a mood stabilizer that she previously did well on for many years but her family is unsure of current compliance
- She has irregular intentional postural tremors of the upper extremities

Further investigation

Is there anything else that you would like to know about the patient?

What new medications were recently started?

- The patient clarified that she had been taking oxycodone/acetaminophen (Percocet) 15 mg/d for the last 3 weeks since her procedure
- Pain levels have improved since and she does not require this medication any longer; hence stopped taking it a few days ago
- It appears that change in sensorium and behavior corresponds to the time of surgery and use of pain medications
- Based on the patient's presentation and recent history, need to rule out a medical cause of observed symptoms
- Ordered complete blood count (CBC), comprehensive metabolic panel, urine analysis, lithium level, thyroid-stimulating hormone (TSH), and free thyroxine (fT4)

What about her history of breast cancer?

- The patient had her last appointment with an oncologist 1 year ago; at that time, was in stable remission
- Given the history of breast cancer may need to order a brain MRI with contrast

What about tremors?

- Reports that tremors have been present for the past year, denies any recent worsening
- Finds it upsetting as it is noticeable by others and people at work comment on it
- Bothered that she needs to hold her coffee cup with two hands for added stability

Question

What would you do for the treatment of a new onset of paranoia?

- Nothing, would wait for lab work to come back, then decide
- Treat the symptoms as the patient is paranoid and required two ER evaluations, and family is extremely worried

Attending physician's mental notes: initial psychiatric evaluation (continued)

- Given that the work-up is being completed on an outpatient basis and will take a few days, decided to start a low dose of haloperidol (Haldol) 2 mg/d to treat her acute psychotic symptoms such as paranoid delusions

- In the past responded well to this medication
- This is a guideline-based reason for not starting with an atypical antipsychotic
- Patient agreed not to drive until her symptoms completely resolved and agreed to take haloperidol (Haldol) in addition to lithium (Eskalith)
- Although upset with her children, was agreeable to involving them in her treatment planning and care

Case outcome: first interim follow-up visit 7 days later

- Lab work showed leukocytosis and urinary tract infection (UTI)
- The patient was started on antibiotics by the primary provider
- Lithium level was in the therapeutic range, 0.9 mEq/L
- Some improvement in confusion and sleep but still having paranoia
- Says she has also been hearing voices
  - She was reluctant to disclose at the time of the first encounter
- Having a hard time focusing and has been forgetting things
- Did not go for a scheduled brain MRI

Attending physician's mental notes: first interim follow-up visit 7 days later

- It appears that the patient is doing better since being off opioids and UTI being treated, but symptoms of psychosis are still clearly persistent, although confusion resolved
- Although able to sleep longer, still having a hard time initiating sleep
- Lithium levels are in the therapeutic range; hence medication non-compliance is not a likely culprit for acute mental worsening
- Patient did not go for a brain MRI, unclear whether there are other possible organic causes of psychosis
- Other labs were normal

Question

Would you increase her current medications or change strategies?

- No, I would wait for the patient to complete the course of antibiotics and re-evaluate
- Yes, I would increase the dose of haloperidol (Haldol) as the patient reports that auditory hallucinations and paranoid delusions continue

Case outcome: second interim follow-up visit at 2 weeks

- Haloperidol (Haldol) was increased to 4 mg/d to treat the residual psychosis
- Patient reports significant improvement in delusions and hallucinations but states that she does not like how the haloperidol (Haldol) makes her feel
- Admits some ongoing paranoid ideation and that her focus is still impaired
- Still unable to work
- Children report that she is doing much better and they are not acutely concerned any longer

Attending physician's mental notes: interim follow-up visit (week 2)

- Appears that the patient has responded well to an increase in the dose of haloperidol (Haldol) but is adamant to change away from this medication
- The patient denies any adverse effects of haloperidol (Haldol) such as akathisia, dystonia, etc.
- No extrapyramidal symptoms (EPS) on physical exam, but intent tremors unchanged from the time of initial visit

Question

What would you do next?

- Provide psychoeducation on the medication with the hope that the patient will stay on the current regimen as it is working
- Stop the haloperidol (Haldol) and see whether patient's symptoms continue to respond
- Cross-titrate haloperidol (Haldol) with an atypical antipsychotic to see whether the patient will be able to tolerate better

Case outcome: interim follow-up visits through 1 month

- Haloperidol (Haldol) was cross-titrated with cariprazine (Vraylar) and the patient is currently on 3 mg/d
- Patient reports further improvement in sleep and resolution of all paranoia and auditory hallucinations
- She is still very bothered with her intent tremors and asking for this to be addressed

Attending physician's mental notes (month 1)

- Cariprazine (Vraylar) is a fairly novel atypical antipsychotic approved for the treatment of schizophrenia and bipolar disorder (BP) – mania and depressed phase
- Besides being a partial D_2/D_3 agonist, cariprazine (Vraylar) also has a high affinity for the serotonin 1_A (partial agonist) and 2_A (antagonist) receptors that has an antidepressant effect
- Cariprazine (Vraylar) has a uniquely potent affinity for dopamine-3 receptor (D_3) that may improve poor cognitive function and alertness that patient has been complaining of
- Although the patient has been on lithium for many years, appears that tremors started only a year ago
- The lithium level is in the therapeutic range – 0.9 mEq/L – and the dose could potentially be lowered, but at risk of a clinical BP relapse
- Tremors appear irregular, intent, rapid, symmetrical, postural, and limited to upper extremities

Further investigation

What else would you like to know when evaluating tremors?

- Current medications: tremors are common side effects of many medications (e.g., stimulants, antidepressants, epilepsy-based mood stabilizers)
  - She is on lithium (Eskalith) and cariprazine (Vraylar), but tremors were present before cariprazine (Vraylar) was started, with no worsening
- No history of familial or essential tremors
- Drinks one cup of coffee daily and 48 ounces of green tea
- Reports that tremors improve with alcohol use, but she rarely drinks given a history of AUD
- TSH performed was within normal limits
- MRI of the brain was ordered, but not completed yet

Question

What would be the most reasonable next step?

- Recommend decrease in caffeine intake and re-evaluate
- Reduce the dose of lithium (Eskalith) and see whether the tremors improve
- Reduce the dose of lithium (Eskalith) and use cariprazine (Vraylar) solely to treat all her symptoms and see whether the tremors improve
- Start propranolol (Inderal) for treatment of tremors
- Start primidone (Mysoline) for treatment of tremors
- Refer to neurology for the treatment of tremors

Case outcome: interim follow-up visits through 3 months

- All of the above may be reasonable options
- Patient was unwilling to reduce the current dose of lithium (Eskalith) given recent decompensation and that it had helped for many years
- Propranolol (Inderal) 40 mg/d was initiated
- Agreed to reduce caffeine intake by cutting out the green tea
- Significant improvement in tremors noted later, but stated that the effect of beta blocker (BB) propranolol (Inderal) wears off after 6–8 hours
- Furthermore, it is making her feel "funny" and she asked for a change in this medication

Attending physician's mental notes (month 3)

- On exam noted that tremors are much improved
- Denies feeling dizzy from propranolol (Inderal) but noted some tiredness and fatigue
- New onset of bradycardia noticed, so EKG will be ordered
- After discussion of bradycardia with the primary care clinician decided to taper off the propranolol and decrease the dose of lithium (Eskalith) to see whether it would help reduce tremors

Case outcome: interim follow-up visits through 6 months

- The patient tolerated a gradual decrease in the dose of lithium (Eskalith) from 900 mg/d to 750 mg/d (level 0.8 mEq/L) and then 600 mg/d (level 0.7 mEq/L) without immediate worsening of her BP1 disorder
- Tremors, although reduced, are still present and appear perhaps not solely related to her lithium level
- She is still quite bothered by tremors and again is asking for help with them
- Patient presents euthymic, sleeping well, able to work and function at baseline again

Question

Do lithium formulation and dosing affect tremors?

- Lithium is available for medical use in the form of lithium carbonate and lithium citrate
- Lithium carbonate is available as immediate-release or slow-release preparation
  - Eskalith is an immediate-release formulation but there is a multi-coated preparation called Eskalith CR which is slower release

- ○ Lithobid is lithium tightly packed in wax and other components to make it dissolve more slowly
- Lithium citrate is an immediate-release liquid version that is considered at times to cause less gastric distress
- Immediate-release lithium is rapidly absorbed and achieves peak serum concentration 1–2 hours after oral administration, while slow-release lithium formulations achieve peak after 4–5 hours
- Some lithium-related adverse effects are related to serum lithium peak time, where lower peaks may afford less tremor
- Slow-release lithium formulations can reduce the rate or degree of severity of lithium-related tremors, upper gastrointestinal cramping, nausea, rash, cognitive dulling, urinary frequency, and neuromuscular slowing as they tend to have lower peak plasma levels
- Occasionally slow-release formulations can increase lower gastrointestinal disturbances (diarrhea) though, compared to immediate-release formulations

Attending physician's mental notes (month 6)

- The patient is currently on the immediate-release formulation of lithium and possibly would benefit from a change to slow-release
- The patient feels comfortable with this
- Decided to stay with bedtime dosing to avoid daily peak plasma levels

Case outcome: interim and multiple follow-up visits through 12 months

- Patient was changed to lithium (Lithobid) 600 mg/d and there was no difference in lithium levels
- Unfortunately, no change in tremors with the transition to the slow-release lithium formulation occurred
- Tremors appear to be mostly independent of lithium level and still are bothersome for the patient
- She agreed to see a neurologist and went for the brain MRI
- Brain imaging showed mild cortical atrophy – unremarkable otherwise
- Prescribed primidone (Mysoline) by neurology, but never started taking it as she read possible adverse effects and did not feel comfortable with the medication
- Will try vitamin B6 1200 mg/d, which can have an effect on tremors
- BP1 remained well controlled with a combination of cariprazine (Vraylar) and a lower dose of lithium (Lithobid)
- Remains well at her baseline level of functioning

Case outcome: interim and multiple follow-up visits through 24 months

- Patient saw some improvement in tremors with vitamin B6 but was bothered by multiple dosing during the day hence stopped taking it
- She asked for lithium (Lithobid) to be discontinued due to possible impact on tremors and felt that her symptoms of BP1 were well controlled on the atypical antipsychotic monotherapy cariprazine (Vraylar)
- She tolerated well her taper from lithium (Lithobid), but again developed UTI that manifested with changes in sensorium and confusion which were quickly recognized and treated with antibiotics
- Patient expressed satisfaction with weight loss and decrease in urinary frequency once off lithium, but tremors still remained the same
- In the end, decided to try primidone (Mysoline) which significantly helped with tremors

Case debrief

- It appears that the patient's initial abrupt presentation with wandering and confusion was a delirious presentation most likely precipitated by UTI and pain medications
- Paranoid delusions and hallucinations persisted even after acute delirium resolved though, and she benefited from the addition of an antipsychotic, suggesting she was likely BP1 with psychosis behind the delirium as well
- In the past, intermittent use of antipsychotics has stabilized her bipolarity
- After resolution of psychosis, the patient was mainly focused on her tremors
- The atypical antipsychotic likely served as a mood stabilizer so that the dose of lithium (Lithobid) was able to be initially decreased and later discontinued without any acute worsening of mood symptoms; however, the patient only had partial improvement in tremors, implying that etiology of tremor is not solely related to lithium and likely essential or familial in nature and a stand-alone disease state
- She continued to follow up with neurology

Take-home points

- Tremors are involuntary, rhythmic, oscillatory movements produced by alternating or synchronous contractions of antagonistic muscles
- Tremor is a common side effect of many psychotropic medications
- The presence of tremors requires careful evaluation before changing treatment or adding medications

- Obtaining detailed history is the first step in the evaluation of intent tremors and it should include the assessment of caffeine intake, use of sympathomimetic agents, presence of alcohol or benzodiazepine withdrawal, history of familial or essential tremors, and other pertinent factors
- Intent tremors are one of the most common reasons why patients stop taking lithium (Lithobid)
- Lithium-induced tremors are generally rapid, symmetric, and indistinguishable from essential or intent physiologic tremors, most prominent with peripheral motor action, such as writing or holding a coffee cup
- Lithium-induced tremors usually present early during the treatment but can emerge later in treatment as well
- Lithium-induced tremors are usually independent of lithium formulation, but higher plasma levels correlate with a greater risk of tremor
- The presence of new, coarse intent tremors should warn physicians of possible lithium toxicity
- Other lithium toxicity signs may include weakness, ataxia, vomiting/ diarrhea, poor concentration, confusion, and lethargy

Performance in practice: confessions of a psychopharmacologist

What could have been done better here?

- Become more aware of side effects associated with older psychotropics before prescribing
  - ○ The patient responded well to an atypical antipsychotic and, eventually, lithium was discontinued without worsening of BP
  - ○ Monotherapy, in general, is the preferred treatment modality as the risk of possible adverse effects decreases
  - ○ Long-term lithium use can have adverse effects on thyroid and kidney functions
  - ○ Long-term antipsychotic use can cause movement disorder or metabolic syndromes

What are possible action items for improvement in practice?

- Psychiatrists should routinely screen for intent and resting tremors after initiating psychotropic medications
- Asking patients to draw a spiral is a useful way to detect and follow tremor severity
- As for treating EPS, clinicians should familiarize themselves with the treatment of intent tremors

Tips and pearls: lithium side effects and management strategies

- When patients present with lithium-induced side effects, watchful waiting is the first-line strategy unless overt toxicity is apparent
- If side effects are still present and bothersome, consider lowering the dose of lithium at the risk of BP relapse
- Some side effects are related to the time of medication administration due to increase in peak levels
- Some side effects are more common with immediate-release formulations (Figure 22.1) and, in clinical practice, slow-release formulations seem to be more used as a way to lower side-effect burden

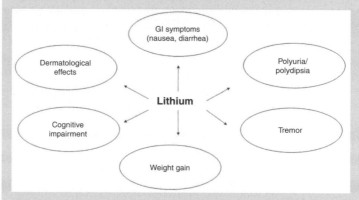

Figure 22.1 Most common side effects of lithium use. Some side effects such as nausea and tremors occur early in the treatment while some can occur later, such as weight gain or organ damage.

Table 22.1 Comparison of pharmacokinetic properties of different lithium formulations

Formulation	Lithium carbonate	Lithium carbonate slow-release	Lithium carbonate packed tightly in wax	Lithium citrate
Brand name	Eskalith	Eskalith CR	Lithobid	-
Dosage form	Capsules	Capsules	Tablets	Liquid
Dosage strength	150 mg, 300 mg, 600 mg	450 mg	300 mg	8 mEq (600 mg)/ 5 mL
Peak serum time	0.5–2 hours	4–12 hours	2–6 hours	15–60 min

Mechanism of action moment

What happens when D₃s are antagonized (Figure 22.2)?

- Dopamine has five receptor subtypes in two different groups – D$_1$/ D$_5$ and D$_2$–D$_4$
- D$_3$s can be localized pre- and postsynaptically
- D$_3$s are present in the ventral tegmental area (VTA) but not usually in the prefrontal cortex (PFC)
- Although many medications may bind to D$_3$s, only two – cariprazine (Vraylar) and blonanserin (Lonasen) – have binding affinity for the D$_3$ that is multiple orders of magnitude higher, compared to dopamine itself, thus allowing them to compete successfully at the binding site
- The blockade of postsynaptic D$_2$ and D$_3$ in limbic regions may contribute to antipsychotic actions of cariprazine (Vraylar)
- Modulation of presynaptic action of D$_3$ via cariprazine's antagonism / partial agonism in the VTA disinhibits the dopamine neurons projecting to the PFC via the mesocortical dopamine pathway, resulting in more dopamine release on D$_1$ receptors
- Increased activity of D$_1$ receptors in the cortex may improve symptoms of depression and negative symptoms of schizophrenia

Mesocortical dopamine pathway

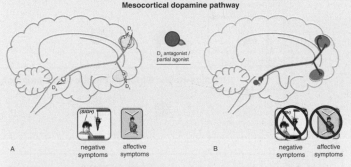

Figure 22.2 Dopamine 3 antagonism / partial agonism in the VTA. (A) Presynaptic D$_3$s detect dopamine and inhibit further dopamine release. These receptors are present in the VTA but not in the PFC. There are, however, postsynaptic D$_1$ receptors in the PFC, which are stimulated by dopamine. Shown here is the mesocortical dopamine pathway, with stimulation of D$_0$s resulting in reduced dopamine release in the PFC. Low levels of dopamine in the PFC are hypothesized to contribute to depressed mood, reduced motivation, and cognitive symptoms, all of which occur in mood disorders, as well as to create negative symptoms in schizophrenia. (B) Antagonism / partial agonism of D$_3$s in the VTA can increase dopamine release in the PFC. Because there are no D$_3$s in the PFC, D$_3$ antagonists / partial agonists have no effect there. Dopamine is free to stimulate D$_1$ receptors, hypothetically improving symptoms of depression.

- Patients with mood disorders and schizophrenia may experience affective "brightening," as well as improvements in energy and motivation

Two-minute tutorial

Treatment of BP

- Many patients with BP1 require combination treatments consisting of atypical antipsychotics and mood stabilizers (Figure 22.3)
- They sometimes additionally take hypnotics, anxiolytics, and antidepressants
- The combination with the most evidence for mania is to use an atypical antipsychotic combined with lithium (Eskalith) or valproate (Depakote)
- Combining with lamotrigine (Lamictal) has been studied less but is often used in practice for the treatment of BP

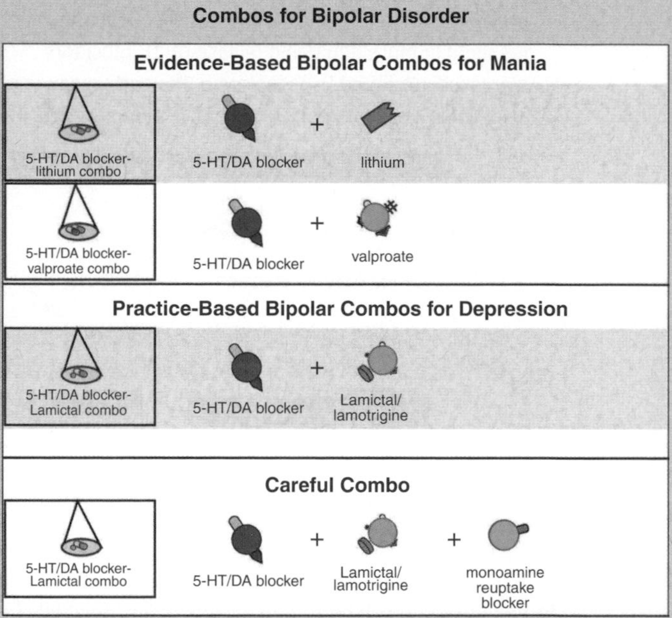

Combos for Bipolar Disorder

Evidence-Based Bipolar Combos for Mania

5-HT/DA blocker-lithium combo

5-HT/DA blocker + lithium

5-HT/DA blocker-valproate combo

5-HT/DA blocker + valproate

Practice-Based Bipolar Combos for Depression

5-HT/DA blocker-Lamictal combo

5-HT/DA blocker + Lamictal/lamotrigine

Careful Combo

5-HT/DA blocker-Lamictal combo

5-HT/DA blocker + Lamictal/lamotrigine + monoamine reuptake blocker

Figure 22.3 Most frequent medication combinations used in the treatment of BP

PATIENT FILE

Post-test question

Lithium-induced tremors can occur with which of the following?
A. Initiation of medication
B. Long-term use of medication
C. Toxicity due to high levels of lithium
D. Concomitant use with antipsychotic
E. All of the above

Answer: E

As discussed previously, lithium-induced tremors most frequently occur early in treatment but can emerge later in treatment as well. Coarse tremors should caution clinician to perform blood work and check lithium levels as worsening tremors could be an initial sign of lithium toxicity. In addition, patients treated with antipsychotics (D_2 blockers) can present with complex tremors from multiple etiologies as antipsychotic use can lead to resting tremors.

References

1. Girardi, P, Brugnoli, R, Manfredi, G, et al. Lithium in bipolar disorder: optimizing therapy using prolonged-release formulations. *Drugs in R and D* 2016; 16:293–302
2. Gitlin, M. Lithium side effects and toxicity: prevalence and management strategies. *Int J Bipolar Disord* 2016; 4:27
3. Goldberg, J, Ernst, C. *Managing the Side Effects of Psychotropic Medications*, 1st edn. Arlington, VA: American Psychiatric Association, 2012
4. Gong, R, Wang, P, Dworkin, L. What we need to know about the effect of lithium on the kidney. *Am J Physiol – Renal Physiol* 2016; 311:F1168–F1171
5. Mago, R, Borra, D, Mahajan, R. Role of adverse effects in medication nonadherence in bipolar disorder. *Harv Rev Psychiatry* 2014; 22:363–6
6. Stahl, SM. Treatments for mood disorders: so-called "antidepressants" and "mood stabilizers. In *Stahl's Essential Psychopharmacology: Neuroscientific Basis and Practical Applications*, 5. Cambridge: Cambridge University Press, 2021, 283–358
7. Volkmann, C, Bschor, T, Köhler, S. Lithium treatment over the lifespan in bipolar disorders. *Front Psychiatry* 2020; 11:377
8. Wilber, ST, Ondrejka, JE. Altered mental status and delirium. *Emerg Med Clin North Am* 2016; 34:649–65

Case 23: Two ladies with bruises

The Question: Is the risk of bleeding with SSRIs clinically significant?

The Psychopharmacological Dilemma: What to do when patients develop bruising from the medication?

Nevena Radonjić

Pretest self-assessment question

Selective serotonin reuptake inhibitors (SSRIs) mainly affect the platelets by which of the following?
A. Decreasing their number (thrombocytopenia)
B. Affecting their adhesive functioning
C. Both A and B

Patient evaluation on intake

- Patient #1
  - A 30-year-old woman planning a pregnancy with a chief complaint of "I have bruises"
- Patient #2
  - A 48-year-old woman with a chief complaint "I am covered with bruises"

Psychiatric history

- Patient #1 has a long history of major depressive disorder (MDD), and has been stable on an SSRI, citalopram (Celexa) 40 mg/d, for many years
- Patient #2 has re-exacerbation of MDD and a history of chronic pain and has recently been started on a serotonin–norepinephrine reuptake inhibitor (SNRI), duloxetine (Cymbalta) 30 mg/d
- Both patients present with sudden onset of bruising without major trauma
- Patient #1 reports that she has recently been taking over-the-counter non-steroidal anti-inflammatory drugs (NSAIDs) for painful menstrual periods
- Patient #2 reports, besides bruising, having mouth sores and taking the NSAID ibuprofen (Advil) 800 mg/d, on as-needed basis for many years for chronic pain
- On physical exam both patients have bruises on the abdomen and lower extremities even from the smallest pressure

Question

What would you do next?

- Hold the SSRI/SNRI and perform a complete blood count (CBC), comprehensive metabolic panel (CMP), and prothrombin time / international normalized ratio (PT/INR)
- No medication change, suggest bruising is not serious, and provide psychoeducation on the potential impact of SSRI/SNRI on platelets and advise avoiding NSAIDs
- Stop the SSRI/SNRI and NSAIDs given adverse effects and consider alternative treatment options

Attending physician's mental notes

- Both patients are doing well on serotonin-enhancing antidepressants
- The serotonin reuptake-inhibiting antidepressants carry warnings about bruising and bleeding side-effect phenomenon
- They are taking NSAIDs which also can create issues with bleeding
- May need to change either the antidepressants or the NSAIDs

Case outcome

- Patient #1 has no medical comorbidities and has developed superficial bruising with concomitant use of SSRI and NSAIDs
  - Obtained blood work showed normal platelet count, normal PT/INR and intact liver function
  - After psychoeducation, patient decided to stay on the citalopram (Celexa) as she has been on the medication for a long time without major adverse effects and finds it very effective for the management of her MDD symptoms
- She was interested to know whether changing from one SSRI to another would make a difference related to bruising
- Also raised concern related to the risk of postpartum hemorrhage given that she is planning pregnancy
  - Patient was advised to discuss painful and excessive periods with her primary care clinican and identify alternative ways to address symptoms given recent bruising
  - Cautious use of NSAIDs was recommended
- Patient #2, besides MDD, has a long history of chronic pain, diabetes mellitus type 2 (DM2), and hypothyroidism, and is not on any anticoagulation therapy
- She developed bruises and mouth sores shortly after initiation of an SNRI, duloxetine (Cymbalta)

- In coordination with her primary care clinician ordered CBC, PT/INR, CMP, antinuclear antibodies (ANA), and erythrocyte sedimentation rate (ESR)
  - Obtained blood work was only positive for ANA and elevated ESR
  - Was further referred to rheumatology for possible Behcet's syndrome
    - Behcet's syndrome is a rare disorder causing blood vessel inflammation in the body and can manifest with various signs and symptoms including mouth sores, eye inflammation, skin rashes, and lesions and genital sores
- Decided to stop duloxetine (Cymbalta) given these adverse effects and although in the past she tolerated the SSRI escitalopram (Lexapro), without any adverse effects, she did not find it beneficial for MDD symptoms
- She continued with supportive psychotherapy only and found a sense of relief as she felt validated with the possible autoimmune diagnosis, given years of nonspecific symptoms and chronic pain

Case debrief

- Both patients developed bruises while on serotonin-enhancing SSRI/SNRI, and had used NSAIDs on as-needed basis
- Blood work was useful to rule out potential thrombocytopenia or liver failure, but was not necessarily the most sensitive indicator of their platelet dysfunction
- While patient #1 experienced adverse effects due to the concomitant use of SSRIs with NSAIDs, appears that patient #2, in addition, also had an underlying medical condition that contributed to the observed excessive bruising
- Both patients were followed carefully in the coming weeks and did not have any further complications or hemorrhage
- These cases highlight the need for clinicians to discuss with patients, at the time of initiation of serotonergic antidepressants, the potential adverse effects on platelet function and the caution needed with the concomitant use of NSAIDs

Take-home points

- Aberrant serotonergic neurotransmission plays a role in the etiology of MDD
- Serotonin also has an important role in hemostasis and blood clotting
- Antidepressants can impact normal platelet functioning allowing increased bruising while treating MDD

- The risk for adverse effects is higher when antidepressants are taken with other medications affecting hemostasis/coagulation or in patients at risk (patients with a history of thrombocytopenia, platelet dysfunction or coagulopathies, acute intracerebral hemorrhage, or on several antiplatelet medications)
- For patients who have experienced adverse effects from medications with high or intermediate levels of serotonin reuptake inhibition (SRI), clinicians might consider medications with low SRI properties, such as mirtazapine (Remeron), bupropion XL (Wellbutrin XL), or trazodone (Desyrel)
- Clinicians should consider previous medical history when prescribing antidepressants, and in patients with higher risk consider medications with lower inhibition of serotonin reuptake

Performance in practice: confessions of a psychopharmacologist

What could have been done better here?

- Was adequate education on the risks of using NSAIDs provided to the patient?
- Improve informed consent practices

What are possible action items for improvement in practice?

- Be aware of the different pharmacodynamic properties of antidepressants and how they may interact physiologically outside the realm of treating just mental and emotional symptoms, by being more aware of potential physical side effects

Tips and pearls

- Psychotropic medications target specific molecular sites that affect neurotransmission
- Classic antidepressants block one or more of the transporters for serotonin, norepinephrine, and/or dopamine, called SERT, NET, and DAT, respectively
- Many antidepressants (SSRIs, SNRIs, serotonin partial agonist / reuptake inhibitors [SPARIs], tricyclic antidepressants [TCAs]) to a certain degree inhibit presynaptic SERTs which is also called SRI
- SERT removes serotonin from the synapse, recycles it into the presynaptic neuron and terminates its signaling
- SERT belongs to sodium/chloride coupled transporters, called the solute carrier SLC6 gene family
- The SLC6 gene family also includes transporters for norepinephrine (NET), dopamine (DAT), γ-aminobutyric acid (GABA [GAT1–4]), and glycine (GlyT1 and GlyT2)

- If a medication binds to an inhibitory allosteric site on SERT it will reduce the affinity of the SERT for its substrate serotonin and prevent serotonin binding
- Besides its localization in the central nervous system, SERT is also present in the periphery on cells in the enteric nervous system, platelets, mast cells, and syncytiotrophoblast cells of the placenta

Two-minute tutorial

The role of serotonin in hemostasis

- Serotonin plays an important role in platelet function and the formation of blood clots
- Platelets maintain low plasma levels of serotonin by sequestering and storing serotonin within the granules within themselves
- When aggregation of platelets starts, serotonin is released into the blood and activates 5-HT$_{2A}$ receptors on the platelet membrane, promoting the change of platelet shape from discoid to spheroid and further enhancing the process of aggregation and clotting
- SSRIs inhibit the SERT on platelets responsible for the uptake of serotonin and down-regulate 5-HT$_{2A}$ receptors
- As a result, intraplatelet levels of serotonin in patients on SSRI are decreased and/or depleted, and the process of platelet aggregation might be affected as they do not have enough serotonin to promote their aggregation or sticking to other platelets
- The best method to evaluate hemorrhagic events in individuals taking SSRIs is still to be determined as there is no readily available test a clinician can order
- However, a platelet aggregation test could be ordered but is still not widely available

Does it matter which antidepressant?

- Antidepressants differ in the degree of inhibition of SRI properties at the SERT sites (Table 23.1) and can be classified as
  - High serotonin reuptake inhibitors
  - Intermediate serotonin reuptake inhibitors
  - Low serotonin reuptake inhibitors
  - Non-serotonin reuptake inhibitors
- Antidepressants with high and intermediate inhibition of serotonin reuptake are associated with an increased risk of hospitalization for abnormal bleeding
- Although the data is limited, antidepressants with low serotonin reuptake inhibition may be associated with a lower risk of bleeding and should be considered in patients at risk

Table 23.1 Different degrees of serotonin reuptake inhibition with different antidepressants

Degree of Inhibition of Serotonin Reuptake

High	Intermediate	Low/None
Paroxetine (SSRI)	Vilazodone (SPARI)	Mirtazapine (NaSSA)
Clomipramine (TCA)	Imipramine (TCA)	Bupropion (NDRI)
Sertraline (SSRI)	Citalopram (SSRI)	Doxepin (TCA)
Duloxetine (SNRI)	Fluvoxamine (SSRI)	Nortriptyline (TCA)
Fluoxetine (SSRI)	Amitriptyline (TCA)	Desipramine (TCA)
Escitalopram (SSRI)	Vortioxetine (SPARI)	Nefazodone (SARI)
	Venlafaxine (SNRI)	Trazodone (SARI)
		Levomilnacipran (SNRI)

NaSSA – norepinephrine antagonist / selective serotonin antagonist; NDRI – norepinephrine dopamine reuptake inhibitor; SARI – serotonin antagonist / reuptake inhibitor; SNRI – serotonin–norepinephrine reuptake inhibitor; SPARI – serotonin partial agonist / reuptake inhibitor; SSRI – selective serotonin reuptake inhibitor; TCA – tricyclic antidepressants

When is caution needed? Who is at risk?

- Patients on SSRIs have an increased risk for upper gastrointestinal (GI) bleeds
  - This risk is even higher when patients are on both SSRIs and NSAIDs
  - Combined use of aspirin with SSRIs increased upper GI risk 12.2 times, while with NSAIDs the risk was only increased 5.2 times
  - Although SSRIs increase the risk of upper GI bleeding, the absolute risk of a serious bleeding event is very small, with a number needed to harm (NNH) in a low-risk population being 3,177, and in a high-risk population, 881
    - NNH suggests here that out of 3,177 patients treated, one will have a serious bleeding event, for example
  - This risk might be decreased with concomitant use of standard acid-suppressing drugs
- Antidepressants may increase the risk of postpartum hemorrhage
  - The risk is small and related to more proximal exposure to delivery
- Antidepressants with high serotonin reuptake inhibition increase the risk for spontaneous intracranial hemorrhage, particularly in the first 30 days of use with concomitant use of oral anticoagulants
- Antidepressants and anticoagulants
  - No association with increased risk of bleed in patients with atrial fibrillation and anticoagulant therapy with either warfarin or rivaroxaban has been noted
  - No difference in risk for serious bleeding in patients on SSRI and low-molecular-weight heparin (LMWH) treated for venous thromboembolism compared to patients only on LMWH

Post-test question

Selective serotonin reuptake inhibitors (SSRIs) mainly affect the platelets by which of the following?

A. Decreasing their number (thrombocytopenia)

B. Affecting their adhesive functioning

C. Both A and B

Answer: B

Although there are rare reported cases of thrombocytopenia with SSRIs, in general SSRIs affect hemostasis by impacting platelet function, and not their number.

References

1. Andrade, C. Selective serotonin reuptake inhibitor use in pregnancy and risk of postpartum hemorrhage. *J Clin Psychiatry* 2022; 83(2):22f14455

2. Anglin, R, Yuan, Y, Moayyedi, P, et al. Risk of upper gastrointestinal bleeding with selective serotonin reuptake inhibitors with or without concurrent nonsteroidal anti-inflammatory use: a systematic review and meta-analysis. *Am J Gastroenterol* 2014; 109: 811–19

3. Brazell, C, McClue, SJ, Preston, GC, et al. 5-Hydroxytryptamine (5-HT)-induced shape change in human platelets determined by computerized data acquisition: correlation with [125I]-iodoLSD binding at 5-HT2 receptors. *Blood Coagul Fibrinolysis* 1991; 2:17–24

4. Dalton, SO, Johansen, C, Mellemkjaer, L, et al. Use of selective serotonin reuptake inhibitors and risk of upper gastrointestinal tract bleeding: a population-based cohort study. *Arch Intern Med* 2003; 163:59–64

5. Halperin, D, Reber, G. Influence of antidepressants on hemostasis. *Dialogues Clin Neurosci* 2007; 9:47–59

6. Jiang, HY, Chen, HZ, Hu, XJ, et al. Use of selective serotonin reuptake inhibitors and risk of upper gastrointestinal bleeding: a systematic review and meta-analysis. *Clin Gastroenterol Hepatol* 2015; 13:42–50.e43

7. Maclean, JA, Schoenwaelder, SM. Serotonin in platelets. In Pilowsky, M, ed., *Serotonin: The Mediator that Spans Evolution*. Boston: Academic Press, 2019, 91–119

8. McCloskey, DJ, Postolache, TT, Vittone, BJ, et al. Selective serotonin reuptake inhibitors: measurement of effect on platelet function. *Transl Res* 2008; 151:168–72

9. Meijer, WEE, Heerdink, ER, Nolen, WA, et al. Association of risk of abnormal bleeding with degree of serotonin reuptake inhibition by antidepressants. *Arch Intern Med* 2004; 164:2367–70

10. Nochaiwong, S, Ruengorn, C, Awiphan, R, et al. Use of serotonin reuptake inhibitor antidepressants and the risk of bleeding complications in patients on anticoagulant or antiplatelet agents: a systematic review and meta-analysis. *Ann Med* 2022; 54:80–97

11. Perahia, DG, Bangs, ME, Zhang, Q, et al. The risk of bleeding with duloxetine treatment in patients who use nonsteroidal anti-inflammatory drugs (NSAIDs): analysis of placebo-controlled trials and post-marketing adverse event reports. *Drug Healthc Patient Saf* 2013; 5:211–19

12. Quinn, GR, Hellkamp, AS, Hankey, GJ, et al. Selective serotonin reuptake inhibitors and bleeding risk in anticoagulated patients with atrial fibrillation: an analysis from the ROCKET AF Trial. *J Am Heart Assoc* 2018; 7:e008755

13. Renoux, C, Vahey, S, Dell'Aniello, S, et al. Association of selective serotonin reuptake inhibitors with the risk for spontaneous intracranial hemorrhage. *JAMA Neurology* 2017; 74:173–80

14. Rudnick, G. *SERT, Serotonin Transporter.* New York: Elsevier, 2007

15. Samuel, NG, Seifert, CF. Risk of bleeding in patients on full-dose enoxaparin with venous thromboembolism and selective serotonin reuptake inhibitors. *Ann Pharmacother* 2017; 51:226–31

16. Song, HR, Jung, Y-E, Wang, H-R, et al. Platelet count alterations associated with escitalopram, venlafaxine and bupropion in depressive patients. *Psychiatry Clin Neurosci* 2012; 66:457–9

Case 24: The lady who was afraid for her kids

The Question: Finding effective treatment for obsessive–compulsive disorder (OCD) in the perinatal period

The Psychopharmacological Dilemma: Differentiating between perinatal OCD and postpartum psychosis

Nevena Radonjić

Pretest self-assessment question

What are the available non-pharmacological treatment options for OCD?

A. Exposure and response prevention (ERP) cognitive behavioral therapy (CBT)
B. Deep transcranial magnetic stimulation (dTMS)
C. Deep brain stimulation (DBS)
D. A and B
E. All of the above

Patient evaluation on intake

- A 26-year-old woman with a history of generalized anxiety disorder (GAD), post-traumatic stress disorder (PTSD), and Attention-Deficit/ Hyperactivity Disorder (ADHD), presenting 3 months postpartum and reporting a higher level of anxiety compared to usual
- In the past 10 weeks has new intrusive thoughts that something bad will happen to her children, which recently have become even more intense over time and harder to dismiss
- Reports that these thoughts are deeply disturbing and affecting her functioning as she is afraid to leave kids unattended now

Psychiatric history

- In mental health care since age 13 when her anxiety became unmanageable and was diagnosed with GAD due to multifocal, uncontrollable worrying
- Reports that at that time she was started on a selective serotonin reuptake inhibitor (SSRI), fluoxetine (Prozac), which was stopped after a brief trial as she started to experience suicidal ideation
- Looking back, she thinks that suicidal ideation was most likely related to her anxiety and not necessarily in connection with the use of the SSRI, nor its side effect
- At that time, she required evaluation in the emergency room (ER), but was discharged home as she was deemed safe

- Described her relationship with food and weight as "complicated" and reports periods of restricting food intake due to body image issues, followed by periods of purging
- As a child was diagnosed with ADHD, inattentive type, but never had a trial of the stimulant as her mother was against it
- Since, she has been intermittently seen by mental health providers, mostly in times of crisis and usually for a few sessions at a time
- Denies any history of suicide attempts or inpatient psychiatric admissions

Social and personal history

- Married, mother of three children, oldest 10 years old, middle child 3 years old, and youngest one 3 months old
- Left school at the age of 18 due to pregnancy, and plans in the future to take her general educational development (GED) test
- Current husband is gainfully employed and supportive
- Patient does not work
- Reports history of intimate partner violence (IPV) prior to this marriage

Medical history

- Negative for a history of head trauma or seizures
- No current medical issues

Family history

- Father has a history of unspecified anxiety disorder
- Older brother has GAD and major depressive disorder (MDD)
- To the best of her knowledge no deaths by suicide in the family history

Medication history

- One short SSRI trial with fluoxetine (Prozac) 10 mg/d, efficacy not established due to discontinuation of medication

Current medications

- Prenatal vitamins
- Vitamin D
- Norethindrone (Camila) 0.35 mg/d

Psychotherapy history

- Intermittently attending supportive therapy in the clinic

Patient evaluation on initial visit

- Reports onset of intrusive anxiety symptoms 1 week after giving birth to her third child
- Denies similar symptoms after previous two pregnancies
- Endorsed high level of anxiety in the past 10 weeks, overall with racing thoughts, and fearing that something bad will happen to her kids
- Reports that, although she knows that these concerns are not reality-based, does not allow anybody else to take care of kids and does not leave them unattended
- Denies any thoughts of self-harm or harm to kids
- Characterizes her thoughts as disturbing and is distressed and seeking help

Question

What does the presence of intrusive thoughts mean clinically?

- Nothing, as intrusive thoughts are normal phenomena experienced by a majority of the general population on an occasional basis, easy to dismiss, and not associated with any further action
- Increases in frequency, intensity, and duration of intrusive thoughts in the postpartum period are associated with the increased risk of postpartum OCD or could be part of a ruminative depressed state

Attending physician's mental notes: initial psychiatric evaluation

- The patient is complex given her premorbid history of well-defined GAD, ADHD, and possibly an eating disorder
- The worsening of anxiety and intrusive thoughts clearly correlate with the time of delivery and are new symptoms for her presently
- The perinatal period is a risk factor for the onset or exacerbation of OCD and postpartum women are 1.5–2.5 times more likely to suffer from OCD vs. the general population
- The prevalence of postpartum OCD is still an area of active research and it is reported to range from 2.7% to 9%
- Perinatal OCD is often present with other psychiatric conditions and this is the case with this patient
- She is currently not on any psychotropic medication
- The priority here is to differentiate between MDD ruminations vs. OCD vs. postpartum psychosis and assess for safety

Question

Is there anything else that you would like to know about the patient?

What about her reproductive history?

- This is her third child from four pregnancies
  - Reports history of one miscarriage
- This was a planned pregnancy, and per the patient, this is to be her last pregnancy
- She is currently using progestin-based contraceptive, norethindrone (Camila), as birth control
- She is breastfeeding and plans to continue so until the baby is 1 year old
- Reports anxiety always being present but never experienced episode like this one before

Perinatal OCD vs. perinatal psychosis?

- Although she is having difficulty falling asleep, once asleep she is able to get around 4 hours of rest
  - Reports that she is able to sleep longer, but gets up to nurse the baby
- On exam she is negative for grandiosity or increase in the goal-directed activity, does not present pressured or talkative, has a cohesive thought process, intact sensorium, no risky behaviors, and no family history of bipolar disorder (BP)
- Denies depressed mood or anhedonia and does not meet criteria for MDD
- Although intrusive thoughts are very disturbing, presents with intact reality testing and is aware that there is no real threat to her children
- Based on obtained history, does not meet criteria for psychosis or BP or MDD, and most likely presents with perinatal OCD as her worry seems to be focused singly on harm befalling her kids rather than an exacerbation of diffuse worrying from her pre-existing GAD

What about a history of trauma?

- Reports that she had a traumatic relationship as a young adult
- Endorsed presence of intrusion reliving symptoms, persistent avoidance, negative alterations in cognition and mood, such as the constant feeling of fear and lack of trust toward others, and marked increases in emotional arousal and reactivity
- Scored 65 out of 80 on PTSD CheckList for DSM-5 (PCL5) and was positive in all diagnostic domains for PTSD
- Reports having a good relationship with her husband and denies any current IPV

What about a possible eating disorder?

- Reports that she has a complex relationship with eating and weight
- Shared having periods of binging followed by purging, either via vomiting or by using a laxative
- Reports that she feels conflicted related to purging as she is breastfeeding
- Current weight is within normal range, but she perceives herself as overweight
- Meets criteria for bulimia nervosa (BN), purging type now

Attending physician's mental notes: initial psychiatric evaluation (continued)

- Although able to take care of her kids, the patient is presenting in distress and suffering due to intrusive thoughts and fears that something bad will happen to her children
- Diagnostically, she appears to meet the criteria for OCD as these thoughts seem not to be driven by MDD, PTSD, or any psychotic process
- She additionally has several comorbidities such as GAD, PTSD, ADHD, and BN that are further complicating her presentation
- Most recent blood work demonstrated lower vitamin D levels, otherwise results unremarkable

Question

What would you do next?

- Initiate SSRI to target GAD, OCD, PTSD, and BN symptoms
- Initiate low-dose atypical antipsychotics such as quetiapine (Seroquel) to promote sleep, and decrease anxiety and intrusive thoughts
- Initiate benzodiazepine (BZ) sedatives in addition to an SSRI to reduce acute anxiety/distress and promote sleep more quickly
- Reach out to the family to obtain more information
- Refer to therapy for support and possibly CBT

Case outcome: interim follow-ups through 2 weeks

- After an in-depth discussion on potential treatment options, the patient agreed to start an SSRI, escitalopram (Lexapro) 10 mg/d, and tolerated without major adverse effects
- She declined any medication that could promote major weight gain such as quetiapine (Seroquel) or mirtazapine (Remeron)

- Additionally, given that she is breastfeeding during nighttime, declined any medication with sedating properties such as the BZ agents
- Escitalopram (Lexapro) is considered compatible with breastfeeding
  - It is secreted into breast milk but in a relatively low amount
  - Its relative infant dose (RID), indicating the extent of drug exposure to the infant while breastfeeding, is 3–6% at most
  - Medications with RID < 10% are considered likely safe for the infant
- Reports that the intensity of intrusive thoughts decreased mildly and that she is feeling 10–20% better overall
- Shared feeling ashamed of her obsessive thoughts and is reluctant to involve her family
- Agreed to start individual therapy

Attending physician's mental notes: interim follow-ups through 2 weeks

- The patient is tolerating SSRI well and is reporting a slight decrease in symptoms
  - Escitalopram (Lexapro) is off-label regarding its use in OCD, PTSD, and BN but is approved for GAD
  - Other SSRIs are approved in these areas and often there is cross-effectiveness when SSRIs are used in comorbid patients
- She is still struggling with intrusive thoughts and is somewhat isolated at home
- She is still the main care provider to her children
- Given her presenting symptoms, it is possible that she will need higher doses of SSRI as the majority of patients with OCD will require moderate to high doses of the medication and a longer duration of treatment
- Hopefully will see a reduction in a wide variety of her symptoms with the SRI approach

Question

What would you do next?

- Encourage the patient to keep therapy appointments and provide psychoeducation and support
- Continue with the current dose of escitalopram (Lexapro) as the medication was recently started
- Given that the majority of patients will need a higher dose for OCD, increase dosing further for the escitalopram (Lexapro)

Case outcome: interim follow-ups through 1 month

- Patient opted to stay with the same low dose of escitalopram (Lexapro) and has started individual therapy
- She reported a further reduction in the intensity and frequency of intrusive thoughts over time
- Noted that her other anxieties significantly decreased as well
- Reports that she is still struggling with inattention and is constantly fidgeting
- Furthermore, very bothered with her physique and that she is again binge eating

Attending physician's mental notes: interim follow-ups through 1 month

- Appears that the patient is responding better than expected to low-dose SSRI and reports now 50% symptom response after 4 weeks
- Noted improvement in functioning and now allowing her parents to take her child to school
- Given her history of ADHD and BN, the patient might benefit from the initiation of lisdexamfetamine (Vyvanse) to target both
  - Lisdexamfetamine (Vyvanse) is approved for ADHD and binge eating disorder (BED)
  - Ideally, BN is phenotypically close to BED in presentation and this stimulant will help

Question

Any concerns related to the use of stimulants while breastfeeding?

- The data on methylphenidate (Ritalin) and amphetamine (Adderall) use during breastfeeding is limited
- RID for lisdexamfetamine (Vyvanse) and methylphenidate (Ritalin) is 1.8–6.2% and 0.2–0.4% respectively
- Given a lower transfer to breast milk and no adverse effects on infants reported, methylphenidate is the preferred stimulant to be used during lactation

What other medication(s) could be useful in the treatment of ADHD and BN?

- Bupropion XL (Wellbutrin XL) is often clinically used off-label for the treatment of ADHD and BN
- It increases synaptic concentrations of the same norepinephrine and dopamine neurotransmitters afforded by the stimulants
- Given that this patient has both, this could be a possible treatment option

- Additionally, a serotonin–norepinephrine reuptake inhibitor (SNRI) might be valuable as the SRI components might treat PTSD, GAD, OCD, BN, and the NRI component of the ADHD

What would you do next?

- Recommend starting d-methylphenidate ER (Focalin XR) in addition to SSRI
- Recommend starting bupropion XL (Wellbutrin XL) in addition to SSRI
- Further increase current SSRI, escitalopram (Lexapro)
- Switch from the current SSRI to an SNRI such as duloxetine (Cymbalta)

Case outcome: interim follow-ups through 2 months

- Patient agreed to increase the dose of SSRI escitalopram (Lexapro) to 15 mg/d, but declined any other treatment options for ADHD and BN
- Reports with further reduction in OCD symptoms and intrusive thoughts, she is becoming more aware of her mood and endorsed feeling quite depressed
- Wonders if SSRI is causing MDD and asks for dose reduction
- Reports that she finds relief from the thoughts that her children will be harmed and has started leaving them with her husband

Attending physician's mental notes: interim follow-ups through 2 months

- The patient responded well in the anxiety domain but is now feeling more depressed
- Denies any worsening in sleep or suicidal ideation, states that she is able to find joy in her children, appetite fluctuates, and is struggling with self-image
- Agreed to decrease in the dose of SSRI back to 10 mg/d as she previously did well on it and feels that high dose is hurting her

Case outcome: interim follow-ups through 6 months

- Although the dose was decreased, the patient missed several follow-up appointments and eventually dropped out of care
- Appears that, similar to previous treatment trials, she only stayed in care while in a more acute crisis
- She was able to benefit from provided support and SSRI, and had a decrease in the intensity of intrusive thoughts

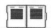

Case debrief

- This patient has a history of ADHD, GAD, PTSD, and BN and presented with a new onset of perinatal OCD
- She responded well to initiation of SSRI and experienced a reduction in intrusive obsessive thoughts that were ego-dystonic to her
- She experienced, however, a worsening of mood and stopped coming to further appointments
- She also stopped attending therapy and was reluctant to try more focused CBT due to required time commitment
- Although she was initially quite distressed with intrusive thoughts, the children's safety was not at risk and she was still able to take care of them as she was not psychotic
- She had untreated ADHD, PTSD, and BN that she was not interested in addressing

Take-home points

- The perinatal (antenatal and postnatal) period represents a period of vulnerability for exacerbation of existing perinatal mood and anxiety disorders (PMADs) or onset of new PMADs
- Several screening scales are easily accessible and validated for OCD detection
  - Obsessive Compulsive Inventory – Revised (OCI-R)
  - Perinatal Obsessive Compulsive Scale (POCS)
  - Yale–Brown Obsessive Compulsive Scale (Y-BOCS)
- Safety is a priority and it is important for clinicians to be able to differentiate between perinatal OCD and postpartum psychosis, which is more dangerous
- Patients with OCD have intact reality testing; intrusive thoughts are ego-dystonic and associated with guilt and shame and rituals are aimed at decreasing distress
- Postpartum OCD is generally associated with a low risk of harm to the infant and is most often treated on an outpatient basis
- In contrast, patients with postpartum psychosis have impaired reality testing and thoughts are ego-syntonic, increasing the risk for unpredictable aggressive and lethal behavior
- Postpartum psychosis has a rapid onset, usually in the first 2–4 weeks after delivery
- Postpartum psychosis represents a psychiatric emergency and almost always requires psychiatric hospitalization and the involvement of social services

Performance in practice: confessions of a psychopharmacologist

What could have been done better here?

- Given history of medication and visit non-compliance post crisis management, interpret this earlier as a focus of psychotherapy to prevent attrition

What are possible action items for improvement in practice?

- Review post-partum-onset psychiatric conditions to improve diagnosis and to better provide front-line strategies in these situations

Tips and pearls

- Increase in anxiety is common in new parents and is considered a normal part of the adjustment to new life roles and circumstances
- However, at times, anxious thoughts can become very intense and distressing and manifest as obsessions – unwanted thoughts, images, urges, and doubts or compulsions – rituals, or checking behaviors, and should not be diagnosed as an adjustment disorder
- Providing psychoeducation to the patient and family is an important part of the treatment plan and there is a need for reassurance as mothers with perinatal OCD tend not to act on their thoughts
- Some patients prefer non-psychopharmacological treatment options and some would benefit from the combination of both medications and psychotherapy
- Psychotherapy using ERP techniques as part of a well-defined CBT approach has shown good effectiveness here
- Approximately 40–60% of OCD patients will have a satisfactory response to SSRI

Neuroanatomy moment

Focus on impulsivity and compulsivity

- Patients can often present with impulsive–compulsive disorders
- In this case, the patient has impulsive disorders such as ADHD and BN, and a compulsive disorder, such as OCD
- The common feature of both impulsivity and compulsivity is the failure to control responses
  - Impulsivity is the inability to stop initiating actions
  - Compulsivity is the inability to terminate ongoing actions

- ○ Impulsivity is mediated by a neuronal circuit loop with projections from the ventral striatum to the thalamus, thalamus to the ventromedial prefrontal cortex (VMPFC) and anterior cingulate cortex (ACC), and from the VMPFC/ACC back to the ventral striatum
  - ▪ This circuit is usually mediated top-down by prefrontal cortex (PFC) glutamatergic neuronal activity, and if this is lacking, impulsivity can occur
  - ▪ Compulsivity is mediated by a loop that projects from the dorsal striatum to the thalamus, the thalamus to the orbitofrontal cortex (OFC), and from the OFC back to the dorsal striatum
  - ▪ If the top-down regulation from OFC fails, compulsivity can then manifest
  - ▪ When it comes to treatment options, exposure therapy may lead to the reversal of abnormal neurocircuitry firing as the improvement in symptoms lasts even after the therapy has been stopped while serotonergic medications suppress abnormal circuitry while the drug is being taken

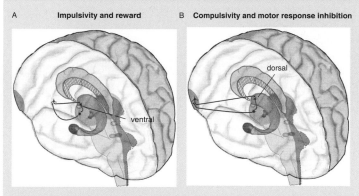

A   **Impulsivity and reward**   B   **Compulsivity and motor response inhibition**

dorsal

ventral

Figure 24.1 The circuitry of impulsivity and reward (A) and compulsivity and reward (B).

Two-minute tutorial

The neurobiology of OCD

- OCD is a multifactorial condition presenting with a clinically heterogeneous phenotype
- Although presenting symptoms can differ, the commonality is the presence of obsessive thoughts and/or compulsive behaviors that impact functioning or cause distress

- Both polygenetic and environmental risk factors play a role in the development of OCD
- Genetic factors increase the vulnerability for OCD while environmental factors such as perinatal events, stress, trauma, and neuroinflammation can trigger the onset of OCD and affect glutamatergic, serotonergic, and dopaminergic neurotransmission
- Neuroimaging studies implicated the cortico-striatal-thalamo-cortical circuit (CSTC) in generating the pathophysiology of the disorder, as noted above
- The CSTC circuit controls movement execution, habit formation, and reward, while the hyperactivity of this circuit manifests with the typical clinical presentation for OCD
- Individuals with OCD also have hyperactivity of the OFC, a brain region involved in reward-guided learning and decision-making, resulting in the inability to control compulsions

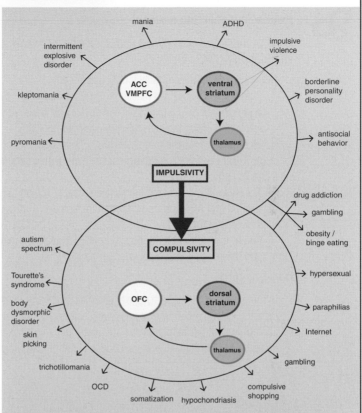

Figure 24.2 Impulsive–compulsive disorder construct. Impulsivity and compulsivity are seen in a wide variety of psychiatric disorders. Impulsivity can be thought of as the inability to stop the initiation of actions and involves a brain circuit centered on the ventral striatum and linked to the thalamus, to the VMPFC, and to the ACC. Compulsivity can be thought of as the inability to terminate ongoing actions and hypothetically involves a brain circuit centered on the dorsal striatum and linked to the thalamus and OFC. Clinicians can use approved DBS and dTMS to introduce electrical currents in order to allow these neural circuits to diminish activity and operate more appropriately, thus lowering OCD symptoms.

Mechanism of action moment

Deep brain stimulation (DBS) and deep transcranial magnetic stimulation (dTMS) for OCD

- DBS is approved for compassionate use in OCD
  - Bilateral electrodes are placed surgically through the skull and powered by a pacemaker-like device and battery that is implanted under the skin near the shoulder/axillae
  - Electricity leaves the battery through the lead wires and into the terminal electrodes and disrupts the hyperactive circuits of OCD
- dTMS is approved for OCD
  - This magnetic treatment increases electrical activity targeting the VMPFC and ACC and does not require surgery, but requires daily sessions at the office
  - Again, this approach improves circuitry activity, normalizing it and lowering OCD symptoms

Perinatal OCD

- In the perinatal period, OCD can present as a new onset of this disorder or exacerbation of a previously existing condition
- The etiology of perinatal onset is still under active research, but the importance of biological and psychosocial factors is recognized

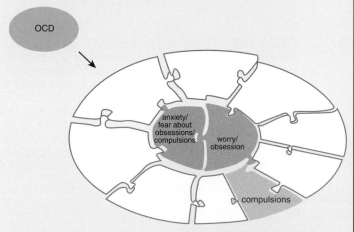

Figure 24.3 OCD. The symptoms typically associated with OCD are shown here and include obsessions that are intrusive and unwanted and that cause marked anxiety or distress, as well as compulsions that are aimed at preventing or suppressing the distress related to the obsessive thoughts. Compulsions can be repetitive behaviors (e.g., handwashing, checking) or mental acts (e.g., praying, counting).

- The DSM-5 diagnostic criteria for OCD are the same as the criteria for perinatal OCD, and currently in the DSM-5 for OCD diagnosis, there is no specifier for "with peripartum onset" like there is for MDD
- Risk factors for perinatal OCDs include
  - Primiparity
  - Close temporal proximity to delivery, usually within the first 4 weeks
  - History of psychiatric comorbidities
  - Family history of mood disorders and substance use disorders
- Typical clinical presentation includes the presence of obsessions and/or compulsions that are time-consuming and affect functioning and family life and that cannot be better explained by another medical, substance-use, or psychiatric condition
- OCD obsessions in the perinatal period often manifest with aggressive thoughts and images of harming the child and contamination obsessions, with neutralizing behaviors such as compulsive cleaning and handwashing
- The specific studies on the course and prognosis of perinatal OCD are so far limited
- OCD often leads to MDD as the new mother develops low self-esteem and feels she is a bad or unsafe parent

Treatment of (perinatal) OCD

- The treatment of perinatal OCD is similar to that in general OCD treatment guidelines and is comprised of pharmacological and non-pharmacological options
- Non-pharmacological options include:
  - CBT with exposure and response prevention (ERP) approaches
  - dTMS
  - DBS
  - Anterior cingulotomy
  - Psychodynamic psychotherapy
  - Meditation-based interventions
- Pharmacological options:
  - SSRIs are the first-line treatment option, and, often, higher doses of SSRIs will be needed with a longer treatment duration for the successful treatment of OCD compared to doses needed in the treatment of MDD or GAD, social anxiety disorder, or panic disorder (PD)
    - Escitalopram – 60 mg/d, not FDA-approved
    - Citalopram – max 40 mg/d due to risk of QTc prolongation with higher doses

- Fluoxetine – 80 mg/d FDA-approved, but up to 120 mg/d used
- Fluvoxamine – 300 mg/d FDA-approved, but up to 450 mg/d used
- Paroxetine – 60 mg/d FDA-approved, but up to 100 mg/d used
- Sertraline – 200 mg/d FDA-approved, but up to 400 mg/d used
  - Second-line treatments include the tricyclic antidepressant (TCA) clomipramine (Anafranil) (dose up to 250 mg/d is approved), SNRIs or the sedating antidepressant mirtazapine (Remeron)
  - For patients who have failed several SSRIs, augmentation with an atypical antipsychotic could be a reasonable pharmacological option

Post-test question

What are the available non-pharmacological treatment options for OCD?

A. Exposure and response prevention (ERP) cognitive behavioral therapy (CBT)
B. Deep transcranial magnetic stimulation (dTMS)
C. Deep brain stimulation (DBS)
D. A and B
E. All of the above

Correct answer: E

Several non-pharmacological treatment options have shown efficacy in the treatment of OCD, with the most evidence available for ERP CBT. Repetitive dTMS is also an effective treatment option for OCD, but largely for patients who responded to SSRI or only failed one SSRI trial, hence it could be best to implement it earlier in the treatment plan. DBS is approved for compassionate use in OCD for those who have failed many treatments and are deemed treatment refractory.

References

1. Abramovitch, A, Abramowitz, JS, Mittelman, A. The neuropsychology of adult obsessive–compulsive disorder: a meta-analysis. *Clin Psychol Rev* 2013; 33:1163–71
2. Abudy, A, Juven-Wetzler, A, Zohar, J. Pharmacological management of treatment-resistant obsessive–compulsive disorder. *CNS Drugs* 2011; 25:585–96

3. Barrett, R, Wroe, AL, Challacombe, FL. Context is everything: an investigation of responsibility beliefs and interpretations and the relationship with obsessive–compulsive symptomatology across the perinatal period. *Behav Cogn Psychother* 2016; 44:318–30

4. Beucke, JC, Sepulcre, J, Talukdar, T, et al. Abnormally high degree connectivity of the orbitofrontal cortex in obsessive–compulsive disorder. *JAMA Psychiatry* 2013; 70:619–29

5. Fairbrother, N, Albert, A, Keeney, C, et al. Screening for perinatal OCD: a comparison of the DOCS and the EPDS. *Assessment* 2021; 10731911211063223

6. Harmelech, T, Roth, Y, Tendler, A. Deep TMS H7 coil: features, applications & future. *Expert Rev Med Devices* 2021; 18:1133–44

7. Hudepohl, N, MacLean, JV, Osborne, LM. Perinatal obsessive-compulsive disorder: epidemiology, phenomenology, etiology, and treatment. *Curr Psychiatry Rep* 2022; 24:229–37

8. Kittel-Schneider, S, Quednow, BB, Leutritz, AL, et al. Parental ADHD in pregnancy and the postpartum period – a systematic review. *Neurosci Biobehav Rev* 2021; 124:63–77

9. McGuinness, M, Blissett, J, Jones, C. OCD in the perinatal period: is postpartum OCD (ppOCD) a distinct subtype? A review of the literature. *Behav Cogn Psychother* 2011; 39:285–310

10. Pauls, DL, Abramovitch, A, Rauch, SL, et al. Obsessive–compulsive disorder: an integrative genetic and neurobiological perspective. *Nat Rev Neurosci* 2014; 15:410–24

11. Pellegrini, L, Garg, K, Enara, A, et al. Repetitive transcranial magnetic stimulation (r-TMS) and selective serotonin reuptake inhibitor-resistance in obsessive–compulsive disorder: a meta-analysis and clinical implications. *Compr Psychiatry* 2022; 118:152339

12. Rădulescu, A, Herron, J, Kennedy, C, et al. Global and local excitation and inhibition shape the dynamics of the cortico-striatal-thalamo-cortical pathway. *Scientific Reports* 2017; 7:7608

13. Sánchez-Meca, J, Rosa-Alcázar, AI, Iniesta-Sepúlveda, M, et al. Differential efficacy of cognitive–behavioral therapy and pharmacological treatments for pediatric obsessive–compulsive disorder: a meta-analysis. *J Anxiety Disord* 2014; 28:31–44

14. Sharma, V, Sommerdyk, C. Obsessive–compulsive disorder in the postpartum period: diagnosis, differential diagnosis and management. *Womens Health (Lond)* 2015; 11:543–52

15. Sit, D, Rothschild, AJ, Wisner, KL. A review of postpartum psychosis. *J Womens Health (Larchmt)* 2006; 15:352–68

16. Speisman, BB, Storch, EA, Abramowitz, JS. Postpartum obsessive–compulsive disorder. *J Obstet Gynecol Neonatal Nurs* 2011; 40:680–90

17. Stahl, SM. *Impulsivity, Compulsivity, and Addiction*, 5th edn. Cambridge: Cambridge University Press, 2021.
18. Starcevic, V, Eslick, GD, Viswasam, K, et al. Symptoms of obsessive–compulsive disorder during pregnancy and the postpartum period: a systematic review and meta-analysis. *Psychiatr Q* 2020; 91:965–81
19. van den Heuvel, OA, Boedhoe, PSW, Bertolin, S, et al. An overview of the first 5 years of the ENIGMA obsessive–compulsive disorder working group: the power of worldwide collaboration. *Hum Brain Mapp* 2022; 43:23–36
20. Zambaldi, CF, Cantilino, A, Montenegro, AC, et al. Postpartum obsessive–compulsive disorder: prevalence and clinical characteristics. *Compr Psychiatry* 2009; 50:503–9

Case 25: The woman whose kidneys could not handle lithium

The Question: How do you manage bipolar I disorder (BP1) over the lifespan?

The Psychopharmacological Dilemma: Finding adequate treatment for elderly patients with bipolar disorder (BP) and kidney failure

James Gilfert

Pretest self-assessment question

At what level of kidney failure should you likely discontinue lithium (Eskalith)?

A. Stage 2 Mild chronic kidney disease (CKD) (glomerular filtration rate [GFR] = 60–89 mL/min)
B. Stage 3a Moderate CKD (GFR = 45–59 mL/min)
C. Stage 3b Moderate CKD (GFR = 30–44 mL/min)
D. Stage 4 Severe CKD (GFR = 15–29 mL/min)
E. Stage 5 End Stage CKD (GFR < 15 mL/min)
F. There is no exact stage when you need to discontinue lithium (Eskalith). Even in Stage 5 CKD or on dialysis, it is possible to be on lithium depending on a cost–benefit analysis
G. Stage 4 and above

Patient evaluation on intake

- A 66-year-old woman with an attempted suicide was brought to the emergency room (ER) after overdosing on "a few hundred" milligrams of clonazepam (Klonopin)
- Was found unconscious, naked, in her neighborhood by neighbors who called an ambulance
- Medical work-up was unfounded initially
- Admitted to the medical unit for 4 days
  ○ Found to be in atrial fibrillation
  ○ Anticoagulated and cardioverted with diltiazem (Cardizem) and atenolol (Tenormin)
- Medically stable by the third day of admission, when psychiatry was consulted given the recent reported suicide attempt

Psychiatric history

- Patient has a history of post-traumatic stress disorder (PTSD) and BP1 since her early 20s
- History of two past suicide attempts
- Reports several hospitalizations going back to her 20s

- History of clear manic episodes lasting weeks, which involve rapid speech, elevated mood, hyperactivity, getting very involved in political demonstrations, and believing she can "make a big difference in politics" to a delusional level
- The patient has been treated by a local psychiatric nurse practitioner who provided the following collateral information
  - The patient has a history of manic and depressive episodes as long as she has known her (at least back to the patient's 40s or 50s)
  - The patient has made four serious suicide attempts
    - She tends to stockpile medications and uses for suicide attempts
  - Previous medication trials include: lithium (Eskalith), lamotrigine (Lamictal), aripiprazole (Abilify), brexpiprazole (Rexulti), cariprazine (Vraylar), olanzapine (Zyprexa), and haloperidol (Haldol)

Social and personal history

- Reports a history of physical and sexual abuse perpetrated by her father growing up
  - Stated that her mother was aware but did not protect her
- Has a bachelor's degree in history
- Used to work as a technician at a hospital in sterile operations but is retired and has income from Social Security
- Married without any children
- Uses a four-prong cane due to unstable gait due to peripheral neuropathy
- Remote history of cannabis, hallucinogen, and stimulant use
  - Denies any current or recent substance use

Medical history

- Hypertension (HTN)
- CKD stage 3
- Peripheral neuropathy
- Glaucoma
- Hyperlipidemia

Family history

- History of alcohol use disorder (AUD) in the family (father and siblings)

Current medications

- Duloxetine (Cymbalta) 60 mg/d, a serotonin–norepinephrine reuptake inhibitor (SNRI)
- Gabapentin (Neurontin) 900 mg/d, a calcium channel-blocking epilepsy medication, pain dampener
- Bupropion SR (Wellbutrin SR) 100 mg/d, a norepinephrine–dopamine reuptake inhibitor (NDRI)
- Atenolol (Tenormin) 50 mg/d
- Diltiazem (Cardizem) 120 mg/d
- Atorvastatin (Lipitor) 40 mg/d
- Aspirin 81 mg/d
- Albuterol inhaler Q4H PRN for wheezing
- Furosemide (Lasix) 20 mg/d
- Multivitamin daily
- Fish oil daily
- Brimonidine and timolol (Combigan) ophthalmic drops
- Erythromycin ophthalmic ointment

Attending physician's mental notes: initial psychiatric evaluation

- The patient on exam appears depressed with the linear thought process, a normal rate of speech, and intact reality testing, denies any current suicidal ideation, and expressed feeling thankful that she is still alive
- Although dysphoric, she endorses feeling "hopeful"
- Previous psychiatric history is consistent with BP1
- Appears that she is currently presenting in a depressive episode of BP1 and is on SNRI and NDRI for bipolar depression, and gabapentin for neuropathic pain and apparent mood stabilization
- Based on the patient's presentation and gravity of the suicide attempt, she meets the criteria for continued inpatient level of psychiatric care and is now admitted on involuntary status to a psychiatry unit

Further investigation

Is there anything else that you would like to know about the patient?

How about lab work?

- Creatinine (Cre) on admission is 1.42; patient's baseline Cre in the past year has been chronically elevated – 1.30 which calculates to a chronic baseline GFR of 45 mL/min/1.73m^2 by the 2021 Chronic Kidney Disease Epidemiology Collaboration (CKD-EPI) formula using creatinine

- Electrolytes and liver function tests are in the normal range
- CBC is unremarkable
- TSH not available
- EKG after stabilization on the medical unit within normal limits, no QTc prolongation

When was the last time the patient was on an approved mood stabilizer?

- Gabapentin (Neurontin) is not approved for BP1 and actually has negative findings
- The patient reports that she did well on lithium (Eskalith) for many years but that medication was stopped once she developed CKD
  - Reports that due to CKD she is not willing to take it again
- Lamotrigine (Lamictal) reportedly led to a rash and had to be stopped
- She tried several atypical antipsychotics with various effectiveness
  - Aripiprazole (Abilify) reportedly led to akathisia
  - Brexpiprazole (Rexulti) was tolerated well but was not helpful with mood symptoms
  - Cariprazine (Vraylar) reportedly led to falls
  - Olanzapine (Zyprexa) led to falls as well
  - Haloperidol (Haldol) reportedly led to acute dystonia
- Due to these past experiences, patient currently declines taking any future antipsychotics

What are evidence-based recommendations for the treatment of bipolar depression?

- Several atypical antipsychotics have been approved for the treatment of bipolar depression, such as lurasidone (Latuda), cariprazine (Vraylar), lumateperone (Caplyta), fluoxetine + olanzapine combination (Symbyax), and quetiapine (Seroquel)
- Although not FDA-approved for the treatment of bipolar depression, lamotrigine (Lamictal) is often used in clinical practice
  - Lamotrigine (Lamictal) is FDA-approved for bipolar maintenance, i.e., to delay entry of a euthymic patient into either depression or mania
- There is limited evidence for the use of lithium (Eskalith), valproic acid (Depakote), and carbamazepine (Tegretol) in the treatment of bipolar depression, but they are used sometimes in clinical practice where lithium (Eskalith) may have the most compelling data

Attending physician's mental notes: initial psychiatric evaluation (continued)

- Patient has been on lithium (Eskalith) in the past with good effect, and it could be a reasonable option given the recent suicide attempt, but she has CKD
  - Lithium (Eskalith) has specific data and approval to lower suicidal activity in BP1
  - Has been shown to decrease suicidal behaviors
    - even if mood stabilization is not achieved
    - even with lower serum concentration levels
- Although lithium (Eskalith) is considered to be the gold standard for the treatment of BP1, its superiority to other medications for bipolar maintenance and depressive states is still debatable
- Were her years of lithium treatment in the past the cause of her CKD?
  - It is clear that lithium (Eskalith) use causes polyuria and nephrogenic diabetes insipidus. It may also cause renal insufficiency (declining GFR), but recent evidence suggests, however, that the risk of renal insufficiency is less severe with lithium than was previously thought. The evidence suggesting that lithium causes chronic renal insufficiency was to some extent the product of confounding by indication. That is, patients with BP who would be treated with lithium (Eskalith) have higher rates of conditions like hypertension, metabolic syndrome, and type 2 diabetes that themselves increase risk of renal insufficiency
  - Modern prescribing practices can minimize the risk of lithium (Eskalith) leading to renal insufficiency. Twice-daily dosing of lithium (Eskalith) can increase the risk of it causing renal insufficiency (dosing just once daily is safer). Keeping lithium trough levels below 1.00 mEq/L can also prevent kidney damage that leads to renal insufficiency
  - Therefore, it is possible that lithium use in the past in this patient contributed to her CKD, but it is difficult to be sure of the extent. It is possible that further treatment with lithium (Eskalith) could worsen her renal insufficiency, but this risk is now believed to be less than formerly thought and can be minimized by dosing lithium (Eskalith) only once daily and avoiding lithium levels above 1.00 mEq/L
- Her GFR (of 45 mL/min/1.73m^2 by the 2021 CKD-EPI formula using creatinine) puts her right at the edge of Stage 3b – Moderate CKD

- For patients in CKD Stages 3a or 3b, the decision whether to use lithium (Eskalith) is made by assessing the risks and benefits, based on this patient's history and findings
  - It may be wise to assess for proteinuria, hematuria, and a more rapid decline in GFR which would suggest not to use lithium (Eskalith)
  - If renal function was to worsen, then discontinuing gives the patient some chance for GFR to recover, but it is not a guarantee
  - For patients in Stage 4 or Stage 5, lithium (Eskalith) should generally be avoided. However, in some cases, if the benefit is high and could outweigh the risks, it may still be continued but afraid the patient may end up on dialysis
- This patient is in a situation in which we could decide either to continue or to stop it. Ultimately, she herself was not willing to consider taking lithium
- Divalproex (Depakote) is FDA-approved for acute mania, and there is evidence of its efficacy in bipolar maintenance and mixed episodes, while its effectiveness in bipolar depression is quite limited
- As the patient declined all atypical antipsychotics, lithium (Eskalith), and lamotrigine (Lamictal), we discussed the possibility of starting divalproex (Depakote) instead, as the least offending agent, albeit with the least depression data

Attending physician's mental notes: psychiatric hospitalization day 5

- Patient agreed to be started on divalproex and was initiated on 500 mg/d of the slow-release formulation
- Other psychotropic medications gabapentin (Neurontin), duloxetine (Cymbalta), and bupropion XL (Wellbutrin XL) had been resumed
  - Guidelines suggest avoiding unipolar antidepressants in BP1 patients as it may destabilize, causing mixed features or rapid cycling, or trigger manic events
    - Will need to monitor for this closely
    - Ideally may be able to use divalprox (Depakote) as a monotherapy
- Initial trough divalproex (Depakote) level 48 hours after the initiation was 19.5 mcg/mL and the dose was increased to 1000 mg/d, ideally to achieve a therapeutic level of 50–125 mcg/mL
- At this time, the patient began reading voraciously and staying up late into the night with new-onset hyposomnia
- Furthermore, she reported diarrhea
- The follow-up trough level after 4 days taking 1000 mg/d was therapeutic at 116.8 mcg/mL

Questions

Was divalproex (Depakote) used appropriately? How to dose divalproex (Depakote)?

- For normal adult patients with no liver impairment, divalproex (Depakote) can be started at 10–15 mg/kg or 500–750 mg/d and increased by 250–500 mg per day every 1–3 days
- Providers titrate the dose for a combination of desired clinical effectiveness and therapeutic blood levels
- It is sometimes dosed even higher initially for rapid symptom control at 20–30 mg/kg in a loading dose
- For this 90 kg (200 lb) patient, that would give a broad range from 900 mg/d to 2700 mg/d
- This patient ended up with a level at the higher end of the therapeutic range while being on 1000 mg/d, most likely due to her age
  - In elderly patients, caution is needed given possible reduced hepatic function with decreased elimination, and recommended starting dose in this population can be 125–250 mg/d
  - The therapeutic dose in this population may ultimately be reached with a dose of 500–1000 mg/d

What is a therapeutic level of divalproex (Depakote)?

- The general range for valproic acid (VPA) is between 50 and 125 mcg/mL of total serum concentration
- The patient was started on divalproex (Depakote ER) 500 mcg/d, and after 48 hours serum VPA level was 19.5 mcg/mL

What is the half-life of divalproex (Depakote)? Was the dose of 500 mg/d subtherapeutic for her?

- No, not necessarily. The half-life of divalproex (Depakote) in the average adult patient is between 9 and 16 hours, so 48 hours is about 3–4 half-lives. By 5 half-lives, drug level should be at a steady state. But, given the extended release formulation which was used, and given her age, the half-life would likely be artificially longer
- Therefore, when the level at 48 hours was drawn, steady state was most likely not reached as yet, in retrospect

What are the most common side effects of divalproex (Depakote)?

- Gastrointestinal (GI) side effects are common with valproic acid formulations
  - Valproic acid, the parent drug of divalproex (Depakote), has the most GI side effects of all preparations

- ○ Immediate-release divalproex formulations have more risk of nausea but less risk of diarrhea
- ○ Extended-release divalproex formulations have more risk of diarrhea and less risk of nausea
  - ▪ This patient had diarrhea, which is what one would expect on the extended-release formulation
- ○ The hyposomnia the patient developed is odd given that divalproex (Depakote) generally also causes sedation as a key side effect, and this raises the worry that she is experiencing breakthrough mania for some reason

Case outcome: psychiatric hospitalization day 8

- Patient stopped taking divalproex (Depakote) after experiencing diarrhea and was not willing to re-try it
- Although its levels were at the higher end, she thankfully did not exhibit any signs of neurotoxicity such as confusion, somnolence, or dizziness, but only reported diarrhea
- A discussion about starting carbamazepine (Equetro) occurred instead and she chose to read some information about the drug and refused to start it
- Over the next few days, the patient's thought process became rambling and tangential, and she displayed marked irritability and grandiosity
- The primary team saw her as hypertalkative to a pressured level of speech, tangential, and it was difficult to interrupt or keep her on task
- Patient declined to start carbamazepine (Equetro) anymore as she had read printed information about its possible drug–drug interactions
- She however agreed to an increase of her gabapentin (Neurontin) to 1800 mg/d
- She remained on the unipolar antidepressant duloxetine (Cymbalta), but the bupropion XL (Wellbutrin XL) was discontinued

Attending physician's mental notes: psychiatric hospitalization day 8

- Appears that the patient has switched to mania pretty quickly despite a therapeutic divalproex level on the psychiatric unit
- One question is whether she may have not been adherent to antidepressants on an outpatient basis, and their reintroduction and consistent use in the hospital is now a force pushing her into mania

- The duloxetine (an SNRI) is probably more worrisome than the bupropion (an NDRI) for causing mania, but the patient stated that duloxetine (Cymbalta) was very beneficial for her neuropathic pain and does not want to stop the medication
- Gabapentin (Neurontin) is not known to be of any clear value as a monotherapy in treating or preventing mania, but in this situation the patient stated that she finds it beneficial for her mood and is agreeable to an increase in its dose. It may also improve neuropathic pain and reduce need for the SNRI later
  - By working with this patient and increasing this dose, ideally a better alliance can be made to effect better psychopharmacological changes later

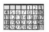

Case outcome: psychiatric hospitalization day 19

- By day 12 of the inpatient psychiatric hospitalization, the patient was still manic and presented with impaired sleep, irritability, grandiosity, pressured speech, and was being intrusive across the unit
- She would walk around the unit so fast that she left her walker behind, and she would assault staff with her walker at other times
- She became hypersexual and inappropriate with some patients and staff
- She began to refer to the resident as "the baby doctor"
- She was unwilling to agree to any medications besides the gabapentin (Neurontin) and duloxetine (Cymbalta) which she is already taking
- On day 13, the attending physician started the legal process for treatment over objection to change her medications

Question

What would you do next?

- Medicate over objection with an atypical antipsychotic
- Medicate over objection with divalproex (Depakote)
- Medicate over objection with carbamazepine (Equetro)
- Medicate over objection with lithium (Eskalith)

Case outcome: psychiatric hospitalization day 19 (continued)

- On day 14, after reading additional information on off-label carbamazepine (Equetro), underlining a lot of text in the informational drug packet, and asking to see its chemical structure, she agreed to start it at 400 mg/d

- On day 17, the dose of carbamazepine (Equetro) was increased to 600 mg/d
- On day 18, the patient reported feeling "drunk as a skunk" and complained of dizziness, tremor, and some unwitnessed falls
- On day 19, a trough carbamazepine level was 16 mcg/mL
  - The normal range of carbamazepine level is between 8 and 12 mcg/mL
  - She is felt to be toxic at this dose

Attending physician's mental notes: psychiatric hospitalization day 19 (continued)

- Carbamazepine (Equetro) commonly has central nervous system (CNS) side effects such as drowsiness, dizziness, and ataxia
  - Ataxia is reported in as many as 15% of cases
- Additionally, carbamazepine (Equetro) can lower sodium levels and further contribute to observed neurological symptoms
- It appears that the patient is again experiencing side effects from mood stabilizer toxicity, and her levels of carbamazepine (Equetro) are seemingly supratherapeutic
- There are no recommended dosing adjustments of carbamazepine (Equetro) in kidney impairment or in older adults
- Kidney impairment can increase the accumulation of toxic metabolites of carbamazepine (Equetro), as can concurrent divalproex (Depakote) use, but that agent was discontinued about 6 days prior to starting the carbamazepine (Equetro), hence it is unclear why the levels are high

Case outcome: psychiatric hospitalization day 31

- Carbamazepine (Equetro) is discontinued on day 20 and then restarted at only 100 mg daily on day 21
- On day 28, the level is 8.4 mcg/mL which is in the middle of the therapeutic range, but the patient was still manic
- After some discussion, the patient agrees to take the atypical antipsychotic olanzapine (Zyprexa) with good initial effects
- Her manic behavior becomes more appropriate, thought process slowly becomes less tangential
- Next she began to sleep more, and slowly had become less irritable and grandiose
- She however complains of vague tremors that are not observable, at the dose of olanzapine (Zyprexa) of 10 mg/d
  - Dose was decreased to 7.5 mg/d, and, by discharge, she was taking only 5 mg/d while still improving symptomatically

- ○ Benztropine (Cogentin) 2 mg/d, an anticholinergic alleviated all tremors
- Duloxetine (Cymbalta) had been decreased to 40 mg/d to decrease its potential in driving her toward mania
- Discharged home with outpatient follow-up at a local clinic after 31 days on the psychiatric unit

Case debrief

- Patient presented after a suicide attempt in what appears to be a depressive episode of BP1
- Like this patient, BP1 patients have a 4–19% lifetime risk of suicide, which is 10–30 times as great as for the general population
- Lithium has a known antisuicide effect, but the patient was reluctant to take it given her history of CKD
  - ○ It would have been a debatable choice to give lithium (Eskalith) at her stage of kidney disease
- Patient was continued on both SNRI and NDRI which may have driven the shift into mania as she had no bona fide mood stabilizer to help her stay euthymic
- Bipolar patients (especially during manic phases) may lack insight into their illness and the need for treatment, which made the management of this case challenging
- During the hospital stay, she had adverse effects from each medication tried, resulting in non-efficacy
- Patient finally agreed to take a low dose of an atypical antipsychotic, and her symptoms improved sufficiently to enable her to be discharged from the hospital

Take-home points

- Prescribers should be aware of the pharmacokinetic changes present in older adult patients and consider them when prescribing medications, as lower doses may provide efficacy in older adults, and normal doses may cause toxicity
- Impact on kidney function
  - ○ Even in the absence of kidney disease, many older adults have a decline in kidney function
  - ○ The patient's creatinine level is important, but it may make sense also to calculate their GFR with a formula such as the CKD–EPI equation
  - ○ This formula takes the patient's age into account
    - ▪ Older patients have a decrease in muscle mass
    - ▪ They produce less creatinine from muscle breakdown

- Their kidneys do not have as much of a job to do in filtering out creatinine, so any increase in creatinine reflects a more significant decrease in GFR in an elderly person
  - Older adults may have decreased clearance of renally metabolized medications, such as lithium (Eskalith), resulting in the need for dose adjustment
  - Furthermore, some guidelines recommend lower target serum levels of lithium of 0.4 to 0.8 mEq/L in older adults
- Impact on liver function:
  - Hepatic function also declines with age even in the absence of liver disease, and dose adjustments may be required for hepatically metabolized medications
- Elderly patients have more fat and less muscle, which can affect the volume of distribution of drugs as well
- Elderly patients are more likely to be on several different medications (polypharmacy) and could potentially have significant drug–drug interactions, thus increasing drug levels artificially and causing toxicity more readily
  - The American Geriatric Society developed the Beers Criteria which list many medications that should be avoided due to potential adverse effects in the elderly
  - Carbamazepine (Equetro) is listed as a medication to use with caution due to risk of causing the syndrome of inappropriate antidiuretic hormone (SIADH) and hyponatremia
    - It has some anticholinergic effects, but these may be more relevant in overdose than at therapeutic levels
  - Medications with anticholinergic effects are generally advised against due to risk of confusion, constipation, and dry mouth
    - Benztropine is a medication that was used in this case temporarily due to worry about resting tremor / EPS caused by olanzapine (Zyprexa)
    - This may be ill advised – however, it improved her tremor
    - The patient was satisfied and therefore more compliant as such
  - Benzodiazepines (not used in this case) are recommended against due to the risk of falls, motor vehicle accidents, respiratory depression, and cognitive impairment
  - Antipsychotics still often need to be used in BP1 and schizophrenia (SP) in the elderly, but do entail risks of stroke and greater cognitive decline in patients with dementia

Performance in practice: confessions of a psychopharmacologist

What could have been done better here?

- The manic episode could have possibly been averted by discontinuing her antidepressants
- The treating team could have pursued treatment over objection earlier in the hospital stay, and the patient could have been started on an atypical antipsychotic that would result in faster stabilization of depressive symptoms and prevented her later mania
- A better understanding of pharmacokinetics would have helped the management of some adverse effects from divalproex (Depakote) and carbamazepine (Equetro) seen during the hospitalization

What are possible action items for improvement in practice?

- Providers need to consider pharmacokinetic changes present in older adult patients when prescribing psychotropic medications
- A good general take-home point is to check in a reference database whether there are any recommended dose adjustments for a given medication in older adults
- Also, consider entering the patient's whole medication list into a drug–drug interaction checker resource that is readily available

Tips and pearls

- Lithium (Eskalith) is purely renally eliminated
- Its dose needs to be lowered whenever kidney function is diminished (Table 25.1)
- In patients with CKD, lithium use carries the risk of further worsening their kidney function
- By recommendations and expert opinion, for any kidney impairment at Stage 3a or worse, lithium (Eskalith) should be used at lower doses and the kidney function more frequently monitored
- It is recommended to avoid all use in Stage 4 or Stage 5, and to avoid use in dialysis unless there are no other treatment options

Table 25.1 Lithium treatment recommendations in different stages of CKD

CKD stage	GFR (mL/min)	Lithium recommendation
Stage 1	$\geqslant 90$	No dosage adjustment
Stage 2 (Mild CKD)	60–89	No dosage adjustment
Stage 3a (Moderate CKD)	45–59	Start low, monitor levels frequently, and weigh the risks of further kidney damage against the benefits
Stage 3b (Moderate CKD)	30–44	Start low, monitor levels frequently, and weigh the risks of further kidney damage against the benefits
Stage 4 (Severe CKD)	15–29	Avoid use, but may still use in special situations
Stage 5 (End Stage CKD)	< 15	Avoid use, but may still use in special situations

Two-minute tutorial

Bipolar disorder

- Bipolar disorder (BP) is a complex, chronic mood disorder
  - Has a lifetime prevalence of 1%
  - Can manifest with manic/hypomanic symptoms, depressive episodes, and/or mixed or psychotic features
- The aggregate lifetime prevalence of BP1 is 0.6%, BP2 is 0.4%, subthreshold BP is 1.4%, and for the bipolar spectrum may be upwards of 2.4%
- Besides mood symptoms, patients with BP often have cognitive symptoms, such as altered reaction time and executive dysfunction, that contribute to disability
- Bipolar depression is a major cause of morbidity and mortality in BP
  - Bipolar patients spend more time depressed than manic
    - Especially BP2 patients
  - Suicide attempts are more common in depressive episodes

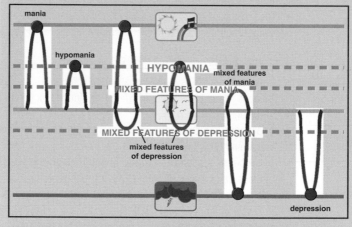

Figure 25.1 Mood episodes. Mood symptoms exist along a spectrum, with the polar ends being pure mania or hypomania ("up" pole) and pure depression ("down" pole). Patients can also experience mood episodes that include symptoms of both poles; such episodes can be described as mania/hypomania with mixed features of depression, or depression with mixed features of mania. A patient may have any combination of these episodes over the course of illness; subsyndromal manic or depressive episodes also occur during the course of illness, in which case there are not enough symptoms or the symptoms are not sufficiently severe to meet the diagnostic criteria for one of these episodes. Thus, the presentation of mood disorders can vary widely.

Treatment of BP

- Providers should have a good knowledge of the evidence-based treatments for BP, including their pharmacokinetic considerations and most common side effects (Table 25.2)
- In many patients with BP1, it can be advisable to use more than one medication if monotherapy does not lead to complete remission, or in the prevention of further mood episodes toward either pole
- Sometimes antidepressants are cautiously used in addition to a mood-stabilizing medication, but most guidelines recommend atypical antipsychotics as first options for bipolar depression
    - Quetiapine (Seroquel), cariprazine (Craylar), lurasidone (Latuda), lumateperone (Caplyta), and olanzapine–fluoxetine combination (Symbyax) are FDA-approved (Table 25.3)
- In some patients, first and second choices may be contraindicated, or patients may be unwilling to take them, so providers need to be aware of alternative options

Table 25.2 Comparison of mood stabilizers

	Lithium	Valproic acid	Carbamazepine	Lamotrigine
Evidence-based indications (* indicates FDA-approved)	Mania* Bipolar maintenance* Less evidence for bipolar depression	Mania* Bipolar maintenance* Less evidence for bipolar depression	Mania* Bipolar maintenance	Bipolar maintenance* Some evidence for bipolar depression
Mechanism of action	Inhibits dopamine and glutamate neurotransmission Increases GABA neurotransmission Neuroprotective effects through BDNF and Bcl-2 Inhibits glycogen synthase kinase 3 (GSK 3) pathway	Increases availability of GABA in CNS. Blocks voltage-gated sodium channels	Blocks presynaptic voltage-gated sodium channels, which inhibits glutamate release. Also blocks muscarinic and nicotinic acetylcholine receptors, NMDA receptors, and adenosine receptors	Inhibits release of glutamate Inhibits voltage-sensitive sodium channels Stabilizes neuronal membranes
Normal starting doses	600–900 mg/d	500–750 mg/d	100–400 mg/d	25 mg/d. 25 mg every other day if also on valproic acid. 50 mg/d if on carbamazepine or other inducing antiepileptics. (See another published resource for details on dosing schedule)
Usual dose range for BP	900–1800 mg/d Titrate to therapeutic blood level	1500–2500 mg/d	600–1200 mg/d Because it induces its own metabolism, may have to increase dose after a few weeks after induction occurs	200 mg/d. 100 mg every other day if also on valproic acid. 300 mg/d if on carbamazepine or other inducing antiepileptics
Normal adult half-life	18–36 hours	9–19 hours	12–65 hours Very variable due to autoinduction	25–33 hours
Therapeutic blood levels	0.8–1.2 mEq/L Sometimes lower (0.6 mEq/L)	50 to 125 mcg/mL	4–12 mg/L	1 to 6 mcg/mL

Metabolism	Exclusively renally cleared	Hepatic by CYP2A6 (minor), CYP2B6 (minor), CYP2C19 (minor), CYP2C9 (minor), CYP2E1 (minor)	Hepatic	Hepatic
Dosage adjustment for renal impairment	CrCl 30 to < 60 mL/minute: starting dose 150–300 mg/d. May avoid use or start even lower at CrCl < 30 mL/minute	None	None, but toxic metabolite levels could rise	None but may dose cautiously in severe impairment
Dosage adjustment for hepatic impairment	None	Not recommended to use in even mild–moderate impairment. Contraindicated in severe impairment	Consider dose reduction	Moderate to severe impairment without ascites: decrease initial, escalation, and maintenance doses by ~25%. Moderate to severe impairment with ascites: decrease initial, escalation, and maintenance doses by ~50%
Dosage adjustment for elderly patients	Choose lower starting dose. May choose lower therapeutic target level such as 0.6–0.8 mEq/L	Max blood level 90 mcg/mL	No specific recommendations but consider dose reduction	No specific recommendations
Drug–drug interactions	Via kidney effects: ARBs, ACEIs, thiazide and loop diuretics, carbonic anhydrase inhibitors. Serotonergic interactions also.	Lithium can increase valproic acid level. Interactions through hepatic metabolism induction or inhibition. Interaction with other CNS depressants	Many, by means of hepatic metabolism induction and inhibition. Interaction with other CNS depressants. Induces its own metabolism	Valproic acid inhibits its metabolism. Carbamazepine and other inducers induce its metabolism. Interaction with other CNS depressants
Monitoring labs	BUN, creatinine, sodium, calcium, TSH, free thyroxine (fT4), bHCG, CBC, EKG	Liver enzymes, bHCG, ammonia, CBC, PT/PTT	CBC with diff, reticulocytes, liver and renal function tests, serum sodium, bHCG, HLA-B*1502 and HLA-A*3101 genotype screening prior to therapy initiation in patients with Asian / South Asian ancestry	Less important

Table 25.2 (cont.)

	Lithium	Valproic acid	Carbamazepine	Lamotrigine
Pregnancy considerations	Cardiac malformations in first trimester. Polyhydramnios, fetal/neonatal cardiac arrhythmias, hypoglycemia, diabetes insipidus, changes in thyroid function, premature delivery, floppy infant syndrome, or neonatal lithium toxicity later in pregnancy	Causes major congenital defects such as neural tube defects, causes intellectual disability	Causes major congenital malformations. Not recommended in pregnancy	Risk of major malformations has not been observed
Breastfeeding considerations	Recommended to avoid breastfeeding. Is present in breast milk. Risk of hypotonia, hypothermia, cyanosis, electrocardiogram changes, and lethargy	Considered compatible with breastfeeding. Is present in breast milk. Theoretical risk of hepatic damage to baby	Is present in breast milk. Considered compatible in breastfeeding with consideration of risks. Has risks of respiratory depression, seizures, nausea, vomiting, diarrhea, and/or decreased feeding	Is present in breast milk. Considered compatible with breastfeeding with consideration of risks. Has risks of apnea, drowsiness, poor sucking, thrombocytosis, and rash
Key side effects	CNS symptoms, tremor, arrhythmia, hypercalcemia, hypothyroidism, nephrogenic diabetes insipidus, polydipsia, polyuria, chronic kidney failure, weight gain	CNS effects, bone marrow suppression, hepatotoxicity, hyperammonemia, encephalopathy, pancreatitis	Blood dyscrasias, arrhythmia, hepatotoxicity, hyponatremia, CNS effects	Aseptic meningitis, blood dyscrasias, Stevens–Johnson syndrome, DRESS, toxic epidermal necrolysis

ACEIs – angiotensin converting enzyme inhibitors; ARBs – angiotensin II receptor blockers; Bcl-2 – B-cell lymphoma 2; bHCG – beta-human chorionic gonadotropin; BUN – blood urea nitrogen; CrCl – creatinine clearance; HLA – human leukocyte antigen; PT – prothrombin time; PTT – partial thromboplastin time

Table 25.3 List of medications used in different phases of BP

Acute mania	Bipolar maintenance	Bipolar depression
Lithium*	Lithium*	Lurasidone*
Divalproex*	Divalproex	Cariprazine*
Carbamazepine*	Carbamazepine	Lumateperone*
Olanzapine*	Olanzapine*	Olanzapine + fluoxetine*
Quetiapine*	Quetiapine	Quetiapine*
Asenapine*	Asenapine*	
Risperidone*	Risperidone	
Ziprasidone*	Lamotrigine*	
Aripiprazole*		
Chlorpromazine*		
Cariprazine*		
Haloperidol		

* FDA-approved medications for the indication

Post-test question

At what level of kidney failure should you likely discontinue lithium (Eskalith)?

A. Stage 2 Mild chronic kidney disease (CKD) (glomerular filtration rate [GFR] = 60–89 mL/min)

B. Stage 3s Moderate CKD (GFR = 45–59 mL/min)

C. Stage 3b Moderate CKD (GFR = 30–44 mL/min)

D. Stage 4 Severe CKD (GFR = 15–29 mL/min)

E. Stage 5 End Stage CKD (GFR < 15 mL/min)

F. There is no exact stage when you need to discontinue lithium (Eskalith). Even in Stage 5 CKD or on dialysis, it is possible to be on lithium depending on a cost–benefit analysis

G. Stage 4 and above

Answer: G

By recommendations and expert opinion, for anything Stage 3a or worse, lithium (Eskalith) should be used at lower doses and have frequent monitoring. It is recommended to avoid use in Stage 4 or Stage 5 and to avoid use in dialysis. Lithium (Eskalith) is sometimes used even in Stage 5 CKD or dialysis in special situations, and this should be done according to a risk–benefit analysis.

References

1. Aiken, CB, Orr, C. Rechallenge with lamotrigine after a rash: a prospective case series and review of the literature. *Psychiatry (Edgmont)* 2010; 7:27–32

2. Dutta, S, Reed, RC. Functional half-life is a meaningful descriptor of steady-state pharmacokinetics of an extended-release formulation of a rapidly cleared drug: as shown by once-daily divalproex-ER. *Clin Drug Investig* 2006; 26:681–90

3. Dutta, S, Reed, RC, O'Dea, RF. Comparative absorption profiles of divalproex sodium delayed-release versus extended-release tablets – clinical implications. *Ann Pharmacother* 2006; 40:619–25

4. Gitlin, MJ. Antidepressants in bipolar depression: an enduring controversy. *Int J Bipolar Disord* 2018; 6:25

5. Gupta, S, Kripalani, M, Khastgir, U, et al. Management of the renal adverse effects of lithium. *Adv Psychiatr Treat* 2013; 19:457–66

6. Hayes, JF, Marston, L, Walters, K, et al. Lithium vs. valproate vs. olanzapine vs. quetiapine as maintenance monotherapy for bipolar disorder: a population-based UK cohort study using electronic health records. *World Psychiatry* 2016; 15:53–8

7. Hong, JSW, Atkinson, LZ, Al-Juffali, N, et al. Gabapentin and pregabalin in bipolar disorder, anxiety states, and insomnia: systematic review, meta-analysis, and rationale. *Mol Psychiatry* 2022; 27:1339–49

8. Kang, MG, Qian, H, Keramatian, K, et al. Lithium vs valproate in the maintenance treatment of bipolar I disorder: a post-hoc analysis of a randomized double-blind placebo-controlled trial. *Aust N Z J Psychiatry* 2020; 54:298–307

9. Kessing, LV, Hellmund, G, Geddes, JR, et al. Valproate v. lithium in the treatment of bipolar disorder in clinical practice: observational nationwide register-based cohort study. *Br J Psychiatry* 2011; 199:57–63

10. Kverno, K, Beauvois, L, Dudley-Brown, S. Lamotrigine rash. *Nurse Pract* 2018; 43:48–51

11. Mathews, M, Gratz, S, Adetunji, B, et al. Antipsychotic-induced movement disorders: evaluation and treatment. *Psychiatry (Edgmont)* 2005; 2:36–41

12. Mowla, A, Boostani, S, Ehsaei, Z. Comparing lithium with valproate for clinical and social status of bipolar disorder patients in inter-episode interval: a retrospective comparative study. *J Neurol Res* 2020; 10:226–30

13. Pigott, K, Galizia, I, Vasudev, K, et al. Topiramate for acute affective episodes in bipolar disorder in adults. *Cochrane Database Syst Rev* 2016; 9:CD003384-CD003384

14. Sachs, GS. Strategies for improving treatment of bipolar disorder: integration of measurement and management. *Acta Psychiatr Scand Suppl* 2004; 7–17

15. Servais, A. Néphrotoxicité du lithium. *Nephrol Ther* 2019; 15:120–6

Case 26: The gentleman who was sober and could not focus

The Question: Do non-stimulants work for Attention-Deficit/ Hyperactivity Disorder (ADHD)?

The Psychopharmacological Dilemma: Treatment of ADHD in patients with a history of alcohol use disorder (AUD) and borderline intellectual functioning (BIF)

Nevena Radonjić

Pretest self-assessment question

Which of the following apply to borderline intellectual functioning (BIF)?

A. Affects approximately 15% of the population
B. Tested IQ levels are in the range of 70–85
C. Does not have a separate diagnostic category in DSM-5
D. Affects school performance and social functioning
E. Can be comorbid with ADHD and autism spectrum disorder (ASD)
F. All of the above

Patient evaluation on intake

- A 48-year-old male with a chief complaint of "Getting angry too fast"

Psychiatric history

- Reports a long history of AUD, sober now for 8 years, and in a supportive living environment
- Attends Alcoholics Anonymous (AA) daily
- On psychological testing, has BIF with an IQ 75
- Wants a general educational development (GED) diploma but now struggles in night school
  ○ Reports difficulty with attention and comprehension, easily gets distracted, forgets to complete homework, and avoids tasks requiring sustained attention
- Complained of frequently interrupting others and having a hard time sitting calmly in a chair
- Reports getting frustrated too quickly and his irritability being a major problem
- Taking now a subtherapeutic tricyclic antidepressant (TCA), doxepin (Sinequan) 50 mg/d, for symptoms of major depressive disorder (MDD) and insomnia, and also an antihistamine, hydroxyzine (Vistaril) 75 mg/d, for anxiety, but still has a depressed mood, impaired sleep, anhedonia, poor focus, and passive suicidal ideation

- Per history, appears that the episode of MDD has been accompanied by anxious distress as he is endorsing restlessness, feeling tense, along with poor concentration due to worry and feeling that something bad will happen
  - This anxiety started at the time of MDD onset
- No history of inpatient stays or suicidal ideation

Social and personal history

- Divorced, remarried, and has 18-year-old son with whom he has close contact
- Is amicable in his relationship with ex-wife
- Sober from alcohol, but is smoking cigarettes half-pack daily and not currently interested in addressing it
- Denies any current cannabis use, used to smoke 3–4 blunts daily for years
- Not utilizing family support

Medical history

- Asthma
- Hypertension
- Successful spinal fusion for neck injury

Family history

- Mother had a history of MDD
- Uncle had paranoia

Medication history

- History of trazodone (Desyrel) trial for sleep several years ago that he tolerated well, prescribed by primary care clinician

Current medications

- Doxepin (Sinequan) 50 mg/d, a TCA, was started while inpatient getting rehabilitation for MDD and AUD
- Hydroxyzine, an antihistamine anxiolytic, 75 mg/d as needed for anxiety
- Albuterol inhaler (ProAir)
- Fluticasone inhaler (Wixela Inhub)

Psychotherapy history

- Attends supportive psychotherapy and group therapy now for AUD

Question

Based on this patient's history and the available evidence, would you consider the diagnosis of ADHD?

- No, as the impaired attention is due to BIF
- No, as the impaired attention is due to MDD
- No, as the impaired attention is due to anxious distress
- Yes, as up to 40% of individuals with BIF have ADHD as a comorbidity

What would your next treatment likely be?

- Better delineate whether the depressive and anxiety disorders are affecting attention
- Better delineate whether ADHD is a true pre-existing comorbidity
- Start a stimulant for the treatment of ADHD
- Start a non-stimulant for the treatment of ADHD

Attending physician's mental notes: initial psychiatric evaluation

- Given the above symptoms, the patient meets the criteria for MDD with anxious distress, and additionally has well-established BIF and AUD in stable remission
- On mental status examination, presents with dysthymia, short attention span, concrete thinking process, and difficulty comprehending abstract constructs
- Both MDD and GAD can affect attention, and the patient is on a relatively low dose of antidepressant doxepin (Sinequan)
- The usual range in which doxepin (Sinequan) has antidepressant properties is between 75 and 150 mg/d as it acts as a serotonin–norepinephrine reuptake inhibitor (SNRI) given its active metabolite nordoxepin
  - It does have antihistamine and anticholinergic effects that may worsen cognition
  - At lower doses (3–6 mg/d) predominantly antagonizes histaminergic H1 receptors
  - At higher doses, it antagonizes α_1 adrenergic and muscarinic M1 receptors
- It appears that there is room to improve symptoms of MDD with anxious distress, and once these are better controlled, can re-evaluate attention and irritability

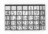

Case outcome: interim follow-ups through 1 month

- Given observed symptoms, the patient was offered an increase in the dose of doxepin (Sinequan) to 75 mg/d for 2 weeks, then 100 mg/d
- Reports now that his mood and sleep improved and he is less worried, but still struggles with irritability and has a low threshold for frustration
- Furthermore, feels discouraged that he will never obtain GED as he has difficulty maintaining his attention

Attending physician's mental notes: interim follow-ups through 1 month

- Inattention appears to be one of the key symptoms affecting patient's functioning now
- Besides difficulty sustaining attention, he has distractibility, poor task vigilance, struggles to finish tasks, and avoids tasks requiring sustained mental effort
- Based on detailed developmental history and clinical assessment, patient had those symptoms in addition to BIF before age 12
- Could consider several ADHD treatment options
  - Certain antidepressants such as bupropion XL (Wellbutrin XL), desipramine (Norpramin), and nortriptyline (Pamelor), although not FDA-approved, are effective in the treatment of ADHD
  - Certain antihypertensives such as guanfacine ER (Intuniv) and clonidine ER (Kapvay) are FDA-approved for ADHD in children as non-stimulants
  - Certain norepinephrine reuptake inhibitors (NRIs) such as atomoxetine (Strattera) and viloxazine ER (Qelbree) are FDA-approved for ADHD
  - Many methylphenidate and amphetamine products are FDA-approved for ADHD
- Here doxepin (Sinequan) is now acting as a serotonin–norepinephrine-enhancing multimodal drug that might help with inattention given its NRI activity, but the studies supporting its effectiveness in ADHD are limited

Question

Which medication is the preferred first choice in the treatment of ADHD in adults?

- Guidelines on preferred medications across different age groups are inconsistent

- Based on a recent comprehensive meta-analysis considering both the efficacy and safety of medications used in ADHD treatment, methylphenidate (Ritalin) is supported as a first-choice medication in children and adolescents, and amphetamines (Adderall) in adults

Which medication is the preferred first choice in the treatment of ADHD in patients with a history of substance use disorder (SUD)?

- Clinicians are generally reluctant to prescribe addictive stimulants to patients with a history of SUD
- Immediate-release stimulants have the highest potential for abuse and long-acting formulations should be considered instead if a stimulant is needed
- Although the effect size of non-stimulant and off-label medication efficacy is lower compared to methylphenidates/amphetamines in adults with ADHD, they can be effective in the treatment of ADHD symptoms without any risk of further addiction

Does ADHD treatment help with SUD?

- Individuals with ADHD have educational underperformance, difficulty sustaining jobs, are more prone to accidents, and engage in riskier behaviors including substance use
- Individuals with ADHD and SUD seem to do less well in substance use programs, although often utilize more treatment
- Hence, treatment of ADHD seems to be essential in patients with SUD to achieve the best possible outcomes

Case outcome: interim follow-ups through 6 months

- Patient declined initiation of stimulant given the risk to his sobriety, and guanfacine ER (Intuniv), a postsynaptic receptor α_{2A} adrenergic agonist, was started instead
  - ○ Guanfacine ER (Intuniv) is FDA-approved for the treatment of ADHD in children
  - ○ Is used off-label in adults
- Compared to clonidine (Catapres), another similar α-adrenergic suppressing medication, guanfacine is more selective for α_{2A} adrenergic receptor subtypes and is weaker in producing overall hypotension and sedation side effects as such
- The dose of guanfacine ER (Intuniv) was titrated over the course of several months from 1 mg/d to 4 mg/d
- Improvement with irritability and in interpersonal relationships developed gradually

- Academic struggles persisted despite treatment of inattention, but he was more consistent with school attendance and less discouraged
- In coordination with the school psychologist, special accommodation was provided for ADHD
- Has maintained sobriety and stayed in supportive living

Case debrief

- This patient presented with a complex psychiatric history
- Besides a history of AUD in sustained remission, he also had BIF, and MDD with anxious distress
- All underlying conditions could negatively impact attention and overall functioning
- Here, the patient already presented in remission of AUD and developed a strong social network via AA, helping him to maintain sobriety
- He benefited from the structure and his supportive living arrangement
- Once his symptoms of MDD and anxious distress were stabilized, the clinician was better able to review his developmental history sufficiently to diagnose premorbid ADHD
- Patients with a history of AUD/SUD and ADHD have better outcomes if ADHD is adequately treated
- He tolerated a non-stimulant and his irritability and threshold for frustration improved, perhaps more than his cognitive symptoms
- Furthermore, ADHD diagnosis was instrumental in providing him with academic accommodations in school as patients with BIF tend not to qualify for educational assistance

Take-home points

- ADHD is associated with an increased risk of adverse health outcomes and many individuals with ADHD have psychiatric comorbidities
- Most individuals with ADHD will not experience severe adverse outcomes associated with ADHD, especially if being adequately treated
- The prefrontal cortex (PFC) represents one of the most evolved regions of the primate brain that helps regulate human-specific adaptations such as cognition, emotion, and behavior
- PFC is likely the site of action of guanfacine ER (Intuniv), an agonist of α_{2A} adrenergic receptors

- Endogenous noradrenergic stimulation of α_{2A} receptors is essential for PFC regulation of behavior, thought, and emotion, as blockade of α_{2A} receptors in the dorsolateral PFC (DLPFC) significantly impairs working memory and behavioral inhibition in animal studies
- Guanfacine ER (Intuniv) is approved for the treatment of ADHD in children but the medication is also used off-label for the treatment of the oppositional defiant disorder (ODD), conduct disorder, pervasive developmental disorders (PDD), motor tics, Tourette's syndrome, and in adults with ADHD

Performance in practice: confessions of a psychopharmacologist

What could have been done better here?

- Patient at the time of initial evaluation presented on TCA doxepin (Sinequan)
- Although this medication is approved for the treatment of MDD, it could have been prudent, given his age and possible anticholinergic adverse effects, to switch to more novel and potentially safer antidepressant medication
- Patient had appropriate resistance toward stimulant use given his history of AUD, but possibly would have benefited more in regard to improving his symptoms of inattention, given the greater effect sizes in outcomes when stimulants are used in ADHD

What are possible action items for improvement in practice?

- Clinicians should screen for ADHD in patients with BIF as it is often comorbid and, if untreated, could negatively impact life quality
- Clinicians should stay up to date with available ADHD treatments and appreciate the efficacy, acceptability, and tolerability of different classes of ADHD medications

Tips and pearls

- Doxepin (Sinequan) is a TCA, now most often used in very low doses (3–6 mg/d) for the treatment of insomnia (Silenor)
- Doxepin (Silenor) has a high antagonistic affinity for the H1 receptor, making it a very selective H1 antagonist hypnotic, while avoiding side effects compared to when this drug is used at much higher doses as an antidepressant
- Doxepin (Silenor) is the only TCA evaluated in randomized controlled trials for the treatment of insomnia in adults and the elderly

- When prescribing TCAs at higher doses, clinicians should routinely obtain EKG in patients over the age of 50, as TCAs can block sodium and potassium channels in cardiomyocytes
  - However, if a low dose of doxepin (Silenor) is being prescribed, EKGs are not warranted
- Doxepin (Silenor) could be a medication of choice in the treatment of insomnia in patients with a history of SUD as it is not a controlled substance, and its efficacy and tolerability are well documented
  - Other non-addictive approved prescription hypnotics include ramelteon (Rozerem)
  - Other possible addictive sleeping pills include
    - Benzodiazepines (BZs) such as temazepam (Restoril)
    - Benzodiazepine receptor agonists (BZRAs) such as zolpidem (Ambien), zaleplon (Sonata), eszopiclone (Lunesta)
    - Dual orexin receptor antagonists (DORAs), such as suvorexant (Belsomra), lemborexant (Dayvigo), daridorexant (Quviviq)

Two-minute tutorial

Symptoms of ADHD

- ADHD is a common disorder with a prevalence of approximately 6%
- ADHD is characterized by inattention (selective attention, and difficulty with sustained attention and problem-solving), impulsivity, and hyperactivity, and is caused by cumulative effects of many genetic and some environmental risk factors (Figure 26.1)
- Core symptoms of ADHD are believed to be mediated by a malfunctioning prefrontal cortex
  - Dorsal anterior cingulate cortex (dACC) – selective attention
  - DLPFC – sustained attention, problem-solving, and working memory
  - Ventromedial PFC (VMPFC) – complex decision-making and strategic planning
  - Orbitofrontal cortex (OFC) – impulsivity
  - Prefrontal motor cortex (PMC) – hyperactivity
  - If any of these are poorly functioning, ADHD symptoms may occur

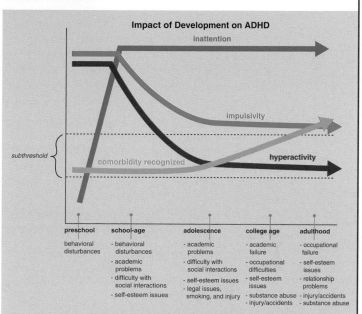

Figure 26.1 Impact of development on ADHD. Consistent with our understanding of neurodevelopment, the evolution of symptoms in ADHD shows that inattention is generally not identified in preschool but becomes prevalent as the patient ages and continues into adulthood. Hyperactivity and impulsivity are key symptoms in childhood, but are less likely to manifest overtly in adulthood, although they may simply be expressed differently. The rates of comorbidities increase over time; this could be due to the fact that the comorbidities were overlooked in children with ADHD or that they truly develop later, consistent with data showing the later onset of other psychiatric disorders compared to ADHD.

The role of dopamine (DA) and norepinephrine (NE) in DLPFC functioning in ADHD patients

- In DLPFC areas, glutamatergic pyramidal neurons receive dopaminergic innervation from the ventral tegmental area (VTA) and noradrenergic innervation from the locus coeruleus (LC)
- When adequately balanced, D_1 stimulation in the DLPFC will reduce the noise in individual glutamate neurons, allowing them to fire in more salient conditions, while noradrenergic α_{2A} receptor stimulation will increase the signal here, resulting in more appropriate prefrontal cortical neuronal firing
  - This allows a network of neurons likely to increase guided attention, focus on a specific task, and control of affect and impulses
- In ADHD, hypothetically, deficient DA input can lead to increased noise within DLPFC cortical glutamate neurons where too many

449

external stimuli are assigned significant salience or valience (too many things to pay attention to all at once), while deficient NE input will cause a decrease in signal resulting in an inability to focus on one stimulus which results in an improper balance (worsening signal-to-noise ratio) that can manifest with symptoms of ADHD

- Pharmacological treatments for ADHD mimic or enhance the beneficial effects of DA and NE on DLPFC glutamate neurons
- Available FDA-approved pharmacological treatments are classified into stimulants (amphetamine and methylphenidate) and non-stimulants (atomoxetine, viloxazine ER, guanfacine ER, and clonidine ER)
- Stimulants are the first-line choice for treatment of ADHD in many guidelines
- Non-stimulants are less effective compared to stimulant medications, but also less likely to be diverted or misused

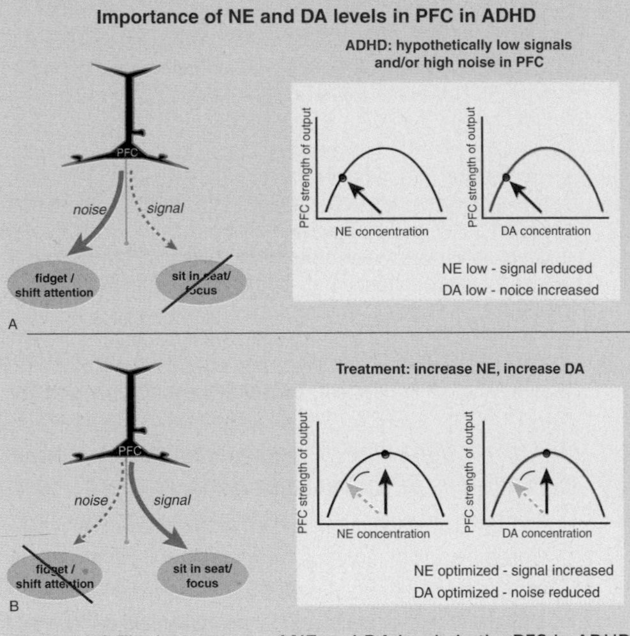

Importance of NE and DA levels in PFC in ADHD

Figure 26.2 The importance of NE and DA levels in the PFC in ADHD. (A) When both NE and DA are too low (on the left side of the inverted U-shaped curve), the glutamatergic network strength of output in the PFC is too low, leading to reduced signal and increased noise. The inability to sit still and focus, together with fidgeting and shifting attention, are often clinical manifestations of this imbalanced signal-to-noise ratio. (B) In order to treat these symptoms, it is necessary to increase strength output by dialing up the concentrations of both NE and DA until they reach the optimal dose (top of the inverted U-shaped curve). This may increase signal, while reducing noise in the cortical system.

Post-test question

Which of the following apply to borderline intellectual functioning (BIF)?

A. Affects approximately 15% of the population
B. Tested IQ levels are in the range of 70–85
C. Does not have a separate diagnostic category in DSM-5
D. Affects school performance and social functioning
E. Can be comorbid with ADHD and autism spectrum disorder (ASD)
F. All of the above

Correct answer: F

BIF is estimated to affect around 15% of the population. Individuals with BIF score on IQ test in the range of 70–85. In DSM-5, BIF is located in the V section under *Other conditions that may be a focus of clinical attention* and it does not have a diagnostic category. Individuals with BIF can have affected school performance and social functioning and often have comorbid ADHD or ASD, which clinicians should screen for.

References

1. Cortese, S, Adamo, N, Del Giovane, C, et al. Comparative efficacy and tolerability of medications for attention-deficit hyperactivity disorder in children, adolescents, and adults: a systematic review and network meta-analysis. *Lancet Psychiatry* 2018; 5:727–38

2. Faraone, SV, Banaschewski, T, Coghill, D, et al. The World Federation of ADHD International Consensus Statement: 208 evidence-based conclusions about the disorder. *Neurosci Biobehav Rev* 2021; 128:789–818

3. Faraone, SV, Radonjić, NV. Neurobiology of Attention-Deficit/ Hyperactivity Disorder. In Tasman, A, et al., eds., *Tasman's Psychiatry*. Cham: Springer, 2023

4. Fernell, E, Gillberg, C. Borderline intellectual functioning. *Handb Clin Neurol* 2020; 174:77–81

5. Katwala, J, Kumar, AK, Sejpal, JJ, et al. Therapeutic rationale for low dose doxepin in insomnia patients. *Asian Pac J Trop Dis* 2013; 3:331–6

6. Khoury, NM, Radonjić, NV, Albert, AB, et al. From structural disparities to neuropharmacology: a review of adult attention-deficit/hyperactivity disorder medication treatment. *Child Adolesc Psychiatr Clin N Am* 2022; 31:343–61

7. Mariani, JJ, Levin, FR. Treatment strategies for co-occurring ADHD and substance use disorders. *Am J Addict* 2007; 16 Suppl 1:45–54; quiz 55–6

8. Rose, E, Bramham, J, Young, S, et al. Neuropsychological characteristics of adults with comorbid ADHD and borderline/mild intellectual disability. *Res Dev Disabil* 2009; 30:496–502

9. Stahl, SM. *Attention Deficit Hyperactivity Disorder and Its Treatment*, 5th edn. Cambridge: Cambridge University Press, 2021.

Case 27: When the music does not stop

The Question: What is the differential diagnosis of new onset of auditory hallucinations in elders?

The Psychopharmacological Dilemma: Finding effective treatment for new onset of musical hallucinations

Nevena Radonjić

Pretest self-assessment question

Which of the following hypnotic medications has the shortest half-life?

A. Zaleplon (Sonata)
B. Zolpidem (Ambien)
C. Doxepin (Silenor)
D. Trazodone (Desyrel)
E. Suvorexant (Belsomra)

Patient evaluation on intake

- An 80-year-old-woman with a history of major depressive disorder (MDD) presenting with a new onset of auditory hallucinations
- Reports that she started hearing classical music a month ago and that it never stops

Psychiatric history

- Patient has a long history of MDD and has been on the selective serotonin reuptake inhibitor (SSRI) sertraline (Zoloft) 200 mg/d with good effect since menopause when she experienced her first episode of MDD, many years ago
- Reports that 3 months ago her primary healthcare provider cross-tapered sertraline (Zoloft) with a selective norepinephrine reuptake inhibitor (SNRI) antidepressant, duloxetine (Cymbalta) 30 mg/d, to target neuropathic pain
- Since, reports worsening of MDD mood symptoms, having daily crying spells, difficulty functioning, impaired sleep, and loss of appetite
- Reports that duloxetine (Cymbalta) was stopped due to worsening of symptoms and she was instead started on a norepinephrine–dopamine reuptake inhibitor (NDRI) antidepressant bupropion XL (Wellbutrin XL)
- A few days later, started hearing music that she initially attributed to radio/TV and only several days later realized that only she can hear it; since then, very distressed and unable to sleep

- Bupropion XL (Wellbutrin XL) was stopped and the patient has been restarted on sertraline (Zoloft), currently on 100 mg/d but still hearing music
- Reports that atypical antipsychotic quetiapine (Seroquel) 25 mg/d was next started for auditory hallucinations, but not effective as yet
- Takes the benzodiazepine (BZ) clonazepam (Klonopin) 0.25 mg/d for anxious distress now
- No history of inpatient stays ever
- No history of suicidal ideation nor suicide attempts
- Never attended therapy

Social and personal history

- Married for 60 years but now widowed, retired, has two sons and a daughter
- Used to work as a teacher's assistant for special needs students
- Stopped smoking more than 30 years ago, no history of other substance use
- Close relationship with children and grandchildren

Medical history

- Type 2 diabetes mellitus (DM2)
- Hypothyroidism
- Hyperlipidemia (HLD)
- Hypertension (HTN)
- Coronary artery disease (CAD)
- Obesity
- Obstructive sleep apnea
- Squamous cell skin cancer

Family history

- Daughter has a history of MDD
- Eldest son – active alcohol use disorder (AUD) and opioid use disorder (OUD)

Medication history

- Was on SSRI sertraline (Zoloft) since perimenopause with good effect until recent medication changes
- Was briefly tried on SNRI duloxetine (Cymbalta) and NDRI bupropion XL (Wellbutrin XL), which were stopped due to either lack of efficacy or possible adverse effects

Current medications

- Sertraline (Zoloft) 100 mg/d, an SSRI
- Quetiapine (Seroquel) 25 mg/d, an atypical antipsychotic
- Clonazepam (Klonopin) 0.25 mg/d, a BZ anxiolytic
- Amitriptyline (Elavil) 50 mg/d, a tricyclic antidepressant (TCA) for pain
- Levothyroxine (Euthyrox) 125 mcg/d, and reports she is euthyroid
- Spironolactone (Aldactone) 25 mg/d
- Carvedilol (Coreg) 25 mg/d
- Losartan (Cozaar) 100 mg/d
- Simvastatin (Zocor) 20 mg/d
- Metformin (Glucophage) 1000 mg/d

Question

Based on this patient's history and available evidence, what do you consider her diagnosis to be?

- MDD with psychotic features
- Psychotic disorder not otherwise specified
- Delirium
- Psychotic disorder due to another medical condition
- Substance-induced psychosis
- Nonpsychiatric auditory hallucinations

What would your next step likely be?

- Blood work and brain magnetic resonance imaging (MRI)
- Increase the dose of the SSRI
- Increase the dose of the atypical antipsychotic
- Start a hypnotic as the patient is unable to sleep and distressed due to the music
- Refer for assessment of auditory function

Attending physician's mental notes: initial psychiatric evaluation

- On mental status exam, she is alert and oriented to self, time, and place; her thought process is coherent, logical, and organized and she does not appear psychotic
- Her sensorium is intact and she does not appear delirious
- Her short- and long-term memory seem accurate
- Her MDD is moderate in severity
  - There has been a reduction in crying spells since she restarted sertraline (Zoloft)

- Will need to see whether auditory hallucinations are present when euthymia is fully achieved to rule out MDD with psychotic features
- Noticeable that she is hard of hearing and has an upcoming hearing assessment
- Given the sudden onset of auditory hallucinations and their nature, i.e., persistent classical music, it is possible that the patient is presenting with auditory hallucinations due to loss of hearing
  - Confirmed it is not tinnitus from the bupropion (Wellbutrin XL) exposure
  - There are no derogatory voices
- Will need to rule out any other acute medical issues or organic processes
- Will also need to rule out substance-induced psychosis, although her history does not suggest any drug use
  - Bupropion (Wellbutrin XL) is typically not sufficiently dopaminergic to create psychosis

Further investigation

Is there anything else that you would like to know about the patient?

- Per family, the patient has no history of substance use or psychosis
- Hearing acuity has shown a steady decline in the past 5 years
- Family did not notice any profound cognitive decline and she is able to function independently
- Her ambulation has been affected by knee pain and now has a history of falls
- Reports that neither clonazepam (Klonopin), a BZ, nor quetiapine (Seroquel), an atypical antipsychotic, are helpful, and that she is struggling to fall asleep due to auditory hallucinations
  - Her symptoms pre-existed their use
- Still taking a low dose of TCA amitriptyline (Elavil) at bedtime for sleep and pain

Case outcome: interim follow-ups through 2 weeks

- The sertraline (Zoloft) dose was increased to 150 mg/d and the patient achieved further improvement in MDD symptoms and was no longer dysphoric, and she is closer to feeling her old self
- To avoid unnecessary polypharmacy that may also drive up side-effect burden, and given no clear benefits from the BZ or atypical antipsychotic, both were discontinued
- Blood work ruled out any acute processes such as infection, electrolyte disbalance, or thyroid dysfunction

- Brain MRI was within normal limits for her age and ruled out any acute pathology
- Hearing assessment demonstrated moderate to severe bilateral loss of hearing and she was diagnosed with bilateral hypoacusis
- Hearing aid was recommended, which she started using a few days prior to this session
- Reports still hearing the same classical music, less noticeable however during the daytime when she is busy and wearing a hearing aid
- Musical hallucinations are especially bothersome at nighttime as they are keeping her up when things are quiet
- Stated that lack of sleep is now significantly affecting her functioning
  ○ Although she is taking TCA amitriptyline (Elavil) for neuropathic pain at bedtime, does not find it helpful for sleep initiation
  ○ Stated the low-dose clonazepam (Klonopin) was initially helpful, but then stopped working and was stopped, as above

Attending physician's mental notes: interim follow-ups through 2 weeks

- Patient responded well to an increase in the dose of SSRI, and is now not depressed but still hearing these complex auditory hallucinations
  ○ These hallucinations therefore seem independent of MDD
  ○ No clear organic cause has been determined
- It is likely that patient is presenting with "musical ear syndrome," the auditory variation of Charles Bonnet syndrome, an uncommon condition in which patients without mental illness, due to visual deprivation, experience visual hallucinations – but in her case the effect is auditory
  ○ Although musical ear syndrome is considered a rare condition, it is most likely underreported due to stigma related to auditory hallucinations
  ○ It is estimated that approximately 2.5% of elder patients with impaired hearing report hearing musical hallucinations when being asked about it
  ○ The underlying mechanism of musical ear syndrome is believed to be sensory deprivation causing spontaneous activity of the auditory system

Question

What would you consider doing next?

- Further increase the dose of SSRI as she was previously euthymic on 200 mg/d of sertraline (Zoloft)
- Restart BZ clonazepam (Klonopin) at a higher dose to target impaired sleep and bedtime anxiety
- Initiate BZ lorazepam (Ativan) instead to promote sleep and reduce bedtime anxiety
- Start non-BZ hypnotic such as zolpidem (Ambien) to promote sleep initiation
- Provide reassurance and psychoeducation on sleep hygiene

Case outcome: interim follow-ups through 6 months

- The dose of SSRI was further increased and she achieved remission of MDD
- She initially responded well to lorazepam (Ativan) 0.5 mg/d at bedtime for anxiety and insomnia
    - Chosen for its shorter half-life than clonazepam (Klonopin)
    - Ideally used to recapture effectiveness
    - It stopped working after a few weeks and she was again up all night
- Instead, non-BZ medication, a benzodiazepine receptor agonist (BZRA) zolpidem (Ambien) sublingual at a low dose of 3.75 mg/d, with a shorter half-life, was started, and she found it effective for sleep induction
    - These medications are sometimes called 'Z' drugs as they start phonetically with the 'Z' sound
        - Zolpidem (Ambien, Intermezzo)
        - Zaleplone (Sonata)
        - Eszopiclone (Lunesta)
- Psychoeducation on the musical ear syndrome was provided and she experienced relief once understanding the cause of the problem
- Appreciation of the impact of sensory deprivation on her auditory system motivated her to use a hearing aid consistently
- With the consistent use, daytime musical hallucinations significantly decreased
- Sleep time remained a problem due to taking the hearing aid off and the low-dose zolpidem (Ambien) was effective
- At this point, the patient was referred back to the primary provider for long-term management of non-BZ for sleep

Case debrief

- This patient experienced an exacerbation of MDD with a switch from SSRI to SNRI
- In addition, she started new onset of auditory hallucinations
- Although there are reported cases of musical hallucinations from medications, in this case, bilateral hearing loss is the most likely culprit
- Patient responded well to an increase in the dose of SSRI and her depressive symptoms resolved
- As the musical hallucinations were the result of sensory deprivation and not a reflection of the psychotic process, the use of antipsychotic medication was not warranted and atypical antipsychotic quetiapine (Seroquel) was stopped
- Temporary use of a BZ sedative was tried with partial effectiveness to lower her agitation and improve sleep, but creates some risk in this elderly patient
- Although the hearing aid helped decrease the intensity of musical hallucinations during the day, she still found them very bothersome at nighttime and had difficulty falling asleep
- Given the level of distress from lack of sleep, zolpidem (Ambien) was initiated at a low dose, and she found it helpful for sleep initiation
  - This medication is a BZRA which is similar to a BZ, but is likely more effective in agonizing the BZ1 subreceptor and enhancing the effectiveness of the brain's sleep centers
- Once the patient understood the cause of musical hallucinations, she was no longer as distressed and was using a hearing aid consistently

 Take-home points

- Auditory hallucinations represent an abnormal perception of sound in the absence of an external auditory stimulus
- Depending on the content, they can be classified as simple (one tone) or complex (elaborate content)
- Musical hallucinations represent a subset of auditory hallucinations with complex content in the form of melodies, music, or songs
- The risk factors for musical hallucinations are elder age, female gender, impaired hearing, social isolation, brain atrophy, and psychiatric history
- This patient had many of the above-mentioned risk factors excluding social isolation

- Treatment of musical hallucinations is focused on the treatment of the underlying condition
- Here patient responded well to the use of a hearing aid and to psychoeducation on the nature of auditory hallucinations

Performance in practice: confessions of a psychopharmacologist

What could have been done better here?

- This patient experienced worsening of depressive symptoms, possibly due to a change of medications, but also likely due to unrecognized hearing impairment
  - The primary provider chose both to use a TCA and to change to an SNRI where likely only one agent was needed
  - Likely only one agent was needed, and unfortunately both were dosed below the therapeutic level allowing for an MDD relapse
  - Possibly, a further increase in the dose of SNRI could have been helpful for both MDD and neuropathic pain, and TCA could have been stopped, decreasing the anticholinergic burden in elderly patient
  - Given her age and medical comorbidities, polypharmacy should be minimized
- Non-pharmacologic interventions for the musical ear syndrome could be tried
  - Psychoeducation as noted above
  - Use of white noise generator or a window fan at night
  - Cognitive behavioral therapy (CBT)

What are possible action items for improvement in practice?

- Clinicians should be aware that impaired hearing could affect mental health in numerous ways
- Collaboration with the primary provider is needed when patients present with hearing impairment, and hearing assessment should be encouraged

Tips and pearls

- With increased age, sleep patterns change
  - Sleep timing phases advance and elder individuals go earlier to bed and rise earlier
  - Total sleep hours may decrease
  - Sleep onset latency is increased
  - The duration of light sleep increases
  - Slow wave restorative deep sleep decreases
  - Rapid eye movement (REM) sleep decreases

- The primary treatment modality for insomnia in elders is use of sleep hygiene skills and CBT as there are no side effects to contend with
- Pharmacological treatment represents adjunctive treatment and should be considered when indicated
- Careful consideration of benefits vs. risks and joint decision-making between clinician and patient are recommended
- All currently available hypnotic drugs carry significant risks in elder patients, and short-term or intermittent use should be recommended
- Here, zolpidem SL (Ambien), an imidazopyridine hypnotic that binds selectively to the α-1 and α-5 subunits of the GABA-A complex, was used
  - It has more specific binding to the BZ1 sub-receptor sites on GABA-A compared to BZs
  - In the elderly, zolpidem (Ambien) in low doses does not alter sleep architecture
  - Randomized controlled trials of oral zolpidem (Ambien) in elders showed effectiveness in improving sleep latency, decreasing nocturnal awakenings, and increasing sleep duration and quality compared to a placebo
  - Most common adverse effects of zolpidem (Ambien) are headache, somnolence, dizziness, and complex sleep behaviors such as sleep driving, sleep shopping, sleep eating, and sleep sex
  - Zolpidem (Ambien) also increases the risk of falls in elder patients, which needs to be discussed with patients and families before the medication is initiated
- Doxepin (Silenor) is an antihistamine when this TCA is dosed from 3 to 6 mg at bed
  - It has approval and studies in the elderly as well

Mechanism of action moment

- Insomnia in patients could have severe consequences as it impacts the quality of life, and daytime functioning, and negatively affects physical and mental health (Figure 27.1)
- Non-BZ drugs otherwise known as BZRA or Z drugs are positive allosteric modulators (PAMs) of GABA-A receptors (Figure 27.2)
- Non-BZ drugs are efficacious in the short-term treatment of insomnia and, long term, unlike BZ, do not seem to cause as much tolerance or as many withdrawal effects when used at appropriate doses

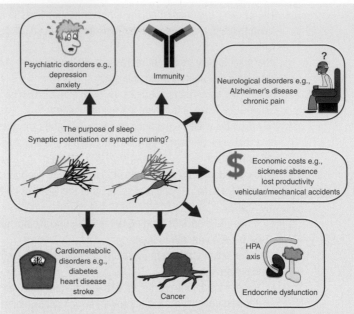

Figure 27.1 Costs of sleep/wake disorders. Disturbances in the sleep/wake cycle can have profound influences on both physical and mental health. From a neuropathological perspective, disruption in sleep may affect synaptic potentiation and/or synaptic pruning. Chronically disturbed sleep can increase the risk of mental illness, cardiometabolic disorders, and cancer, as well as disrupt immune and endocrine function. HPA axis: hypothalamic–pituitary–adrenal axis.

- They tend not to ruin sleep architecture or promote as much respiratory suppression
- There are three medications (but several preparations) in this group that differ in the length of half-lives
  - Zaleplon (Sonata)
  - Zolpidem SL (Intermezzo)
  - Zolpidem (Ambien)
  - Zolpidem CR (Ambien CR)
  - Eszopiclone (Lunesta)
  - R,S-zopiclone (Stillnox) is not available in the US

GABA$_A$ PAMS – "Z Drugs"

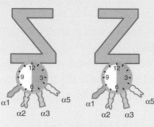

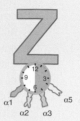

R,S-zopiclone
(Stillnox not in US)

eszopiclone
(Lunesta)

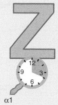

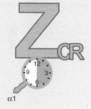

zaleplon
(Sonata)

zolpidem
(Ambien)

zolpidem CR
(Ambien CR)

Clocks below each drug represent its half-life

Figure 27.2 Z drugs include racemic zopiclone (not available in the United States), eszopiclone (Lunesta), zaleplon (Sonata), zolpidem (Ambien), and zolpidem CR (Ambien CR). Zaleplon (Sonata), zolpidem (Ambien), and zolpidem CR (Ambien CR) are selective for GABA-A receptors that contain the α_1 subunit; however, it does not appear that zopiclone or eszopiclone have this same selectivity.

Two-minute tutorial

Impact of impaired hearing on mental health

- According to the World Health Organization (WHO), normal hearing is defined as an averaged hearing threshold of 25 dB or less in the frequencies of 0.5, 1, 2, and 4 kHz in the better-hearing ear
- Approximately 1.3 billion people have some form of hearing impairment and it is estimated that close to 500 million people have disabling hearing loss
- Given the aging of society, the incidence of age-related hearing loss is on the rise

- It is estimated that, after the age of 60, hearing thresholds decline each year by 1 dB even in individuals without any otological problems
- Although highly prevalent, hearing loss is often undetected and untreated in elder individuals
- Individuals with age-related impaired hearing are at higher risk for psychological distress and a decrease in life quality (Figure 27.3)
- Impaired hearing increases the risk of anxiety and depression, especially in women
- Hearing loss is associated with frailty, falls, and increased risk of incident hospitalizations

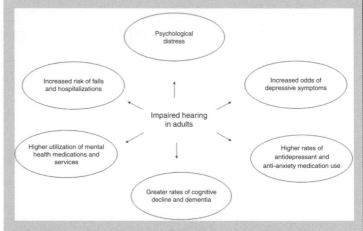

Figure 27.3 Impact of age-related hearing loss on mental health

Impact of impaired hearing on cognition

- Hearing loss has been linked to the acceleration of cognitive decline and increased rates of dementia
- Neuroimaging studies demonstrated that older individuals with hearing impairment compared to individuals with normal hearing had accelerated volume declines in the whole brain and a decrease in the volume of the right temporal lobe
- Mild hearing impairment increases the risk for dementia 1.9 times, while severe hearing impairment increases the risk of dementia 5 times
- Golub et al. (2019) demonstrated that even subclinical hearing loss is inversely correlated with cognitive performance, raising the question of whether the current hearing threshold of 25 dB should be revisited

- Retrospective cohort study analyzing the association between the use of a hearing aid and the time of diagnosis of hearing loss-associated AD/dementia, depression or anxiety, or injurious falls showed delayed onset of these diagnoses with the use of a hearing aid
- Further studies are needed to show whether this relationship is causal, and if so, proven hearing loss could represent a modifiable risk factor to reduce risk or delay the onset of dementia
- Clinicians should hence encourage hearing restoration in their patients

Musical hallucinations

- Auditory hallucinations are a prominent feature of many psychiatric disorders and are commonly present in schizophrenia (SP) (75%), bipolar disorder (BP) (20–50%), PTSD (40%), and MDD with psychotic features (10%)
- Auditory hallucinations, however, are not only the hallmark of psychiatric disorders but can be the result of hearing loss, sleep disorders (hypnagogic and hypnopompic hallucinations), epilepsy, brain lesions, or substance use, and certain hallucinations can be present even in the absence of any well-documented pathology
- Musical hallucinations represent complex auditory hallucinations and are usually melodies of well-known music from the past, such as religious, folk, or pop songs heard during childhood and adolescence
- Musical hallucinations are usually associated with ear disease
- Conditions associated with musical hallucinations include:
  - Psychiatric disorders (MDD, obsessive–compulsive disorder [OCD])
  - Structural brain lesions (cerebral atrophy, temporal lobe lesions, epilepsy, brain tumors, vascular origin)
  - Medications (amphetamines, bisphosphonates, bromocriptine, BZs, carbamazepine, dipyridamole, ketamine, marijuana, opioids, paracetamol, pentoxifylline, phenytoin, prazosin, propranolol, ranitidine, TCA, tramadol)
  - Systemic illnesses (Lyme disease, listeriosis)

Treatment of musical hallucinations

- Given that musical hallucinations are fairly rare, treatment protocols are lacking
- At times, musical hallucinations can disappear without an intervention

- If the level and intensity of musical hallucinations are not distressing, psychoeducation and support should suffice
- The treatment should be focused on the identification and management of the primary condition
- For patients who are distressed by musical hallucinations, pharmacological treatment can be considered
- Given the heterogeneity of the disorders causing musical hallucinations, distinct etiological groups respond differently to treatment
- If the musical hallucinations are caused by a substance or medication, the offensive agent should be removed
- For patients with hypoacusis (sensorineural hearing loss), treatment of hearing impairment and coping strategies can result in the improvement of symptoms
- Antidepressants and antiepileptics can be successful in the treatment of musical hallucinations depending on their etiology, and generally the use of antipsychotics is discouraged
- Although the use of anticholinesterase inhibitors in individual cases has been successful, the data so far is limited

Post-test question

Which of the following hypnotic medications has the shortest half-life?

A. Zaleplon (Sonata)
B. Zolpidem (Ambien)
C. Doxepin (Silenor)
D. Trazodone (Desyrel)
E. Suvorexant (Belsomra)

Answer: A

Sleep medications exert their effect via different neurotransmitter systems. Zaleplon (Sonata) and zolpidem (Ambien) are BZRA drugs and also PAMs of GABA-A receptors, with a half-life of 1 hour and 2.5 hours respectively, and are effective in the initiation of sleep. Doxepin (Silenor) in low doses 1–6 mg/d predominantly acts as a histamine H1 receptor antagonist and has a half-life of 6–8 hours. Trazodone (Desyrel) works to reduce arousal in insomnia via blockade of the serotonin, norepinephrine, and histamine with a half-life of 7–10 hours. Suvorexant (Belsomra) is a dual orexin receptor antagonist (DORA) of both orexin 1 and orexin 2 receptors, that improves both initiation and maintenance of sleep, with a half-life of 12 hours.

References

1. Abad, VC, Guilleminault, C. Insomnia in elderly patients: recommendations for pharmacological management. *Drugs Aging* 2018; 35:791–817

2. Alvarez Perez, P, Garcia-Antelo, MJ, Rubio-Nazabal, E. "Doctor, I hear music": a brief review about musical hallucinations. *Open Neurol J* 2017; 11:11–14

3. Bigelow, RT, Reed, NS, Brewster, KK, et al. Association of hearing loss with psychological distress and utilization of mental health services among adults in the United States. *JAMA Network Open* 2020; 3:e2010986

4. Choong, C, Hunter, MD, Woodruff, PW. Auditory hallucinations in those populations that do not suffer from schizophrenia. *Curr Psychiatry Rep* 2007; 9:206–12

5. Ciorba, A, Bianchini, C, Pelucchi, S, et al. The impact of hearing loss on the quality of life of elderly adults. *Clin Interv Aging* 2012; 7:159–63

6. Cosh, S, von Hanno, T, Helmer, C, et al. The association amongst visual, hearing, and dual sensory loss with depression and anxiety over 6 years: the Tromsø study. *Int J Geriatr Psychiatry* 2018; 33:598–605

7. Evers, S, Ellger, T. The clinical spectrum of musical hallucinations. *J Neurol Sci* 2004; 227:55–65

8. Golub, JS, Brickman, AM, Ciarleglio, AJ, et al. Association of subclinical hearing loss with cognitive performance. *JAMA Otolaryngol Head Neck Surg* 2020; 146:57–67

9. Jan, T, Del Castillo, J. Visual hallucinations: Charles Bonnet syndrome. *West J Emerg Med* 2012; 13:544–7

10. Kumar, S, Sedley, W, Barnes, GR, et al. A brain basis for musical hallucinations. *Cortex* 2014; 52:86–97

11. Lin, FR, Ferrucci, L, An, Y, et al. Association of hearing impairment with brain volume changes in older adults. *Neuroimage* 2014; 90:84–92

12. Lin, FR, Metter, EJ, O'Brien, RJ, et al. Hearing loss and incident dementia. *Arch Neurol* 2011; 68:214–20

13. Mahmoudi, E, Basu, T, Langa, K, et al. Can hearing aids delay time to diagnosis of dementia, depression, or falls in older adults? *J Am Geriatr Soc* 2019; 67:2362–9

14. Newsted, D, Rosen, E, Cooke, B, et al. Approach to hearing loss. *Can Fam Physician* 2020; 66:803–9

15. Prommer, E. Musical hallucinations and opioids: a word of caution. *J Pain Symptom Manage* 2005; 30:305–7

16. Singh, A, Karasin, J, Madhusoodanan, S. The sound of music: a rare case of auditory Charles Bonnet syndrome in an elderly male. *Ann Clin Psychiatry* 2019; 31:107–10

17. Stahl, SM. *Disorders of Sleep and Wakefulness and Their Treatment: Neurotransmitter Networks for Histamine and Orexin*, 5. Cambridge: Cambridge University Press, 2021.

18. Stahl, SM. Does treating hearing loss prevent or slow the progress of dementia? Hearing is not all in the ears, but who's listening? *CNS Spectr* 2017; 22:247–50

19. Trott, M, Smith, L, Xiao, T, et al. Hearing impairment and diverse health outcomes: an umbrella review of meta-analyses of observational studies. *Wien Klin Wochenschr* 2021; 133:1028–41

20. Völter, C, Götze, L, Dazert, S, et al. Impact of hearing loss on geriatric assessment. *Clin Interv Aging* 2020; 15:2453–67

21. Waters, F, Blom, JD, Jardri, R, et al. Auditory hallucinations, not necessarily a hallmark of psychotic disorder. *Psychol Med* 2018; 48:529–36

Case 28: The man who tried to get it right

The Question: Obsessive–compulsive personality traits or obsessive–compulsive disorder (OCD)?

The Psychopharmacological Dilemma: Risks vs. benefits of taking selective serotonin reuptake inhibitors (SSRIs)

Amanda Stallone and Muslim Khan

Pretest self-assessment question

Which SSRI has the longest half-life and least likely chance of producing withdrawal upon cessation?
A. Citalopram
B. Escitalopram
C. Fluoxetine
D. Fluvoxamine
E. Paroxetine
F. Sertraline

Patient evaluation on intake

- A 69-year-old man referred by geriatrics for longstanding obsessive–compulsive personality traits

Psychiatric history

- Obsessive–compulsive personality traits started in adolescence
    - Including perfectionism with preserved ability to complete tasks, excessive work at expense of other obligations, is overly conscientious, is a poor delegator, is a miserly spender
    - For years, symptoms appear to be subthreshold of disorder level for obsessive-compulsive personality disorder (OCPD)
- Around age 40, became more anxious, agitated, and ruminative about work and while at work
- Now constantly worried about making a mistake, thus worsening his underlying personality traits
- Started to engage in excessive research at work to alleviate his fixation on mistakes and worries regarding trivial details
    - These actions helped him overcome his worries to feel better temporarily
    - Once he had solved one exaggerated mistake, he would move on to the next and repeat the cycle again as anxiety and agitation would rise
- Patient fixates on his alleged work mistakes and reports that he cannot forget them because he is worried about the potential implications

- Appears to have developed OCD in his 40s
  - ○ "Ruminations" may be patient's obsessions
  - ○ Obsessions are undone by worrying or engaging in excessive research
  - ○ Can panic when undoing defense is thwarted
- Now admits to major depressive disorder (MDD) symptoms
  - ○ Including poor sleep, dysphoric mood, decreased interest, decreased energy, and increased guilt / feeling worthless
- Feels he has had similar minor episodes throughout his life but believes this is the first major episode
- No history of suicide attempts
- No history of violence
- No previous psychiatric admissions

Social and personal history

- Recently retired as a permit and contract negotiator
- Married with four grown children
- No stress at home or financial stress
- Does not use caffeine products, cigarettes, or drugs
- Drinks 2–4 shots of alcohol with dinner every night

Medical history

- Allergy to penicillin
- No acute medical conditions
- Chronic medical conditions include hypertension (HTN) and gastroesophageal reflux disease (GERD) and migraine headaches

Family history

- Patient's mother has MDD and generalized anxiety disorder (GAD)

Medication history

- Psychiatric medications now prescribed by the patient's primary care clinician (PCC)
- History of SSRI use with escitalopram (Lexapro) 20 mg/d, which had a moderate effect on OCPD, OCD, and MDD
- Symptoms progressed (increasing attention to detail, increasing ruminations, and time spent researching have become more disruptive to daily activities) and the patient was next switched to another SSRI, fluvoxamine (Luvox)
  - ○ Experienced negative side effects (sedation and diarrhea) and a poor therapeutic trial
- Was then switched to a third SSRI, paroxetine (Paxil) 30 mg/d

Current medications

- Paroxetine (Paxil) 30 mg/d (SSRI)
- Zolpidem (Ambien) 10 mg/d (benzodiazepine receptor agonist [BZRA])
- Alprazolam (Xanax) PRN 0.25 mg/d (benzodiazepine [BZ])
- Melatonin PRN before bed
- Valerian PRN before bed

Psychotherapy history

- Patient sees a psychologist every other week for therapy
  - The therapy described by the patient appears to be supportive/ dynamic

Patient evaluation on intake

- Longstanding history of perfectionism and excessive work ethic
- Worsening obsessions vs. ruminations starting at age 40, no identifiable psychosocial trigger
  - OCPD symptoms include perfectionism, excessive work at the expense of other obligations, overly conscientious, poor delegator, miserly spender
  - OCD symptoms include obsessions about previous mistakes at work, which are alleviated by excessive research
    - Panic and anxiety follow if the patient cannot complete the research
  - No perceptual changes, delusions, or (hypo)mania noted
- Dysphoric mood became restricted and constricted
  - Poor sleep, dysphoric mood, decreased interest, decreased energy, and increased guilt / feeling worthless
- Longstanding compliance with psychotherapy
- Has tried three SSRIs
- Compliant with medications and tolerating current medications well but is not yet responding
- Denies paroxetine (Paxil) side effects
- Good insight regarding his symptoms and is motivated for treatment

Questions

How do the σ_1 agonist properties of fluvoxamine (Luvox) impact its side-effect profile?

- Besides its activity on serotonin transporter (SERT), fluvoxamine (Luvox) binds at σ_1 site

- The physiological function of σ_1 is still unknown, but it is believed it mediates anxiolytic properties and has therapeutic activity in both psychotic and delusional depression
- However, it may contribute to increased sedation and fatigue and twice-daily dosing is usually needed
- Fluvoxamine CR (Luvox CR) makes once-daily administration possible as possibly less peak-dose sedation

How does valerian work?

- Valerian (*Valeriana officinalis*) is a herb sold as a dietary supplement in the US
- It is often found in over-the-counter (OTC) products as a mild sedative or a sleep aid
- The proposed mechanism of action is an increase of GABA in the synaptic cleft
- The usual dose of valerian is 600 mg/d
- The most common side effects of valerian are headaches, dizziness, pruritus, and gastrointestinal disturbance

Attending physician's mental notes: initial psychiatric evaluation

- Patient is likely experiencing mild to moderate symptoms of three disorders that have amassed to increase his psychosocial distress
    - Premorbid OCPD
    - Later-onset OCD
    - And now MDD
- Psychosocial stressors and MDD escalate OCPD, and now unfortunately OCD
- OCPD and OCD symptoms are likely now sufficiently severe to have caused disruptions to his quality of life, resulting in mild to moderate MDD
- Safe and amenable to continue outpatient treatment with follow-up psychotherapy from his outpatient psychologist and medication prescription from his PCC

Question

What are the fundamental differences between OCPD and OCD?

- OCD is characterized by obsessions/preoccupations and compulsions
- OCPD is characterized by rigidity in many areas and a tendency toward list/order keeping and often perfectionism
- OCD is ego-dystonic
- OCPD is ego-syntonic

Attending physician's mental notes: initial psychiatric evaluation (continued)

- Given OCD features, patient will likely need a higher-dose SSRI and for a longer duration when compared to treating MDD and other anxiety disorders
- Partial response to SSRIs in the past is reassuring for the possibility of remission if he can tolerate larger doses
- Meets criteria for OCPD, OCD, and MDD, all of which could respond to an SSRI

Question

Is there anything else that you would like to know about the patient?

What kind of work does he do?

- Recently retired as a permit and contract negotiator
- Works part-time as a high school track and field official
- Volunteers once a week at a local library

What is his family and support structure like?

- Lives at home with his wife
  - Wife also recently retired
- Four grown children live 1 hour away
- Many of the patient's friends have recently moved away to warmer climates for retirement

Case outcome: re-consultation 3 years after initial visit

- Patient took paroxetine (Paxil) 40 mg/d and was experiencing a good response
- At some point, his paroxetine was switched back to escitalopram (Lexapro)
- After the medication change, OCD symptoms began to worsen in a pattern like the patient's initial presentation to our consultation team
- Different context was noted compared to his initial presentation
  - He is now concerned about perceived mistakes in his personal life and their ramifications, rather than previous perceived mistakes at work prior to retirement
- No MDD symptoms are present now
- Rates current OCD symptoms as 5/10 in severity vs. 8/10 at his initial presentation, with 10 being the most severe
- Patient stopped escitalopram (Lexapro) and restarted paroxetine (Paxil) 40 mg/d 3 weeks before this evaluation which may partially account for his improving symptoms now

- Eight sessions into cognitive behavioral therapy (CBT) exposure and response prevention (ERP) protocol which is likely helping as well
- Currently taking paroxetine (Paxil) 40 mg/d, zolpidem (Ambien) 10 mg/d, trazodone (Desyrel) PRN 100 mg/d, and alprazolam (Xanax) PRN 0.25 mg/d
- New medical history of renal cancer status post-resection

Question

What would you do next?

- Leave SSRI as is and wait for the effect
- Increase SSRI dose for better effect
- Change to a selective serotonin–norepinephrine reuptake inhibitor (SNRI)
- Change to a tricyclic antidepressant (TCA)
- Augment with a 5-HT$_{1A}$ partial agonist such as buspirone (BuSpar)
- Augment with an atypical antipsychotic

Attending psychiatrist notes: re-consultation 3 years after initial visit (continued)

- Patient appears better compared to his initial presentation but worse than his recent baseline
- Now has moderate perfectionism-type OCD, which should respond well to treatment
- Ongoing longitudinal OCPD traits continue and may not be easily modified
- There is no MDD
- Patient amenable to outpatient treatment with his PCC and psychologist, with ongoing consultation here
- Lethality risk appears low

Case outcome: reconsultation 6 years after initial visit

- Patient taking increased paroxetine (Paxil) at 50 mg/d now
- Current medications include trazodone (Desyrel) 50 mg/d as well
- Achieved remission of OCD with the increased SSRI dose above
  - Has occasional fleeting symptoms that he is able to dismiss but these may be his OCPD and he is better able to challenge these thoughts via CBT
- Patient notes that, with the SSRI dose increase, he began to suffer from erectile dysfunction (ED)
- Updated medical history is now significant for prostate cancer
  - Previously only had minor difficulties with ED, now worse

- Has essentially lost all erectile function since beginning paroxetine (Paxil) 50 mg/d
- Patient concerned with the chance of regaining sexual function vs. an OCD relapse if he were to lower the paroxetine (Paxil)
  - Interested in learning about alternate therapeutic options for ED

Question

What would you do next?

- Nothing, as OCD, OCPD, and MDD are remitted
- Lower the SSRI and restart CBT
- Change to another SSRI
- Lower SSRI dose and augment with an atypical antipsychotic or a 5-HT$_{1A}$ partial agonist
- Change to a serotonin partial agonist / reuptake inhibitor (SPARI)

Attending psychiatrist notes: re-consultation 6 years after initial visit

- Patient is euthymic at today's visit; OCD has been in remission for the past 2–3 years
- Patient reported no sexual dysfunction with the now lower 40 mg dose of paroxetine (Paxil)
- Considered possible pre-existing sexual dysfunction due to prostate cancer and aging contributing to worsening sexual function vs. true side effects from the SSRI, but ED resolved with the lower SSRI dose suggesting a clear side effect exists
- Paroxetine (Paxil) in addition to serotonin reuptake inhibits nitric oxide synthase, which can contribute to reported sexual dysfunction as well

Case outcome: re-consultation 7 years after initial visit

- Patient was taking paroxetine (Paxil) at 40 mg/d with good response
- OCD remains in remission on SSRI dose above, but again experiencing intolerable ED despite lower SSRI dosing
- Patient continues to use CBT skills to manage occasional OCPD symptoms
- Patient still concerned about possible OCD relapse when switching medications, but would like to try
- Patient remains in remission for his prostate cancer
- Began vilazodone (Viibryd), a SPARI, at 10 mg/d for 7 days, then increased to 20 mg/d, because it is known to have fewer sexual side effects than the SSRIs. Taken with food to ensure absorption
- Reports full return of good sexual function

Attending psychiatrist notes: re-consultation 7 years after initial visit

- Patient is euthymic at today's visit; OCD has been in remission for the past 3–4 years
- Patient reports the full return of sexual function after discontinuation of the 40 mg dose of paroxetine (Paxil)
- Remains in remission at the 20 mg/d dose of vilazodone (Viibryd)

Case debrief

- A 68-year-old male, recently retired negotiator referred by geriatrics for longstanding symptoms of OCD and OCPD
- OCPD traits throughout his life: perfectionism, excessive work at expense of other obligations, overly conscientious, poor delegator, miserly spender
- At age 40 became more anxious, agitated, and ruminative, which then interfered more with his psychosocial functioning
- Began experiencing MDD symptoms as well
  - Including poor sleep, dysphoric mood, decreased interest, decreased energy, and increased guilt / feeling worthless
- History of SSRI use with escitalopram (Lexapro) 20 mg/d which had a moderate effect on OCPD, OCD, and MDD
- OCD symptoms progressed and the patient was next switched to another SSRI, fluvoxamine (Luvox)
  - Experienced negative side effects (sedation and diarrhea) and a poor therapeutic trial
- Was then switched to a third SSRI, paroxetine (Paxil) 30 mg/d, eventually increased to 40 mg/d with good response
- At some point, his paroxetine (Paxil) was switched back to escitalopram (Lexapro) and patient experienced a relapse of OCD symptoms
- Patient switched back to paroxetine (Paxil) 40 mg/d, eventually increased to 50 mg/d with remission of OCD symptoms
  - Experienced sexual dysfunction from paroxetine (Paxil), but chose to continue due to fear of relapse
- Several years later, sexual dysfunction side effect was no longer tolerable, and patient was switched to vilazodone (Viibryd)
- Patient remains in remission at 20 mg/d dose of vilazodone (Viibryd) and experienced complete return of sexual function

Take-home points

- OCPD and OCD are different but can co-exist
- Until OCD is treated, it is unclear how much OCPD plays a role

- OCPD and OCD can affect psychosocial dysfunction and often lead to MDD
- Often, the use of serotonergic agents can simultaneously treat OCD, OCPD, and MDD
- As the higher dose of SSRI is needed for OCD treatment, the clinician needs to consider possible side effects and provide psychoeducation to patient

Performance in practice: confessions of a psychopharmacologist

What could have been done better?

- Patient only had three medication changes in 6–7 years with his PCC
- Likely should have told the patient in order to advocate better, or we should collaborate more often
- CR formulation of fluvoxamine (Luvox CR) might have decreased side effects and the patient might have benefited from the medication

What are possible action items for improvement in practice?

- Research available agents with serotonergic potential that may help treatment-resistant OCD

Tips and pearls

- OCD often requires high SSRI doses, as previously discussed in Case 24
- OCD often requires high SSRI doses over several weeks to become effective
- Interestingly, SSRI may help lower traits associated with OCPD or avoidant personality disorder
- OCPD may respond to serotonergic treatments and can certainly respond to CBT and psychodynamic psychotherapy approaches

Mechanism of action moment

- OCD is felt to be a psychiatric disorder that often needs a high level of serotonergic enhancement in the brain in order to lower these anxious symptoms
- Certain SSRIs and the TCA clomipramine (Anafranil) are FDA-approved and most often used, but other psychotropics have serotonergic potential and can be used in more treatment-resistant cases
- Medications with serotonergic potential:
  - SSRIs (fluoxetine, sertraline, paroxetine, citalopram, escitalopram, fluvoxamine)

- 5-HT$_{1A}$ partial agonists (buspirone)
- SPARIs (vilazodone, vortioxetine)
- SNRIs (venlafaxine, desvenlafaxine, duloxetine, milnacipran, levomilnacipran)
- TCAs (imipramine, amitriptyline, clomipramine)
- MAOIs (phenelzine, tranylcypromine, selegiline)
- SARIs (trazodone, nefazodone, mirtazapine)
- Atypical antipsychotics (especially lumateperone, aripiprazole, brexpiprazole)

Two-minute tutorial

SSRI pharmacodynamics: are they all the same?

- Although all SSRIs share the core feature of acting as serotonin reuptake inhibitors, they also have unique properties
  - Fluoxetine (Prozac) has norepinephrine-reuptake inhibition (NRI) and 5-HT$_{2C}$ antagonist actions that can lead to disinhibition of norepinephrine and dopamine resulting in activating effects, such as an increase in energy and decrease of fatigue. It has marked CYP450 2D6 inhibition
  - Sertraline (Zoloft) inhibits dopamine transporters (DATs) and, similar to fluvoxamine, binds to σ_1 c receptors but with lower affinity; DAT inhibition is considered to be weak but might explain some of the observed activating effects, and Sertraline (Zoloft) is often combined with NDRI bupropion, for further increase of DAT and boosting of dopamine. It has mild CYP450 2D6 inhibition
  - Paroxetine (Paxil), as discussed above, has weak NET inhibition, mild anticholinergic M1 actions, and inhibits nitric oxide synthase; anticholinergic activity might promote slight sedating effect of paroxetine. It has marked CYP450 2D6 inhibition
  - Fluvoxamine (Luvox), as previously discussed, binds to σ_1 receptor and likely has the highest affinity for inhibiting SERT
  - Citalopram (Celexa) is a mix of R and S enantiomers; racemic citalopram has more antihistaminergic properties and may have milder CYP450 2D6 inhibition
  - Escitalopram (Lexapro) seems pharmacodynamically cleaner without much CYP450 2D6 inhibition, antihistamine, or anticholinergic burden
- When choosing an SSRI, individual characteristics of the patient need to be taken into account – patients with atypical MDD features might benefit from activating medications such as fluoxetine or sertraline, while patients with agitation might tolerate well "sedating" SSRIs such as fluvoxamine or paroxetine

- Patients with numerous medications / polypharmacy could benefit from escitalopram or sertraline given the fewer CYP450-mediated drug interactions and the "cleanest" profiles, which might reduce the burden of side effects

SSRIs pharmacokinetics: how about all those CYPs and half-lives?

- SSRIs differ in how they are metabolized
  - Fluoxetine (Prozac) is a CYP2D6 substrate that remarkably inhibits CYP2C19, CYP2D6, and CYP3A4; it's the SSRI with the longest half-life, of 4–6 days
  - Paroxetine (Paxil) is a CYP2D6 substrate and a major inhibitor, with the shortest half-life of all SSRIs at 21 hours
  - Sertraline (Zoloft) is a CYP3A4 and CYP2B6 substrate, with a half-life of 26 hours
  - Fluvoxamine (Luvox) is metabolized in the liver via CYP isoenzymes; shows biphasic elimination with a mean half-life of about 15–28 hours
  - Citalopram (Celexa) is a CYP3A4 and CYP2C19 substrate, with a half-life from 24 to 48 hours
  - Escitalopram (Lexapro) is metabolized the same as citalopram, with a half-life from 27 to 32 hours, but has minimal CYP450 inhibition

SSRIs: what about withdrawal or discontinuation syndrome?

- Antidepressant discontinuation syndrome often occurs in clinical practice (20% of patients) and should be discussed with patients when the dose of medication is being reduced or medication changed
- Patients should be advised not to quit any psychotropic that inhibits SERT abruptly, especially those with shorter half-lives
- Discontinuation syndrome is characterized by flu-like symptoms, insomnia, nausea, imbalance, sensory disturbances (parasthesias sometimes called *zaps* by patients), and hyperarousal
- When possible and indicated – such as with SSRIs with a short half-life, such as paroxetine (Paxil) – slow taper and use of CR formulation could decrease the incidence of withdrawal symptoms
  - The short half-life SNRIs (venlafaxine and desvenlafaxine) also are more prone to discontinuation syndrome
- With longer half-life SSRIs such as fluoxetine, little to no taper may be needed and medication can be stopped
- If the doses of the SSRI are low, or if the patient has not taken the SSRI chronically, then a faster taper might be considered

- If symptoms of withdrawal are bothersome and still present, a slower and more gradual taper is recommended
- Sometimes a low dose of long-half-life fluoxetine (10 mg) is added to the discontinuation-prone short-half-life SSRI for a few weeks and then the problematic SSRI is again tapered slowly. The fluoxetine is then discontinued last. This is often called an *SSRI Detox* and may alleviate the discontinuation syndrome

Post-test question

Which SSRI has the longest half-life and least likely chance of producing withdrawal upon cessation?

A. Citalopram
B. Escitalopram
C. Fluoxetine
D. Fluvoxamine
E. Paroxetine
F. Sertraline

Answer: C

As noted above, the SSRI with the longest half-life is fluoxetine and, as such, it has relatively few SSRI withdrawal side effects

References

1. Hadley, SK, Petry, JJ. Valerian. *Am Fam Physician* 2003; 67:1755–8
2. Hemeryck, A, Belpaire, FM. Selective serotonin reuptake inhibitors and cytochrome P-450 mediated drug–drug interactions: an update. *Curr Drug Metab* 2002; 3:13–37
3. Montejo, AL, Prieto, N, de Alarcón, R, et al. Management strategies for antidepressant-related sexual dysfunction: a clinical approach. *J Clin Med* 2019; 8:1640
4. Rothmore, J. Antidepressant-induced sexual dysfunction. *Med J Aust* 2020; 212:329–34
5. Stahl, SM. *Stahl's Essential Psychopharmacology: Neuroscientific Basis and Practical Applications*, 5. Cambridge: Cambridge University Press, 2021
6. Therrien, F, Markowitz, JS. Selective serotonin reuptake inhibitors and withdrawal symptoms: a review of the literature. *Hum Psychopharmacol* 1997; 12:309–23

Index of drug names

Index of case studies